Heart Sense for Women
unlocks the mysteries of a woman's heart health.

Discover:
• Why women—particularly women over 45—are at
greater risk for heart disease
• Why "textbook" symptoms and early warning signals
may not appear in women until it's too late
• Why women's intuition may be more reliable than
a doctor's prescription
• Why emotional factors may sometimes outweigh medical ones
• What women can do to spot trouble and prevent heart attacks
• What a woman should do if she is diagnosed with heart disease
• The 12 heart-healing food groups

. . . and much, much more

According to cardiologist Dr. Sinatra, the key to preventing heart disease
is through the Four Pillars of Health, which are a healthy diet, nutritional supplements, an active lifestyle, and emotional well-being. You can
assess your own risk level by taking Dr. Sinatra's self-test. For women
already diagnosed with heart disease, Dr. Sinatra explains the available
options—from stress management to medical and natural solutions. A
pioneer in vitamin research, he formulates his own vitamins and supplements for heart patients. He is one of only a few doctors truly qualified
to give advice on the best vitamin/nutritional supplements for those
recovering from heart problems.

STEPHEN T. SINATRA, MD, is a board-certified cardiologist, certified
bioenergetic analyst and certified nutrition specialist who has helped
patients prevent and reverse heart disease using conventional medicine as
well as complementary nutritional and psychological therapies at his
New England Heart and Longevity Center in Manchester, Connecticut.
The author of four previous books, he is also the editor of the *Sinatra
Health Report*, a monthly newsletter, and has a successful website,
DrSinatra.com. He lives in Manchester.
JAN SINATRA, RN, MSN, is a cardiac nurse and psychotherapist. Research
editor for the *Sinatra Health Report*, she is also on staff at the New
England Heart and Longevity Center.
ROBERTA JO LIEBERMAN is an award-winning medical writer, editor, and
journalist who specializes in heart health, women's health, and holistic
health.

D0441861

Heart Sense

for Women

Your Plan for
Natural Prevention
and Treatment

BY STEPHEN T. SINATRA, MD,
JAN SINATRA, RN, MSN, AND ROBERTA JO LIEBERMAN

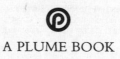

A PLUME BOOK

To our mothers, Patricia E. Sinatra, Margaret Pew, and Gloria Messineo,
who have valiantly and bravely faced heart disease, breast cancer,
and osteoporosis over the years. Their courage has taught us much about faith,
hope, and love—and the invincible power of the human spirit.
With love, Steve, Jan, and Bobbie

PLUME
Published by the Penguin Group
Penguin Putnam Inc., 375 Hudson Street, New York, New York 10014, U.S.A.
Penguin Books Ltd, 27 Wrights Lane, London W8 5TZ, England
Penguin Books Australia Ltd, Ringwood, Victoria, Australia
Penguin Books Canada Ltd, 10 Alcorn Avenue, Toronto, Ontario, Canada M4V 3B2
Penguin Books (N.Z.) Ltd, 182–190 Wairau Road, Auckland 10, New Zealand

Penguin Books Ltd, Registered Offices: Harmondsworth, Middlesex, England

Published by Plume, a member of Penguin Putnam Inc. This is an authorized reprint of a hardcover edition published by LifeLine Press, An Eagle Publishing Company. For information address LifeLine Press, One Massachusettes Avenue NW, Washington, DC 20001.

First Plume Printing, September 2001
10 9 8 7 6 5 4 3 2 1

Ⓟ REGISTERED TRADEMARK—MARCA REGISTRADA

The Library of Congress has catalogued the hardcover edition as follows:
Sinatra, Stephen T.
    Heart sense for women: your plan for natural prevention and treatment / by Stephen T. Sinatra, Jan Sinatra, and Roberta Jo Lieberman
    p.   cm.
    Includes bibliographical references and index.
    ISBN 0-89526-285-1 (hc.)
    ISBN 0-452-28271-3 (pbk.)
    1. Heart disease in women—Popular works.   I. Sinatra, Jan.   II. Lieberman, Roberta Jo.
III. Title.
    RC672.S553 2000
    616.1'2'0082—dc21   00-038063

Printed in the United States of America
Original hardcover design by Julie Lappen

CONTENTS

455,000 men. The increase in deaths from CHD in four years was almost 5.5 percent for women but less than 3.5 percent for men.

Heart attacks, angioplasties, and bypass surgeries are all on the rise for the female gender. No longer is coronary artery disease a male-dominated concern; I have seen dozens of women in their twenties, thirties, and forties develop premature heart disease.

What's behind this silent epidemic? For the last several decades, cardiologists advised women on the prevention of heart disease with data and guidelines established from studies almost exclusively of men. This meant misdiagnosing women and treating them incompletely, ineffectively, or even too late. Simply put, "the rules" for men with heart disease often do not apply to women. We now know there are two significant differences between men and women when it comes to heart disease:

❖ As he ages, a man's risk of CHD rises predictably, in a steady line, while most women are protected by natural estrogen production for the first two-thirds of their lives.
❖ Starting around age forty-five, female hormone production declines. After menopause, it can drop precipitously, leaving women extremely vulnerable to heart disease.

The risk of coronary heart disease in women *quadruples* as menopause approaches. As a result, a woman will be just as likely as a man to develop heart disease and, unfortunately, if so, even more likely to die from it. Complicating matters further, clinical signs of heart disease are often "atypical and unreliable" in women—which is a doctor's way of saying that he's often blind-sided by CHD in women.

During the childbearing years, women are generally not as

PREFACE TO THE PLUME EDITION

Heart disease is the number one killer of women in America today. In fact, a woman is six times more likely to die of heart disease than breast cancer, even though breast cancer gets most of the publicity and research funding. Can you imagine a march on Washington, D.C., to protest lack of funding for research into heart disease in women? It doesn't happen, yet half a million die of coronary heart disease every year!

Consider these facts:

❖ Coronary heart disease (CHD) accounts for 45 percent of all deaths in women, more than all forms of cancer combined. More than double the number of women die each year from cardiovascular disease than from breast, uterine, cervical, and ovarian cancer, and maternal deaths associated with childbirth.

❖ 40 percent of women who have a heart attack die within the following year, versus about 20 percent of men.

❖ In 1991, the American Heart Association reported that 479,000 women died from heart disease, compared with 440,000 men. In 1995, CHD claimed the lives of 505,000 women compared with

vulnerable to heart disease as men, and there seems to be no compelling reason to even think about it. Around age forty-five, as a woman's hormones begin their march toward menopause and natural protection against heart disease cascades away, she may be increasingly vulnerable to the effects of risk factors that she had been getting by with for decades. These include weight gain (just 10 to 15 pounds can be significant), low HDL ("good" cholesterol) levels, and even slightly elevated blood pressure.

In many ways, a man's situation is easier: Since it is well known that men are at risk for heart disease, their level of awareness is higher. For a woman, that awareness is more complex, more subtle, and not as easy to achieve or maintain.

There are no tell-tale physical warning signals that let a woman know she has entered the territory of heart disease risk. The symptoms of menopause come well after she should be taking steps to protect herself; they vary in intensity from woman to woman; and most women do not see them as signaling an increased risk of heart disease.

Your forty-fifth birthday or the appearance of your first menopausal symptoms should be a signal to pay special attention to protecting your cardiovascular health. Ideally, of course, you should be shaping your behavior throughout your entire adult life to prevent heart disease, but it is never too late to start. *Only 31 percent of U.S. women do not have at least one major risk factor for cardiovascular disease.* An awareness of these risks—most of which can be reduced or even eliminated—is essential to every woman interested in her health and well-being.

It's Never Too Late to Create Health

For most women, heart disease does not have to be a natural consequence of growing older, nor is it an unavoidable illness. Despite the "estrogen factor," heart disease is primarily a *lifestyle* disease. Just like men, how women live their lives has a tremendous influence on whether or not they will be at risk. *It is never too late to begin changing your lifestyle to help yourself avoid heart disease.* Every step you take, no matter how small, will help. And since the best heart disease prevention starts in childhood, if you do have children or grandchildren, this book may help you set them on a path toward avoiding heart disease, the number one killer of *both* men and women. It is my hope that this book can become the springboard for a better quality of life for women—and the men and children, sisters and brothers, that make up our family networks.

The greatest gift a doctor can give a patient is to put her on the road to healing. Never before have we had so many healing tools at our disposal, from advanced nutraceuticals to an evolving understanding of the role of lifestyle choices in creating health. In this book, I'm going to share with you the fruits of my twenty-five years in medicine and research. Along the way, I will—

❖ Help you identify the risk factors for coronary heart disease and give you the tools to assess your unique risk profile.

❖ Offer you creative choices about how to help prevent heart disease and heal your heart if you have risk factors or signs of CHD. For instance: Should you consider estrogen replacement therapy (ERT)? I'll lay out your choices clearly.

❖ Provide solutions you can bring to your personal physician, so he or she can become your partner, rather than an authoritarian figure who does things to you and tells you what to do.

❖ Show you how to recognize when something is medically wrong with your heart or cardiovascular system and how to trust your own intuitive wisdom, no matter what your physician or family members might be telling you.

The roots of heart disease often stretch all the way back to childhood. These include the cumulative effects of an unhealthy diet, sedentary lifestyle, cigarette smoking and alcohol, as well as emotional and psychological factors. I'll discuss each of these in greater depth and offer strategies for overcoming them no matter where you are in the process. Regardless of age, from your teens and twenties through menopause and beyond, I want you to *think prevention.*

Heart Sense for Women is for you and every woman in your life—mother, sister, daughter—regardless of health status. I will tell you what works and what doesn't, both in the conventional realm, which can indeed be lifesaving, as well as the latest and most effective alternative and complementary methods. It's about blending the best of both worlds—a truly integrative approach.

To recap the seriousness of the situation, nine out of ten women do not realize the enemy they have in heart disease, and only half of all women understand that their risk for heart disease increases dramatically after menopause. You must be aware of these facts before it is too late. I offer you a road map, a guide, to give you the strength to reverse heart disease if you have it now, the wisdom to prevent it in the future, and the courage to take a stand for your own health.

—Dr. Stephen T. Sinatra
June 2001

INTRODUCTION

Unlocking the Mysteries
of a Woman's Heart

An Emotional Epiphany

Twenty years ago, after I completed my cardiology training and began my education in psychotherapy, a woman in her twenties named Christine came to see me. She kept passing out—literally having episodes of near sudden death. Her electrocardiogram showed arrhythmia—rhythm disturbances in her heartbeat, a potentially fatal abnormality. Despite the seriousness of her condition, her health was not her first concern. All she could talk about was her feelings of agony and guilt during a painful divorce and her financial struggle to take care of her son. Beyond resuscitating her, I did not know how else to help.

Christine was sent to a clinic in Boston to determine whether she was a candidate for potent anti-arrhythmia heart medications. Her laboratory tests indicated that she was, but she refused to take the drugs, convinced that the stress of the divorce and concerns about her son were the causes of her heart problems. The doctors in Boston did not agree, expecting her to drop dead at any time without the medications.

The cardiologists in Boston sent Christine back to me with a suggestion that I put her on some heavy duty cardiac medications. I realized that, despite our best intentions, she wouldn't take the drugs. Christine was caught in the middle of a bitter divorce and she felt overpowered. She confided in me that her husband was using his personal connections and professional influence to gain custody of their young son. The male doctors who had advised her to take the heart medications were giving her the same kind of controlling messages she was getting from her husband. Once I understood this, I decided that my best intervention was to support her refusal to take the medication, no matter what the other physicians had recommended.

"Don't take the drugs if you don't want to," I told her. Christine was shocked! But I believe it was the right advice, because more often than not heart problems *are* more than medical problems: they are problems *of the heart*, of the fullness of our emotional life. In the end, she was right. After her divorce was finalized and she had the confidence that she could provide for her son, Christine's dangerous arrhythmia stopped without any drugs or further treatment. Now, twenty years later, she is still my patient, and she has had no further episodes of arrhythmia.

Christine's case shows how ill-equipped conventional medicine can be when it comes to dealing with heart disease in women. Instead of acting as her partners in healing, Christine's male cardiologists were authoritarian, and totally ignored the emotional dimensions of her illness. They insisted on using powerful, dangerous drugs instead of exploring other possibilities. And, most importantly, they had refused to listen to Christine's intuitive knowledge of her own body, which turned out to be medically correct.

Over my twenty-five years of practice as a cardiologist, I have learned more about heart disease from patients like Christine than from many of my medical colleagues who fail to see beyond what is taught in medical school and published in the mainstream journals. I prefer to learn from my patients. And one thing I have learned is that while heart disease is the leading cause of death among American women—one out of three American women die of heart disease—women's needs are still too often ignored, misunderstood, and poorly treated by conventional medicine.

Most women intuitively understand the importance of the emotional and psychological aspects of heart disease in ways that most men, and certainly most cardiologists, do not. For years, my wife Jan and I have conducted stress and illness workshops for cardiac patients. Even though the majority of my patients are men, most of the participants in the workshops are women, because women are more in touch with and more willing to deal with the emotional dimension of cardiovascular illness. And because of that they have a distinct and powerful advantage to overcoming heart disease.

I've also found that the spiritual dimension is just as strong a factor as the emotional and psychological perspectives in preventing and healing heart disease. I've seen what many other physicians and healers have also seen—especially in women—regardless of the illnesses being treated: that spiritual commitment, whether it be expressed through family connection, meditation, prayer, or other means, plays a crucial role in healing.

I realized early in my career that because heart disease in women hadn't been studied and was poorly understood, a specialized approach was needed—one that would take into account the unique nature and biology of women. I also realized, from listening to my female patients and their insights, that treating heart

disease effectively meant more than just focusing on a pump mal-
function—it meant treating the *whole* person.

Mainstream (also called Western or conventional) medicine is
based on the assumption that the body can best be "cured" through
outside interventions by a physician or surgeon. As a result, our pre-
vailing model of medicine has become mainly rescue- and crisis-
oriented, geared to intercede with treatment only after something
has gone wrong. Its treatments are analogous to home or auto
repair: diagnose the malfunctioning part and then repair it, often
through a process of trial and error. Sometimes this approach works,
but more often than not it means repeated trips back to "the shop"
for additional rounds of treatment.

While this medical model can be lifesaving for many acute
illnesses and conditions (such as heart attacks, infectious diseases,
emergencies, and traumatic injuries), it has proven to be limited
and ineffective for a surprising number of other health conditions.
Patients are often subjected to powerful drugs and/or painful surgical procedures, both of which carry inherent risks. All too often
this method fails to address the underlying medical condition,
which eventually recurs.

Diagnostic Dilemma

Many people, including doctors, long believed that a woman having a heart attack would perceive her symptoms in the same way
that a man would. But now, thanks to more recent research, we
know better. A woman's symptoms, both for a heart attack and for
earlier signs of heart disease, can be very different and far more
subtle than a man's. Because so many physicians are still unaware
of women's unique heart attack symptoms, they are more often
misdiagnosed as anxiety, stress, or indigestion.

Three decades ago, the ratio of people admitted to coronary

care units was roughly nine men to every woman. Unfortunately this was not because women *required* less treatment but because they *received* less treatment. In days past, women's pain was often written off by physicians as anxiety or "all in your head." More often a woman with chest symptoms or shortness of breath was sent home with a pat on the head and a prescription for Valium, or maybe an antidepressant. Add to this the always present pressure for physicians to keep medical costs down and not to admit anyone to a hospital without a great deal of hardcore evidence, and you have a real treatment dilemma—especially if you're a woman.

Even today, when a woman goes to her health care provider for an assessment of her symptoms, she may find herself caught up in a diagnostic dilemma. Because her symptoms are often less definitive or dramatic than those of her male counterpart, her doctor may disregard them or fail to order follow-up tests.

Anytime a *man* over forty years of age with arm or chest pain comes into the ER, the decision is easy… admit him. But with a woman, the symptom may be discomfort in the chest that mimicks indigestion, or it might be in her back, jaw, or teeth. Or, it might show up as severe fatigue. Cardiologists call these confounding cardiac signs "atypical," meaning they do not fit the "textbook" picture of what they're expecting.

Even after twenty-five years as a cardiologist, and being aware of the unusual symptoms displayed by many women, I still find that coronary artery disease (CAD) in women often presents itself like a complex mystery, where following the "clues" is still one of the most difficult challenges that I face. That's why I want you to become familiar with the symptoms of heart disease—so you can gain control of your health, implement alternative methods of treating your heart, and prevent a more serious event such as a heart attack.

Toward a New Model of Medicine

Complementary and alternative therapies—also increasingly called integrative medicine—are grounded in the ancient wisdom that *the body is capable of healing itself.* As a result, treatments do not attempt to "cure" medical problems by suppressing symptoms, but rather gently assist the body in returning itself to health and balance.

Essential to this viewpoint is the idea that the body is not separate from the mind, emotions, or spirit—all actively affect your daily health. This, we have come to realize, can be a double-edged sword: while a positive attitude can help heal you when you are sick, a negative mindset can sometimes increase your vulnerability to disease if your mental state is unbalanced or in distress. Alternative medicine is oriented toward finding ways to support the *whole* person, not just the ailing organ or system.

Groundbreaking research by Dr. Candace Pert helped forge a whole new field in this realm called *psychoneuroimmunology.* She discovered that receptor molecules called neuropeptides provide a two-way link between the brain and immune system which gives us a "thinking" immune system that is continuously informed and influenced by our emotional health.

Prevention Before Intervention

Where conventional medicine is based on aggressive intervention, alternative medicine is geared to *prevention.* In the case of natural healing, "interventions" are usually aimed at lifestyle (diet, nutritional supplements, stress reduction), either to help remedy a medical problem or to prevent one. The alternative approach also aims to detoxify the body of excessive amounts of sugar, caffeine, saturated fats, animal petrochemicals, and environmental toxins such as pesticides, which can depress the immune system and cause health problems.

This approach addresses not only the biochemistry of a disease condition (as does conventional medicine), but also explores the person's energy and mind/body dynamics. It recognizes the musculoskeletal system as a barometer of overall emotional and physical condition: muscle, joint, and bone pain (such as tightness and other problems) are seen as indications of disruptions in the physical or emotional state of the individual.

Perhaps most significant, alternative medicine is not "practiced upon" or "done to" the patient. Rather, the client is an active participant in her own treatment, and one who collaborates with the healer to distinguish which interventions are helpful and which treatments are not. This integrated approach seeks to empower each woman so that she can accept some responsibility for her own recovery and subsequent health.

"C'mon Doc... There Must Be a Pill For This!"

I hear statements like this every day. And, although some of them are made in good humor, the truth is that many of my patients expect the medical establishment to have a "quick fix" for them. Pause for a moment and examine your own attitudes about health care. Are you looking to take a cholesterol-lowering drug so you can keep eating the way you always have? Do you resist making dietary and lifestyle changes and watching your fat intake? Would you prefer to take a pill to reduce your blood pressure rather than lose weight or take an honest look at what it is that is really making you hyper-tense? Are you still looking for that miracle drug or cure to "make" you stop smoking? When it comes to weight loss, are you looking for a better television remote control instead of investing in a good pair of walking shoes? Are you still waiting until science comes up with another "magic bullet" (like the Fen-Phen disaster) to help you drop those extra pounds, instead of watching your diet or starting an exercise program?

As far-fetched as it may sound, many of my patients still express disappointment—sometimes even anger—when there's no "quick-fix," offsetting many years of poor lifestyle choices with a drug that can be added to their morning routine, like brushing their teeth.

Don't get me wrong. Traditional treatments such as medication are valid players in an integrated strategy to overcome cardiac problems, but they should *never* be the primary players. Relinquishing your health care needs to "insurance-only" covered services is a form of giving up active participation in your own care. In a way, you become a passive, "fix me" recipient, vulnerable to getting only what today's over-regulated, profit-motivated health care providers determine to be the most appropriate options for you.

Learn to trust yourself to make informed decisions and take personal responsibility to expand your choices. This may mean spending some of your own money—or making a request for funds—in the name of your own healing. It may mean stepping out into the unknown and declaring that *you are worth it*. It takes courage to leap into something new without knowing how things will work out. But I can assure you—the rewards can be enormous and life-changing.

Bioenergetics

Besides being a physician, I am a certified psychotherapist, and use an approach called *bioenergetics,* a type of body-oriented psychotherapy that addresses the physical changes and damage to the body that can occur as a result of unresolved emotional pain and trauma. In the bioenergetics view (and as I have seen in my own practice and those of my colleagues), emotional trauma, psychological conflict, and psychic pain can disrupt and damage the very structure and function of our bodies' musculoskeletal, circulatory, and internal organ systems. This often leaves us vulnerable to chronic physical problems or illnesses, including heart disease. The damage can be halted and even reversed through various therapeutic techniques.

Consequently, one of the cornerstones of my approach to heart disease (and health in general) is to address the psychological and emotional factors that affect the heart. In *Molecules of Emotion* Candace Pert states, "All honest emotions are positive emotions." I agree with Dr. Pert wholeheartedly, and in the following pages we will explore some of the ways in which you can use your own emotions and intuition to prevent or even help heal heart disease.

I will show you how to reclaim a healthy heart and to avoid being one of the victims of heart disease. My "prescription" for you will not only save your heart but will also enhance your overall health and vitality. The four pillars of my program are really quite simple: (1) a Mediterranean-type diet, (2) nutritional supplements, (3) daily exercise, and (4) stress reduction. Following this program, you will lower your blood pressure, break up the plaques in your arteries, strengthen your heart, and renew your independence. This book will teach you how to explore and strengthen your emotional and spiritual connections to prevent or heal heart disease and inspire you to take charge of your heart health. You can't lose!

SECTION I

Women and Heart Disease:
Getting to the Heart of the Matter

CHAPTER ONE

Why Women Are at Risk:
Learn the Language of Your Heart

Warning: Heart Disease Can Strike at Any Age

In all my years of medical school, I never saw a woman admitted to the coronary care unit. It wasn't until I was a resident and cardiology fellow in the mid–1970s that I began to see women—of all ages— with signs of heart disease on a regular basis. Most often women's symptoms were misdiagnosed or overlooked by physicians using conventional methods. But after years of treating female heart patients, a pattern of "atypical" situations that seemed "typical" for women became apparent. It opened my mind and forced me to "think outside the box" when it came to diagnosing and treating heart disease in women.

You Could Have One at Eighteen

In July 1977 I had just completed my fellowship in cardiology and for the first time was in charge of fellows (MDs training in their area of specialty), residents, and interns. An eighteen-year-old girl came into the emergency room with chest pain and other classic symptoms of a heart attack. Because she was so young, my residents insisted that her symptoms could not be serious. They wanted to send her home.

I looked at her hospital chart and saw that she was taking birth control pills with high levels of estrogen and that she was a heavy smoker. Red flags! Both are known risk factors for heart attacks. That was enough for me to admit her to the hospital that day even though my residents and interns thought I was crazy— no other doctor they knew would have done that. But her serum enzymes and electrocardiogram confirmed a heart attack, and that night my partner, Dr. Arthur B. Landry, put an emergency pacemaker into her heart to save her life.

This opened my eyes (and, I hoped, the eyes of my colleagues) to the fact that women of all ages can be at high risk for a sudden heart attack.

You Could Have One at Forty

Nancy was a forty-year-old attorney from Florida who "had it all"— a high-profile job and two young children. In 1990 her world changed dramatically. In the space of a few months she divorced her husband and moved back to her home state of Connecticut with her fourteen-month-old baby boy and five-year-old girl to be closer to her parents. Her dad had Alzheimer's, and her mom needed help caring for him. On top of that, she took a job with a new law firm as a medical malpractice defense attorney. Talk about pressure!

In retrospect, Nancy says: "I probably did it all wrong, doing all of those things at once: new job, new home, divorce, plus a baby." Yet things went along pretty well for about a year, despite her hectic single-mother lifestyle. Nancy, a trim and fit one hundred pounds, never smoked or drank and thought of herself as the picture of health. Her only apparent risk factor for heart disease was her somewhat elevated cholesterol (Nancy told me that she was very fond of red meat in those days). But a heart attack was unthinkable. Then, in January 1992, her father entered a nursing home, and one week later, with no warning, Nancy suffered a massive heart attack.

"One night, when I had planned to be home for a quiet evening with my kids, I felt tightening chest pain, clenching jaw, left arm tingling, cold sweats. Although I didn't realize what was going on, I went to the emergency room, but by then the signs had gone away. Luckily, I had a good doctor who wouldn't let me go home—even though I tried. Then the pain started again, and he called for a cardiac evaluation, which indicated that I'd had a heart attack. I ended up having a cardiac catheterization [angiogram] and staying in the hospital for a week."

I first met Nancy a few years later, when she came to my office for evaluation with a specific interest in cardiovascular-disease prevention. While her physicians had given her top-notch care that probably saved her life, no one had questioned her about her lifestyle and stress factors. To me the pattern was clear: obvious risk factors—ignored by Nancy and her doctors—had precipitated Nancy's heart attack. Those same risk factors—still present—could easily cause another one, perhaps fatal, if left unchecked.

Few forty-year-old women stop to think that they might be at risk for heart disease; they may even be in denial about the subject. Or they may ignore or misinterpret the warning signs, such as chest discomfort, shortness of breath, or heart-rhythm disturbances. Nancy's story shows how women can overlook the warning signs of their own impending heart attacks.

You Could Have One at Seventy

I'll never forget Myrtle, a seventy-year-old woman born of what we lovingly call "strong New England Yankee stock." She and her husband have a busy country veterinary practice, and Myrtle is very involved in the community—rides horseback, plays a delightful violin and a mean fiddle. But when it came to her health, she got a runaround that almost cost her her life.

It was the day before Valentine's Day. Myrtle had been rehearsing all day on her violin for an upcoming church performance when she began to realize that something just wasn't right with her. Both of her arms were heavy, and she felt like she might be coming down with the flu. As she packed up her instrument to rest, she told her husband Harvey of her plan to cancel her part in the Valentine's Day program if she didn't feel better by morning. She tried to rest after dinner, until she became aware of a sharp pain across her back; even her hours of practice could not account for this symptom.

It was almost 9 PM by the time they got to the emergency room of their small local hospital to seek medical attention. There, an electrocardiogram and routine blood tests showed nothing out of the ordinary. The attending doctor asked her quizzically, "What makes you think that there's something wrong with your heart?" The staff remarked on the outstanding state of her health and her exceptionally active lifestyle and cited this as evidence that she was in great shape!

Myrtle was not convinced. She had what she called a premonition. As much as she wanted to go home with Harvey, she asked to be admitted to the hospital. Though her symptoms had subsided, she just didn't feel safe, and she felt intuitively that it might be her heart.

The ER doctor resisted, but he agreed to call her internist, who listened thoughtfully to her concerns and trusted her instincts. He knew Myrtle well and reassured the ER staff that she wouldn't be there if she didn't think it was necessary. He suggested that they should do as she asked.

Myrtle was given a room on an intensive care step-down unit, with an intravenous line and a cardiac monitor for good measure. The next morning, her own doctor reviewed all of her tests and had to concur with the ER physician: there was no evidence that anything was wrong with her heart. Even when the morning EKG showed a few subtle changes, it was nothing on which to base a diagnosis. Harvey ate lunch in Myrtle's room, but she wasn't very hungry. It was agreed she would remain under observation until late afternoon and then return home. Her husband went off to attend to his veterinary practice... and then it happened—*wham*!

The pain in her back was sharp and strong this time. Myrtle hit her call light and called out to the nurses— "I'm having a heart attack!" Her monitor must have gone haywire because at almost the same instant she heard "Code Blue" on the overhead, the staff rushed in, scrambling to save her life.

"The next thing I know, I was floating up by the ceiling, watching everyone in the room working on me, and trying so hard to revive me. I realized what was going on. I had a decision to make. All I know is that I said to myself up there, 'Oh no! I'm not going without Harvey!'"

Her next awareness was of being back in her own body, hearing the doctors and nurses explaining to her what had happened. They told her that as soon as her blood pressure was back to normal, she could be given an intravenous clot buster. They explained the risk of stroke, but Myrtle knew she had to take the chance. She gave her consent.

Harvey had been miraculously delayed in his office. Her trusted life companion rushed back to her side in time to help make the next important decision. The doctor felt that they had a short window of time while Myrtle was stable enough to move to a larger medical facility. Myrtle was transferred by helicopter to a university hospital where doctors performed an emergency angiogram.

Myrtle was lucky. Other women may not be so fortunate. A physician reluctant to admit an apparently healthy patient or who takes a "let's wait and see" attitude can miss the start of a domino effect that can lead, frankly, to death by heart attack. I wish I could say that these three case histories represent anomalies, but as you will see, they are not isolated events.

Ignoring the Signs Can Be Dangerous to Your Health

Denial can be a woman's greatest enemy when it comes to coronary heart disease. Although we are all prone to brush off the signs, for women such denial is more insidious because it is supported by the common attitude that "I'm a woman, I can't have heart disease." Women also mistakenly attribute heart disease symptoms to arthritis or musculoskeletal problems, anxiety, or emotional upset. Women may also ignore their symptoms because from an early age, they have learned to bear pain—in the form of menstrual cramps, pregnancy, and childbirth. As a result, they tend to deal with almost any pain or discomfort, often with little or no complaint, much longer than a man would. This delay in diagnosis is one of the major reasons women tend to have more advanced heart problems when they finally do get treatment.

As we saw with Nancy, a number of physical and psychological factors may conspire to lead a woman—and her physicians—to ignore even the most clear-cut symptoms of a heart attack. I have listened to all-too-many histories that confirm this: Women whose heart attacks begin while they are entertaining or at work, and who don't go to the hospital until the last guest has gone home or the presentation is complete; women who become sick, dizzy, nauseated, and feel "funny" sensations in their chests during times of emotional stress, such as weddings, funerals, and holidays, but attribute the sensations to anxiety and don't go to the emergency room until the next day. So, the first thing for women to understand is which body sensations may be their warning signs.

What Are the Signs?

For both men and women, *shortness of breath and sudden fatigue* can be early warning signs of coronary insufficiency, which means that the heart isn't getting enough blood. When blood supply to the key coronary arteries feeding the heart becomes blocked or reduced and the heart muscle can't get enough oxygen, it's called *ischemia*.

For most men, the initial symptom of heart disease is a myocardial infarction (MI) or heart attack, an episode of ischemia so long in duration that heart muscle damage has occured. For the majority of women, the initial symptom is *angina*. Angina is what I call an "economic state" in which there is a temporary imbalance between the demand for oxygen in the cells of the heart muscle and the supply of oxygen to that muscle. Cardiologists also call it *cardiac insufficiency*—as the major cardiac blood vessels become clogged with plaque, not enough blood (and oxygen) can get through to the heart.

If angina (also called a "heart cramp") is not relieved and lasts long enough, then the ischemia can often lead to permanent muscle destruction, just as if your foot would turn blue if you tightened a tourniquet around your leg for too long. Once the process of ischemia has gone unrelieved and cell death begins (this can start in as soon as four minutes), the individual is said to be having a heart attack. Myocardial (myo = muscle, cardio = heart) infarction (infarct = cell death) means that precious heart muscle is dying and will be replaced with scar tissue over the next four to eight weeks.

A woman's experience of angina is more often *a dull, aching discomfort* frequently beneath the breastbone rather than the sharp, crushing pain more common in men. And her *pattern* of symptom experience is different as well. Men's angina usually strikes after exercise or exertion, and improves with rest; in women, angina often comes and goes with no obvious cause (see "Symptoms of Angina or Heart Attack in Women" on page 22) and may not improve with rest. Because of this, a woman's angina symptoms are many times mistaken as gastrointestinal. There are a lot of antacid commercials out there, and the media have us all programmed to associate gastric symptoms with stomach problems. But the truth is that *GI distress can also be one of the most commonly disregarded signs of cardiac disease.* All too often, I have seen women—and men—fail to seek medical attention for this seemingly innocuous discomfort; thinking that if they could just "burp" they would feel better—only to suffer permanent damage to their heart.

More often, however, women experience chronic, lower-grade symptoms of angina instead of the sudden, dramatic signs that grab a man's attention and that of his medical team. Rather than a sudden onset of shortness of breath, a woman may experience *chronic breathlessness*, or awaken in the middle of the night with *difficulty catching her breath* (this can also be a case of a benign condition called coronary artery spasm, as we shall see in Chapter 8). *Sudden unexplained, generalized fatigue* is another symptom of heart

Women Don't Show "Textbook" Symptoms

ONE OF THE MORE FREQUENTLY overlooked cardiac symptoms is indigestion or GI fullness—that feeling that if you could "just burp" you would feel more comfortable. More often, women with this symptom, or even frank symptoms of a heart attack, are not given the benefit of routine screening with standard diagnostic procedures. This is because men frequently manifest "textbook" symptoms, but women more often experience atypical symptoms, which can lead doctors astray and condition them to not recognize the possible signs of women's heart disease.

disease more common for women, as the heart struggles to meet its energy requirements.

As I mentioned, women may also suffer from *abdominal discomfort* or *nausea and vomiting*, another pattern less typical for men. Or they may experience *pain or pressure radiating into the jaw or neck*, a symptom rarely reported by men. In fact, her jaw pain may be such an unfamiliar symptom for heart disease that a woman may make an appointment down the road with her dentist instead of immediately seeing her medical doctor or going to the emergency room. Both women and men often report *pain in the left arm or elbow* with or without experiencing *chest pain*. Women may also experience *dizziness*, *unexplained lightheadedness*, or even *blackouts* as symptoms of an impending heart attack.

Diagnosing Barbara

Such was the case in diagnosing Barbara, a fifty-six-year-old woman with back pain just below her left shoulder blade that radiated to her shoulders. Barbara also experienced nausea and weakness. All in all, a classic picture for atypical angina and possibly an evolving heart attack. One problem for me was that her EKG was normal. But my biggest problem ended up being Barbara herself. Because her symptoms had subsided and she knew that her cardiogram did not show any changes, and because she felt that she was not at risk for a heart attack, she refused to be admitted to the hospital. It took me a while, but I finally convinced her to stay in the hospital to be on the safe side, and to rule out a problem with her heart.

It was a lucky decision on her part. Within a few hours her symptoms returned, and by then her cardiogram gave us the evidence we needed. The "reciprocal changes" that emerged made the diagnosis for us: an evolving posterior wall myocardial infarction (MI); that is, a heart attack that is happening on the back wall of the heart, an area that is trickier to pick up on the electrocardiogram. Because Barbara was already in the Coronary Care Unit, she had an intravenous line in place and was carefully monitored. We were able to act swiftly to treat her, saving precious heart muscle and preventing major damage.

When Chest Pain Matters

Although atypical chest pain is often a pretender when it comes to diagnosing heart disease, it can also be significant, depending on the individual woman's health history. I try to resist asking my patients about chest pain *per se* because many significant physical signs of cardiac problems may not be perceived by the individual as "pain." I can often get a clearer diagnostic picture by asking about various sensations such as chest heaviness, pressure, tightness, achiness, or soreness.

Chest pain with certain characteristics can be a strong indication of reduced blood flow to the heart (ischemia). The problem is

---

Symptoms of Angina or Heart Attack in Women

Chest (middle, left, or right side) discomfort, pain, or pressure

Back discomfort

Pain or tingling of jaw, elbow, or arm (more often the left arm)

Throat tightness

Shortness of breath

Indigestion or a feeling that if you could "burp" the feeling of fullness would resolve

Nausea, vomiting

Lightheadedness with exertion, dizziness, or vertigo

Disproportionate sweating with activity

Sudden profound fatigue

that symptom profiles for diagnosing this type of heart disease in
women are based on studies of men. And contributing to the disparity, these profiled men are young, but the women who are now
being found to have ischemia are mostly elderly. Making a diagnosis based on younger models may be highly inappropriate because
the older the woman, the more likely she is to have a cardiac event
with or without recognizable symptoms. Data from the landmark
Framingham investigations suggested that overall women have a
higher incidence for a *silent heart attack.*

Wake Up to the Risk of Silent Heart Attack

Depending on which evaluation tool is used, the silent heart attack
may actually represent one-third of all coronary-related events in
women. At the time of the heart attack, the symptom is perceived
as vague or unimportant, or attributed to something else, therefore
delaying or even neglecting treatment. I use the word "silent"
when a patient has no perception of a physical symptom during a
heart attack.

A real-life example of a silent heart attack is Florence, an eighty-
four-year-old woman I had been caring for for twenty years. She was
the last surviving sibling in her family of six brothers and sisters. She
came to my office one day with extreme fatigue and shortness of
breath, which had been worsening over the past few days.

We started with an EKG which failed to give us the information we needed to figure out why she was so exhausted and struggling to breathe. The problem was that Florence denied having any
symptoms typical of a heart attack, such as chest discomfort, nausea,
or dizziness. Had I not performed an echocardiogram to evaluate
her for possible congestive heart failure, I would have missed the
diagnosis: Florence had had a silent heart attack. With the echocardiogram I could visualize the back wall of her heart moving in a

sluggish manner; it was no wonder her heart was failing to keep up the pace. Once we had that information, we could hospitalize her and treat her quickly and effectively. In many cases, however, hindsight is truly 20/20. Many people can recollect a day they *did* have a symptom, but they failed to attribute that symptom to a problem with their heart—usually because it was vague, mild, or atypical.

Diabetes and the Silent Heart Attack

Having diabetes can increase your chances of having a silent heart attack because diabetics are less likely to experience chest wall pain due to desensitized nerve endings, a condition called *diabetic neuropathy*. Women—and men—who have diabetes must be especially alert to shortness of breath or unusual fatigue with or without exertion, as these may be their only warning signs of heart disease. There are more women diabetics than men, another reason the silent heart attack is more common in women.

Because the signs of heart disease and even heart attack can be so difficult to recognize and interpret, it is beneficial to evaluate your heart health and to gain awareness of your individual risk. In the next chapter, I've set up some questions that will enable you to quickly evaluate your risk for coronary heart disease. With this information in hand (and I suggest that you make it part of your medical record and show it to your personal physician as well as your cardiologist), you and your doctor will be able to make more informed decisions should any of the subjective signs of "heart trouble" surface in the future.

While no one is completely immune to heart disease, this is probably the disease over which we have the most control, especially in terms of prevention. A healthy respect for your cardiovascular system can be the springboard to a whole new level of health, vitality, and longevity. By taking the test in the next chapter, checking out the "New Millennium Risk Factors" in Chapter 3, and taking to heart my diet and lifestyle recommendations throughout the remainder of this book, you will be able to identify your specific risks for heart disease and be on your way to a personal action plan.

What to Do When You Are Diagnosed With Heart Disease—A Guide for Women

GET PAST THE GRIEF AND MOVE INTO ACTION. Once you are past the initial shock of your diagnosis and have done whatever it takes to express your emotions and release your sadness, fear, and anger, it's time to move into action. Actions, such as modifying your eating habits, increasing exercise, losing weight, and taking nutritional supplements, can reverse your heart disease, reduce your risk of early mortality, and perhaps even forestall the need for surgery, invasive testing, and potent medication.

GET A GOOD SUPPORT SYSTEM. Whether it's with a spouse, friend, or parent, find someone with whom you can share your genuine feelings and express yourself freely. This is a time to reach out to others for support and guidance. Just taking in the presence and support of someone who loves you will begin the healing process. Only then can you begin to free up the energy to move on to the important lifestyle modifications you will need to integrate—and help you view the diagnosis as a chance for a new lease on life. There really can be opportunity in crisis.

JOIN A CARDIAC REHABILITATION PROGRAM. Call your local hospital and ask if there is a cardiac rehabilitation program available. There you will be counseled by professionals who will educate you about the heart, how it works, and how to take care of it. Supervised exercise prescriptions, nutritional counseling, and peer support are key components of the rehab programs that can get you back on track and functioning within safe guidelines. Peer support is crucial and supporting one another is uplifting. You will be associating with a group of heart patients motivated toward recovery—a good "reference group" for you to identify with throughout your recovery.

PUT THINGS IN A POSITIVE PERSPECTIVE. Use this time as a learning experience and appreciate the new information you are receiving as a result of your heart disease—about your body, soul, and spirit. Think about your relationships, your dreams, and your place in the world. Put things into perspective. When you take your mind off the negativity of the diagnosis, place your whole heart into the healing process, and take responsibility for yourself, you become more proactive in your healing. I have watched the adjustment process bog down and become maladaptive when patients *get stuck* in any of the response stages. Many of my patients, after moving through a period of disbelief to acceptance of their diagnosis, become trapped there, obsessing on their situation until it begins to take on a life of its own. Those who become waterlogged in this swamp of self-pity are unable to move forward into action, becoming stuck as "victims" of their diagnosis while their loved ones scurry around trying to "make them" get well. But I am in awe when I watch others who have been able to "reframe" their experience with a diagnosis of heart disease and push forward onto a road less traveled, where they actually live in a more fully integrated, intimate way with themselves and others.

TRY A NEW ACTIVITY. When you get clearance from your rehab nurse or physician to increase your exercise level to a moderate level, consider trying a new form of activity... like dancing. Walking and dancing are exceptional and fun forms of exercise that will strengthen the heart—literally and figuratively—and will also help with weight loss. All of these lifestyle changes are important. Try to accept your illness, reframe it, and look for the positive things that are happening to you because of it. You may find you need to put your life in order, heal old relationships, and start taking care of yourself. This might include reevaluating your priorities to see just where you are spending your precious time and energy.

DORIS: A SUCCESS STORY. A case in point is Doris, who came to see me for a second opinion about her heart disease diagnosis. When Doris found out that she had serious heart disease, she was able to immediately reframe the experience as a chance to take better care of herself. She began to take more responsibility for her lifestyle and made major modifications. For example, she reduced her intake of alcohol, initiated a low-impact exercise program, and started losing weight. Although Doris was initially in disbelief about her diagnosis, she was able to mobilize a support system where she could share her feelings and "talk things out." She said that during this process she became "more spiritual" and began to pray more often. She worked on her personal relationships, reaching out to others, and becoming much closer to her family then ever before. Now Doris sees life from a different perspective, reaching out to others with her new awareness. She describes it as achieving a new level of "aliveness." And, most importantly, she has hope for the future, confident that she will be able to figure out solutions to her problems when they arise. Doris dug deeply into her emotional and spiritual self and found the strength to deal with her illness.

It may sound strange but people like Doris can testify to the fact that life really can begin again after a diagnosis of heart disease.

CHAPTER TWO

Are You at Risk for Heart Disease?
Take the Test

You are probably familiar with some of the traditional risk factors for heart disease, such as genetics and family history, smoking, obesity, physical inactivity, body shape, and high cholesterol. But you may not know that these risk factors (and there are more) are *cumulative*—the more you have, the greater your risk.

Take pencil and paper in hand as you read through this chapter, and check off your points in each category. If you're not sure of a particular answer, take your best guess—the risk factors will average out. (You can answer all of the questions most accurately by getting a simple blood test: ask your physician for your total cholesterol, LDL-cholesterol, HDL-cholesterol, and triglyceride levels.) By the end of the chapter, you will know all fifteen risk factors and you should have a fairly good idea of your general risk of heart disease.

Risk Factor 1: Age

Advancing age is a risk factor for both women and men. Aging itself puts people at risk of developing more diseases. Often, our immune systems weaken, and the incidence of cancer, heart disease, and neurological disorders increases. Due to the natural protection afforded by estrogen, women typically develop symptoms of heart disease about ten years later than their male counterparts. But aging often brings with it rising cholesterol, a greater likelihood of a sedentary lifestyle, and rising rates of hypertension, obesity, and diabetes—especially among women, making a woman's *overall health* usually worse than a man's when she develops heart disease.

These factors, plus the presence of other conditions—known as *co-morbidities*—mean that a woman's *overall condition* is generally more serious at the onset of heart disease and puts her at a higher risk of dying. And the older a woman is, the more likely she is to develop heart disease: in fact, *one out of every three women age 65 or older will develop heart disease.*

But as an anti-aging specialist, I do not believe that these effects of aging are inevitable—that's where a healthy lifestyle comes into play.

Age up to 35	❑ 1 point
36 to 45	❑ 2 points
46 to 55	❑ 3 points
56 to 64	❑ 4 points
65 years plus	❑ 5 points

Risk Factor 2: Anatomy

Because a woman's body is different from a man's, she is exposed to different—and in many cases more severe—risks for heart disease. For example, a woman's heart is smaller and the inside diameter of her arteries are narrower. Smaller arteries can become blocked more easily, which may make women more susceptible to vessel damage from the same risk factors. Smaller vessels may also account in part for women's higher mortality from heart attacks and greater likelihood of complications and death after bypass surgery and angioplasty.

Men	❑	**0 points**
Women	❑	**2 points**

Risk Factor 3: Cholesterol

Cholesterol is one of several types of blood fats, or lipids. It is a yellow, waxy material manufactured by the liver and also found in many foods. Contrary to the impression created by media and advertising publicizing only its dangers, cholesterol is a natural substance that the body needs in order to function properly. It is a critical component of the cell membrane of every cell in your body and is a basic building block for several hormones, including estrogen. Cholesterol is also a key ingredient in nerve conduction and skin "waterproofing."

By now, most people know that a higher-than-normal level of cholesterol in the bloodstream is a risk factor for heart disease, and that there are several kinds of cholesterol. The two most important types when it comes to heart disease are known as LDL and HDL. LDL or low-density lipoprotein is commonly called "bad" cholesterol because it is the type that accumulates inside artery walls and clogs arteries with plaque, signaling coronary artery disease (CAD). In contrast, HDL or high-density lipoprotein is considered "good" cholesterol because it acts like a dump truck, scooping up excess LDL from the bloodstream and trucking it to the liver for elimination. HDL may also help remove some of the LDL deposits from artery walls. Low LDL and high HDL work together to constitute healthy cholesterol levels.

Natural estrogen acts to lower LDL and raise HDL, which is why premenopausal women are protected from cholesterol risks in ways that men are not. After menopause (whether naturally occurring or surgically produced via total hysterectomy), estrogen production drops and, frequently, LDL "bad" cholesterol levels rise and HDL "good" cholesterol levels fall.

An elevated LDL level poses less of a threat to a woman if her HDL levels are high. In other words, a low HDL level is generally more of a heart disease risk for a woman than a high LDL level. The Framingham Study has shown that even small decreases in HDL after menopause significantly increase a woman's risk of coronary artery disease. The Lipid Research Clinics Follow-up Study found that after age, *HDL level was the most accurate predictor of risk for coronary artery disease in women.*

Even though a high HDL can help overcome high LDL, lowering LDL cholesterol levels can still have a positive overall effect. The Hoffman Heart Institute of Connecticut's Lipid Education Service on coronary heart disease and postmenopausal women released the following on the importance of LDL reduction in both men and women:

❖ Lowering LDL cholesterol reduced major coronary events by one-third in both women and men, young and old
❖ Lowering LDL decreased death or heart attack recurrence by 46 percent for women and 26 percent in men who had a previous heart attack
❖ Few women with prior heart attacks are currently achieving LDL goals

Here are the low, normal, and elevated ranges of cholesterol levels for healthy people without heart disease:

TOTAL CHOLESTEROL (MG/DL)

Desirable	less than 200	❑	1 point
Borderline high	201 to 239	❑	3 points
High	more than 240	❑	5 points

LDL (BAD) CHOLESTEROL (MG/DL)

Desirable	less than 130	❑	1 point
Borderline high	130 to 159	❑	3 points
High	more than 160	❑	5 points

HDL (GOOD) CHOLESTEROL (MG/DL)

Ultra protective	more than 90	❑	-5 points
Very protective	more than 70	❑	-3 points
Protective	more than 50	❑	0 points
Moderate risk	36 to 49	❑	3 points
High risk	less than 35	❑	5 points

Don't know your cholesterol level	❑	3 points

Risk Factor 4: Triglycerides

Triglycerides are another important type of blood lipid. Your body uses triglycerides directly for energy or stores them as fat—"love handles" of fat around the waistline are the hallmarks of triglyceride storage. Most of the fat in your diet is triglycerides, either manufactured in the liver or metabolized from the food you eat. It is known that high triglycerides contribute to atherosclerosis and that they promote the development of coronary artery disease. But the role of triglycerides in heart disease is not understood as well as the role of cholesterol, and the results of research have not yielded clear results.

However, research based on the Framingham Study has shown that *for women over the age of fifty, elevated triglyceride levels are a strong predictor of coronary artery disease.* It's known that estrogen lowers triglycerides, and that women's triglyceride levels rise after menopause, along with their LDL levels.

Elevated triglycerides is a risk factor that can be reduced or eliminated by a combination of diet, exercise, and weight loss. The best approach is a diet moderate in carbohydrates (50 percent) with healthy fats (35 percent) and protein (15 percent).

Normal	**less than 160**	❑ **0 points**
Borderline high risk	**more than 160**	❑ **2 points**
High risk	**more than 200**	❑ **3 points**
Dangerously high risk	**1,000**	❑ **5 points**
Don't know		❑ **2 points**

Risk Factor 5: Early Menopause

If you went through a natural menopause before age forty or menopause before age forty-five induced by surgery, illness, or medical treatment, you will lose the natural protective effects of estrogen at an earlier age than most women.

No menopause	❑ **0 points**
Natural menopause after age 40	❑ **1 point**
Natural menopause before age 40	❑ **2 points**
Surgical/chemical menopause	
before age 45	❑ **3 points**

Risk Factor 6: Diabetes

When I was eight years old, my mother was diagnosed with insulin dependent diabetes at the age of thirty-eight. As a young boy and adolescent, I fearfully witnessed my mother struggle with severe swings in her blood sugar levels and attacks of hypoglycemia, diabetic shock, and ketoacidosis. Even as a medical student, I observed many of the day-to-day complications of her diabetes such as advancing osteoporosis, blindness, diabetic neuropathy, and even angina.

Cardiovascular disease is *the* major complication of diabetes, resulting in increased incidence of heart attack, stroke, peripheral vascular disease (PVD), and congestive heart failure. The cardiovascular effects of diabetes, whether insulin dependent or non-insulin dependent, occur more frequently in women than in men.

At present, at least twelve million Americans are afflicted with non-insulin dependent diabetes. Research also suggests that another twenty-five million are at risk of developing this condition. Because of the damage diabetes does to the blood vessels over time, all diabetics have a higher-than-normal risk for coronary artery disease and other cardiovascular diseases. This risk is even greater for diabetic women, whose risk of dying from coronary artery disease is three to seven times higher than for non-diabetic women (in contrast, diabetic men who face coronary artery disease have a death rate two to three times higher than non-diabetic men.)

Diabetes tends to elevate total levels of blood cholesterol and lower blood levels of HDL ("good") cholesterol, further adding to risk. Adult-onset diabetes is largely the result of being overweight, and because more women are overweight, women are more likely than men to develop this heart-threatening condition.

Indeed, diabetes is such a powerful risk factor that it overwhelms the protective effect of estrogen, even among women of childbearing age, making them just as likely as men to develop heart disease. This alone is a good enough reason for a woman to take control of her risk factors for diabetes, especially weight and dietary habits.

Not a diabetic	❏ **0 points**
Diabetic	❏ **5 points**

Risk Factor 7: Genetics and Family History

For as long as I can remember I have treated entire families plagued with heart disease, often starting at very young ages. Genetics has long been implicated in heart disease and, although researchers did not always know the specific mechanism, it has long been obvious that the more first and second generation blood relatives (such as parents or siblings) you have with heart disease, the higher your own risk will be.

Predisposition for risk can be traced back through several generations. The distinction between genetics and family history, however, gets murky at times and there is a great deal of overlap. While we don't really know if there is a specific gene for heart disease, it is important to realize that your family history of heart disease goes well beyond whose genes you may have inherited.

Family members share more than genetics. Families create networks for socialization, learning, bonding, and belonging. Behaviors, value systems, and personality traits are also learned in the home from your family. For example, families often share habits such as how often and how much to eat. Children are highly influenced by the food choices of their parents or care providers, so if you grew up eating a diet high in saturated fat, that's probably the same diet you're eating yourself and serving your kids. Unless you make a conscious effort to do otherwise, you and your family will probably perpetuate the eating habits of your parents.

Families often highly value—or devalue—healthy habits such as an enthusiasm for exercise or taking vitamin supplements, as well as bad habits such as smoking and consuming excess alcohol and fatty foods. For instance, children of parents who smoke are more likely to adopt that behavior whether they use cigarettes out of habit or as a way of dealing with the stress of life. If you watched a parent light up when he or she felt stressed out, then you may have added that learned behavior to your own repertoire of coping skills.

Some families value hard work—or even overwork—as an honorable activity. In many families, there is little conversation about what you're feeling, but a great emphasis on what you are doing or accomplishing. This can lead to adult behavior that focuses on perfectionism and pushing beyond physical limits.

Shared beliefs, attitudes, habits, and behaviors can protect you from developing heart disease—or predispose you to increased risk. Even if you got a "bad dose" of unfavorable genes, it's still quite possible to "reframe" your genetic predisposition so that it can work for, not against, you.

No heart disease in your family	❑ **0 points**
At least one first or second generation	
relative (such as a parent or grandparent)	
with heart disease	❑ **3 points**

Risk Factor 8: High Blood Pressure

High blood pressure or hypertension is more common in men early in life, but after the age of fifty-five, *more women than men develop it and in surprisingly high numbers.* The terms hypertension and high blood pressure refer to the excessive force of contraction of the left ventricle as well as the heightened resistance in the walls of the arteries as blood is pumped and circulated throughout the body. The additional shear force exerted by the blood against the arteries (when high blood pressure is present) begins to weaken and break down the cellular walls, making it easier for toxic substances such as LDL "bad" cholesterol to form dangerous deposits that embed themselves into the smooth muscle of these arterial walls. This is why high blood pressure is a major cause of heart attack, stroke, and congestive heart failure. To get a sense of just how widespread this dangerous risk factor is, look at these statistics:

❖ In the U.S. alone, an estimated fifty million adults suffer from hypertension, including more than 50 percent of those over sixty and 64 percent of those over seventy.
❖ Of this total, 45 percent of American women between the ages of forty-five and sixty-four, and more than 70 percent of women older than sixty-five, have mild to severe hypertension.
❖ For African Americans, 35 percent will develop high blood pressure and 20 percent will die as a result of hypertension—twice the incidence as Caucasians. The prognosis is worse for women: African American women with high blood pressure have an increased incidence for the development of heart failure.
❖ High blood pressure accounts for an estimated 28.3 million annual visits to a physician's office.

The Nurses' Health Study—which began in 1976 when 122,000 female nurses were asked to fill out a questionnaire about their health and diet habits, and which is updated every two years—found that hypertensive women between the ages of thirty and sixty-five have a risk of coronary artery disease three-and-a-half times higher than normal. And a study by the Chicago Heart Association, which followed up its subjects over fifteen years, found that middle-aged white women with relatively mild hypertension had a death rate from coronary artery disease almost five times higher than women with normal blood pressure. Other research has shown that hypertension is an even *more* serious risk factor for African American women (see "Solving the Riddle of Hypertension in African American Women" on page 192).

One study showed that among 16,759 women between the ages of eighteen and fifty-four, those with hypertension had three times the normal risk of a heart attack. Yet another study indicated over twenty-five years of follow-up that hypertension accounted for more than forty-five percent of heart attacks and sudden deaths among women aged forty to fifty-nine.

What can you do to lower these numbers and protect your heart? My basic "four pillar" program (discussed in depth in Section II)—includes diet, exercise, weight loss, and nutritional supplements. I do, however, prescribe medication when appropriate, including beta blockers, calcium channel blockers, or other "anti-hypertensive" agents. For some patients, emotional release is integral in lowering blood pressure because stressful emotions such as anger or denial may lie at the heart of the problem.

Normal	less than 130/less than 80	❑ 0 points
Borderline	140/90	❑ 2 points
High	more than 150/95	❑ 5 points
Don't know my blood pressure		❑ 3 points
African American woman (in addition to the above)		❑ 1 point

Risk Factor 9: Insulin Resistance

Insulin is a hormone produced and secreted by your pancreas to help you break down and use sugar and carbohydrates from the food you eat. But when too much insulin cruises around in your bloodstream for too long, as it does if you have been on a high-carbohydrate/low-fat diet, specialized receptor cells that help to metabolize sugar begin to shut down. As a result, excess carbohydrates can't be broken down and are stored as fat. This is insulin resistance.

It reminds me of the fairy tale about the boy who cried wolf. After a while, when no wolf appeared, the townspeople stopped responding to the boy. Well, in insulin resistance, the body cries "carbohydrates!" instead of "wolf!," and after a while the body becomes less responsive in utilizing insulin to break down the sugars and carbs. But, something must be done with this extra sugar and carbs. Since they cannot be completely burned up, the body dumps them into stockpiles as stored fat. This is a key concept: *you can gain weight on a diet that is too low in fat and too high in carbohydrates.* In addition, you'll probably feel fatigued and lethargic much of the time. That is why I have nicknamed these low- and no-fat dietary hoaxes as "wolves in sheep's clothing." Much research has shown that overweight people (as well as non-insulin dependent diabetics) who consume large quantities of carbohydrates subsequently overproduce insulin.

Over time, insulin resistance leads to a cascade of unfavorable events including higher blood pressure, carbohydrate cravings, weight gain, and premature heart disease—it's a vicious cycle:

CARBOHYDRATE CRAVING → CARBOHYDRATE OVERLOAD → HIGH BLOOD SUGAR → HIGH INSULIN → FAT STORAGE → MORE CARBOHYDRATE CRAVING

When insulin levels rise and fall steeper and faster, like a roller coaster at an amusement park, blood sugar levels also fluctuate, creating the vicious cycle above. Carbohydrate cravings, increased body fat, a decrease in levels of HDL, and high triglyceride levels are the hallmarks of insulin resistance.

Excess insulin may play a major role in hardening of the arteries, high blood pressure, and hyperlipidemia (increased fat in the blood).

Research indicates that insulin resistance is on the rise and may affect as much as 25 percent of the population. The American

Diabetes Association reports that insulin resistance, which is related to excess abdominal fat (also called centralized fat or visceral obesity), may contribute to as much as 60 percent of the cardiovascular disease in women and 25 percent in men. While excess hip, waist, and thigh fat has not been correlated with any major health problems, Pierre Depres, PhD, Director of the Lipid Center at Laval University in Quebec, reports that insulin resistance is associated with how much fat is located in the abdominal cavity.

Be alert for these warning signs for insulin resistance:

❖ weight gain or increased body fat, especially around
  abdomen (lower belly)
❖ unrelenting carbohydrate cravings (regardless of menstrual cycle)

Carbohydrate-restricted diet	❑ **0 points**
Approximately 50 percent of calories	
from carbohydrates	❑ **1 point**
A lot of carbs in diet, like pasta,	
potatoes, rice, and cereals, but not every day	❑ **3 points**
High-carb diet (carbs are essential to my	
diet and I'm not giving them up!)	❑ **5 points**

Risk Factor 10: Body Shape

The shape of your body and where you carry excess weight also affects your risk of heart disease. Women who are round and put on weight in the middle (around the waist and abdomen) have what is called an "apple" shape and are at higher risk than women who accumulate excess pounds on their hips and buttocks (called a "pear" shape). Apple body types are more likely to develop high blood pressure and adult-onset diabetes, and have high triglycerides, high levels of LDL "bad" cholesterol, and low levels of HDL "good" cholesterol, all of which raise risk of coronary artery disease. A person of the apple body type is also more likely to develop insulin resistance.

Normal shape	❑ **0 points**
Pear shape	❑ **3 points**
Apple shape	❑ **5 points**

Risk Factor 11: Physical Inactivity

The evil twin of obesity is a sedentary lifestyle. The two often go together like chips and dip. About one-fourth of American women are considered couch potatoes. In recent years, scores of research studies have validated the positive effects of exercise on health, from lowering your risk of chronic conditions that range from heart disease and osteoporosis to breast cancer and Alzheimer's disease. But how much exercise is enough?

The good news is that you don't have to become an elite athlete or marathon runner to reap the benefits of exercise. Even everyday activities, like running up and down the stairs at your office instead of taking the elevator, parking your car in the farthest space at the grocery store, and carrying your own groceries can make a difference. And the research now shows that brief bouts of exercise—fifteen minutes at a time—are just as beneficial, if not more so, than longer stretches of activity. So start small and realize that it's easier than you think to exercise!

I'm very active	❑ **0 points**
I'm reasonably active	❑ **3 points**
I'm a couch potato	❑ **5 points**

Risk Factor 12: Poor Diet

There is no question about it: you are what you eat. Do you swing by the drive-through at your local fast-food outlet more than a couple times per month? Do you keep a stash of your favorite chips, crackers, or other junk food in your desk for nibbling? If your diet is high in refined white flour, partially hydrogenated oils, and animal protein and fat, you'll be putting additional strain on your cardiovascular system. If, on the other hand, fruits and vegetables are a big part of your daily diet, along with whole grains and "healthy" fats like olive and flaxseed oil (much like a Mediterranean diet), then you'll be doing your heart a big favor.

I'm a health nut when it comes to diet	❑ **0 points**
I eat a reasonably healthy diet	❑ **2 points**
I may not be a "junk food junkie," but	
I rarely eat enough fresh fruits and vegetables	❑ **4 points**
My diet is unhealthy	❑ **5 points**

Risk Factor 13: Smoking

I can't imagine that anyone doesn't know that smoking is a major risk factor for heart disease. Many people associate smoking with an elevated risk for lung cancer, but the truth is that heart disease is the major threat: *smokers die from heart disease almost three times more often than they die from lung cancer.*

Smokers in general have twice the risk of heart attack as non-smokers. And people who smoke twenty or more cigarettes a day are more likely to suffer a heart attack than those who smoke less than ten or none at all. Smokers are also more likely to experience sudden cardiac death.

The basis for the harmful effects of cigarettes on the heart is nicotine's effect on the arteries. Nicotine causes blood platelets to stick together, contributing to plaque formation and increasing the risk of a blood clot to the heart. Smoking also causes a buildup of carbon dioxide and carbon monoxide that not only directly injures the vessels, but also starves them of the oxygen.

There is also research showing that the buildup of nicotine and carbon monoxide distorts one's perception of pain by increasing the pain threshold, making it more difficult to recognize symptoms of a cardiac event. So, not only does smoking contribute to heart disease and clot formation, it also decreases the likelihood that you will recognize early symptoms of distress signals from your heart.

Smoking also lowers blood levels of protective HDL "good" cholesterol and raises the blood levels of dangerous LDL "bad" cholesterol, causing a distinctive type of damage to the lining of the arteries, especially the coronary vessels. The cardiovascular damage from smoking accelerates when a woman smokes while she takes birth control pills: a woman who takes high-estrogen birth control pills *and* smokes may have a heart attack risk up to 39 times higher than a woman who does not smoke.

The Nurses' Health Study found that premenopausal women who smoke have at least three times the risk of a heart attack as non-smoking women, and a recent study from Norway showed that women who smoke have six times the risk of heart attack as non-smoking women. In contrast, men face a three-fold increase in heart attack risk from smoking. Fortunately, it's never too late to call it quits. Research registry data suggests that the benefit from smoking cessation pertains to postmenopausal as well as younger women.

In the past, men have always smoked more than women, but this seems to be changing: a study in the early 1990s showed that among high school seniors, more girls smoked than boys. One study predicts that in the 2000s, rates of smoking, and deaths and illness among women from smoking—especially among younger women—will match or exceed those of men.

I've never smoked   ❏ **0 points**

I quit smoking more than five years ago   ❏ **1 point**

I'm a light smoker (2 to 3 cigarettes a day)	❏ **3 points**
I'm a heavy smoker (1 pack+ a day)	❏ **5 points**
I'm a heavy smoker on birth control pills	❏ **7 points**

Risk Factor 14: Weight

Being overweight holds greater heart disease risks for women than it does for men. An eight-year research study conducted by JoAnn Manson, MD, at Harvard Medical School found that among obese women, up to 70 percent of their coronary artery disease was the result of being overweight. The study also found that even women who were moderately overweight had a risk of developing coronary artery disease up to 40 percent higher than women of normal weight.

I prefer to use the term "overweight" rather than the medical term "obese," because most women believe that obesity means enormously overweight—fifty, sixty, seventy pounds, or more. In fact, you are considered "obese" if you weigh between 20 to 30 percent more than your ideal weight. This means that if your ideal weight is 125 pounds and you are 25 pounds overweight, as are many women, you are in the lower range of obesity.

Yet even maintaining "normal" weight may not eliminate these risks. A recent study by Walter C. Willett, MD, at Harvard University found that middle-aged women with body weights at the upper end of the normal range have an increased risk of coronary artery disease. Women who gained even modest amounts of weight after the age of eighteen were also found to face a similar increased risk.

Women tend to be more overweight than men, which raises the risk of heart disease. Excess weight also raises the level of triglycerides (fats) in the blood and increases the likelihood that a woman will develop high blood pressure or non–insulin-dependent adult onset diabetes, all of which increase the risk of heart disease.

Normal weight	❑ **0 points**
Slightly overweight	❑ **1 point**
Overweight	❑ **3 points**
Extremely overweight	❑ **5 points**

Risk Factor 15: Stress/Emotional Factors

A high-stress lifestyle is now considered a risk factor for heart disease. Often, a sudden high-stress event can be the trigger for a heart attack. Your body is most vulnerable when you hear shocking news, such as the sudden, unexpected death of a loved one. If you have recently gone through a divorce or loss of a loved one, lost a job or started a new one, your body is being flooded with stress hormones, such as adrenaline and cortisol, that can weaken your cardiovascular system.

Give yourself one point for any line you check off.

STRESS FACTORS

Stressful events within the last year in your life:

❑ **Death of a loved one (including a pet)**
❑ **Divorce**
❑ **Loss of job**
❑ **Serious illness (yours or a loved one's)**
❑ **Other emotionally traumatic event**

EMOTIONAL FACTORS

Don't neglect the emotional component of heart disease. Twenty-five years of clinical experience have proven to me that the way people deal with their emotions—especially fear and anger—can either hurt or protect their hearts. Those who make sincere efforts to experience positive emotions recover more quickly from illness. Here is a brief "Emotional IQ" quiz as it relates to heart health;

again, give yourself one point for each question you check off.

❑ Are you aggressive, short-tempered, and sometimes hostile or cynical?

❑ Do you tend to avoid confrontation and bury your feelings of anger and sadness?

❑ Are you driven by achievement and performance?

❑ Are you frequently overcommitted and have a difficult time saying "no"?

❑ Do you ever suspect that you suffer from depression?

❑ Do you have a strong desire to be in control of events and other people?

❑ Do you feel a deep internal state of anxiety or restlessness?

❑ Are you unhappy with your body image or "performance" in any area of your life, such as a parent, spouse, or employee?

❑ Do you feel that your life is driven by forces that you cannot control?

Scoring

Add all your points and see where you stand with regard to heart health.

0 TO 10 POINTS—Congratulations. You are at extremely *low* risk for heart disease. You can stay that way by continuing your healthy lifestyle and paying attention to changes that accompany the aging process.

11 TO 25 POINTS—All in all, your heart and cardiovascular system are in fine shape and your risk of heart disease is probably low. With a few changes, your heart health can still be improved.

26 TO 35 POINTS—You have many of the risk factors for heart disease which require your attention. You need to look at your lifestyle and become aware of being productive without being self-destructive. Take charge of your life.

36 TO 45 POINTS—You are perilously close to the danger zone. You must take steps to change your lifestyle *now*. You must take serious responsibility for your health.

46 OR MORE POINTS—You are at extremely *high* risk for heart disease. I encourage you to take my recommendations to heart and to work with a capable, compassionate physician who can help put you and your heart on the road to health.

Risk Factor Recap

	LOWER RISK	HIGHER RISK	HIGHEST
Age	*Premenopausal*	*Postmenopausal*	
Coronary Anatomy	*Male*	*Female*	
Cholesterol/ triglycerides	*Low*	*Borderline/ High*	*High*
Diabetes	*No*	*Yes*	*Yes*
Early Menopause	*No*	*Yes*	*Yes*
Genetics/ Family History	*No family history*	*Family history*	
High Blood Pressure	*Normal*	*Borderline/High*	*High*
Fasting Insulin Level	*less than 10*	*15 to 20*	*more than 20*
Obesity	*Normal weight*	*Slightly Over*	*Over-weight*
Physical Activity	*3 times/week+*	*Some*	*"Couch Potato"*
Diet	*Mediterranean*	*Mixed*	*"Junk Food"*
Smoking	*No*	*Light*	*Heavy*
Stress	*Low-stress lifestyle*	*Moderate stress*	*Recent high stress*

CHAPTER THREE

Beyond Cholesterol: New Millennium Risk Factors

The last years of the twentieth century saw the emergence of a new set of risk factors for heart disease. After reviewing the "traditional" risk factors in the last chapter, you may be wondering how there could possibly be any more! But with scientific advancements we are now able to know the—sometimes subtle—reasons why people with "normal" blood profiles and no obvious risk factors turn up with serious heart disease.

These "new millennium" risk factors may be cutting edge today, but they will be mainstream tomorrow. With this new information doctors can zero-in on your type of problem and point the way to a very targeted solution. Fortunately, any of these risk factors can be detected with a blood test and most are extremely responsive to diet therapy and nutritional supplements—lifestyle changes that can help you steer clear of surgery and medication.

Because risk factors are cumulative, you need to be aware of how to recognize these new ones—especially because these new risk factors have been found to be more prevalent in women. Remember: more than two risk factors can produce an increase in your risk of heart disease.

Let me list for you the new millennium risk factors; then I'll discuss each one in more detail:

HOMOCYSTEINE—a dangerous amino acid that promotes free-radical oxidation and premature vascular disease

OXIDIZED LDL—a deadly form of cholesterol and an agent in plaque formation

FIBRINOGEN—a clot-promoting substance in the blood

LIPOPROTEIN A or Lp(a)—a small cholesterol particle that causes inflammation and clogging of the blood vessels

C-REACTIVE PROTEIN (CRP)—an antibody-like substance that reflects the presence of an old or previous infectious agent in the bloodstream

SERUM FERRITIN—most often reflects levels of iron in the body

Homocysteine: Move Over, Cholesterol

Historically, cholesterol has been at center stage when it comes to risk factors for coronary artery disease (CAD). But like a cunning understudy, homocysteine has been waiting in the wings, awaiting its chance to share the limelight with the darling of all metabolic risk factors. There is now evidence that the two may even work as a team to "plaque up" the lining of your arteries and cause vascular disease.

The message of homocysteine was first delivered back in 1969, when Dr. Kilmer McCully proposed that vascular damage and disease were often the result of high homocysteine levels in the blood. Like many great scientists and inventors, McCully was years ahead of his time. His ideas were not accepted by the medical community. In fact he was asked to leave Harvard because of his dedication to getting the word out on homocysteine and heart disease.

Over the last several years, multiple studies have vindicated Dr. McCully's work and confirmed the connection between high homocysteine levels and artery disease, including coronary atherosclerosis, peripheral vascular disease, and carotid artery disease. In fact, some researchers now propose that 42 percent of strokes, 28 percent of peripheral vascular disease (which causes cramping in your legs), and approximately 30 percent of cardiovascular disease (i.e., heart attacks, bypass, angioplasty, angina, etc.) are directly related to excessive levels of homocysteine, an amino acid produced by ineffective protein metabolism.

Make Sure You Get Your B's
So how does one end up with high homocysteine? The classic set-up is a high consumption of certain foods, especially red meat but also wild game, poultry, ricotta cheese, avocado, and sunflower seeds. These foods are rich in methionine, an essential amino acid. But without enough B-vitamin support on board—specifically folate, vitamin B6, and vitamin B12—your body cannot break down methionine effectively, and the treacherous amino acid homocysteine will be formed.

If you do not take in enough B vitamins, and you frequently enjoy red meat, you may be at risk of developing excess homocysteine. No one's put the brakes on this "bad guy" amino acid, and the result is rampaging free radical oxidation in your body. Homocysteine is considered "unfriendly" to cellular membranes, and many researchers believe that excess homocysteine sets the stage for high levels of cholesterol to infiltrate the blood vessel walls, clogging them with plaque.

In my view, homocysteine is just as dangerous as oxidized LDL "bad" cholesterol. Both are key players in an inflammatory process that arises from free radical oxidation. High levels of free radicals are associated with an increased risk of the clotting events seen in peripheral artery disease, thromboembolism, and stroke. There is also evidence that high levels of homocysteine are a predictor of future cardiac events if you have angina.

Many people don't get enough fresh fruits and vegetables and have serious dietary deficiencies of folate, vitamin B6, and vitamin B12. Just think about how often you are actually able to get the recommended five to nine servings of fresh fruits and vegetables in your day. I know I can rarely accomplish that! Researchers are increasingly concerned that serious vitamin deficiencies exist in our population. And such deficiencies can be aggravated by the effects of caffeine or alcohol, which cause excessive urination and wash out precious B-vitamins from your body.

However, in addition to lack of B vitamins, high homocysteine can be hereditary. A rare genetic enzyme defect in the body can cause high homocysteine levels and cause a life-threatening heart problem in children and adults. Recent research suggests that up to 5 percent of the population may have inherited this enzyme defect, and there is also growing evidence that those with low folate levels are susceptible to these genetic factors.

Because of this new genetic data, the evaluation of homocysteine levels should become standard in preventive cardiology, especially for anyone with a family history of heart disease. So far, the data is remarkably consistent, and research indicates that elevated homocysteine is associated with increased vascular risk—including recurrent heart attack and death. Homocysteine may be a factor in up to 28 percent of the population at risk for premature coronary artery disease. For women the results are even more dramatic: In 1998, the *Journal of the American Medical Association* released the results of a study of 80,000 female nurses who had been tracked for fourteen years since 1980. They reported that those who consumed far more than the recommended daily allowance of B6 and folate were about one-half as likely to develop heart disease than those who took less than the RDA.

Study participants received their folate and B6 primarily from cereals and multiple vitamins. The women on high vitamin programs consumed, on average, 700 micrograms (mcg) of folate daily—almost 4 times the RDA of 180 mcg. And the average of 4.6 mg of daily B6 was close to three times the RDA of 1.6 mg. Good dietary sources of folate include dark-green leafy vegetables, beans, legumes, oranges, and orange juice.

One study, published in the July 1997 *New England Journal of Medicine*, looked at the prognostic value of homocysteine levels in 587 patients with known heart disease. After a follow-up period of 4.6 years, only 3.8 percent of patients with homocysteine levels below 9 micromoles per liter (umol/L) had died, compared with 24.7 percent mortality—a six-fold increase—for those with homocysteine levels of 15 umol/L or more. This study confirmed that high homocysteine levels were strongly related to recurrent heart attack and death. Although homocysteine levels greater than 17 umol/L have been associated with severe and premature arterial disease, research has also shown that concentrations approximately 10 percent above the upper limit of normal (10 umol/L) are associated with a significant increase in the risk of heart attack. In a more recent study, it was determined that women with a history of high blood pressure and high homocysteine demonstrate an alarming twenty-five times higher incidence of heart attack and stroke (more about this later).

Researchers estimate that folate supplementation could lead to the annual prevention of 20,000 to 50,000 premature coronary deaths. Several well-designed clinical trials are under way to further evaluate this issue. Meanwhile, the USDA now requires cereals to be fortified with folate because it is also known that higher levels (200 to 400 mcg) decrease the incidence of neural-tube defects in the first trimester of pregnancy. This level of supplementation, however, may be inadequate to reduce cardiovascular risk; just to be safe, I recommend 800 mcg folate and 20 mg vitamin B6 per day for both women and men.

Keep in mind that prolonged exposure to ultraviolet light, oxidation, and excessive heat can break down folate molecules, rendering them inactive and ineffective. So, you may be eating all the right foods, but cooking them at high temperatures will reduce optimal benefits. Worse yet, the precious B vitamins you take in can be lost if you take birth control pills and consume caffeine, alcohol, or diuretics such as Lasix.

I sometimes encounter women who have high homocysteine levels in the face of excellent B-vitamin support. This is when I call in one of the following reinforcements:

BETAINE OR TRIMETHYLGLYCINE (TMG)—500 to 1,000 mg/day enhances a metabolic process called methylation, taking harmful homocysteine and turning it into a more beneficial amino acid. Broccoli, spinach, and beets also support the methylation process. You can find TMG or betaine at health-food stores.

S-ADENOSYLMETHIONINE (SAM-e)—200 to 400 mg/day will also reduce homocysteine levels and has the added benefit of working as a natural antidepressant. It is also available at most health-food stores.

Oxidized LDL: No Friend of Yours

You are no doubt familiar with LDL—low-density lipoprotein, the infamous "bad" cholesterol that we don't want to see on our lipid profiles. But LDL's bad behavior doesn't stop there. The story of how LDL gets into even deeper trouble involves the cells lining your blood vessel walls (endothelium).

Every time you eat or take a breath, the cells of your body undergo oxidation, a normal metabolic process that inevitably leads to the formation of free radicals. While this process is necessary for life, there's a fine line between just enough and too much free radical activity. Free radicals are trigger-happy molecules with an unpaired electron looking to "steal" another electron from the next molecule down the line. This can set off a chain reaction that can alter essential enzymes, proteins, and even DNA.

For example, when you eat highly unsaturated fatty acids like corn oil or margarine (which are actually more susceptible to oxidative damage than saturated fats), their breakdown products form excess free radicals. Without sufficient antioxidants present to "sponge up" the free radicals, they can run roughshod throughout your cardiovascular system, setting you up for heart disease.

Free radicals are encouraged by activities such as smoking, jogging, or running long distances such as three miles or more, or exposure to radiation, pollutants, allergens, and heavy metals like cadmium or aluminum. These molecular marauders have been incriminated not only in coronary heart disease but in the aging process itself! And the heart is the most susceptible of all organs to undergo premature aging triggered by free radical oxidation.

How can you counter free radical activity and interrupt the oxidation of LDL? The good news is that the heart and vascular system are receptive to the benefits of targeted phytonutrients, antioxidants, and nutritionals. Research suggests that fresh, colorful fruits and vegetables are rich in antioxidant properties (via carotenoids and flavonoids) that can prevent the oxidation of LDL and, therefore, heart disease. Carrots, tomatoes, spinach, black and green teas, and even a small amount of red wine all have proven antioxidant qualities. You can also protect yourself by making sure you are getting plenty of vitamins C, E, and B-complex; the mineral, selenium; and nutritionals, alpha lipoic acid and coenzyme Q10. (See nutritional supplements in Chapter 5.)

As free radicals cause an increase in oxidized LDL, they enhance yet another unwanted byproduct called *lipid peroxides*. This results from oxidation of the fats that we eat and can be a major risk factor in the onset of heart disease.

One of the best ways to keep your blood vessels healthy is to avoid unhealthy fats in the first place. Limit the amount of saturated fat in your diet; common sources are red meat, whole milk, and butter. But you also need to be aware of the many oxidized rancid oils that can be found in animal and dairy products such as hard cheeses, margarine, or even mayonnaise. When these fat-containing foods are left open to air, even briefly, they become oxidized on their exposed surfaces. I'm sure you have noticed that even the pulp of a fresh apple, once bitten into, will turn brown quickly if left on the counter. Less dramatic changes can be seen on the surface of mayonnaise or butter (look carefully for a darker yellow on the surface before you use these products, especially those in deli counters or salad bars). Be mindful about scraping away any areas that are "off-color." Keep them wrapped or covered as much as possible.

And be aware of oxidation when purchasing meats from the market. Many meats are stored in glass cases that are opened frequently. Note the color of the meat surface, especially beef. If there are areas of browning on the red meat, it's already oxidized! Don't buy these rancid meats, even if it means changing grocers. The same storage rules apply to other meats. Keep them covered even while defrosting, and avoid consuming "freezer-burned" items, victims of yet another oxidative process.

Your body is in a continuous battle between free radicals and its own protective antioxidant defense systems. What you choose to eat either supports that battle or undermines it. To support your troops, it is best to consume monounsaturated oils like olive oil or almond oil, or omega-3 oils found in flaxseed, grapeseed, fish, and soybean products like tofu. At the same time, avoid what are called *trans fatty acids*—the killer fats—such as in margarine. Check the ingredients for the term "partially hydrogenated"—that's your trans fatty acid in disguise.

Another way to reduce lipid toxins in your body is to take antioxidants, natural chemicals that neutralize free radicals before they do their damage. When your body has sufficient antioxidant support—either from its own natural antioxidants and/or supplemental antioxidants—then you have oxidative protection. But, if your body is losing the battle, resulting in a siege from free radical damage, then you are in a state of oxidative stress that will result in excessive free radical damage, setting up the cascade for oxidized LDL and the threat of plaque development, coronary artery spasm, and eventually heart disease.

There is evidence that a breakdown of the cells lining your coronary arteries from free radical activity and oxidized LDL is the most sensitive and predictive marker for heart disease. This can be from many causes, including a diet high in saturated fats, smoking, and other factors such as high blood pressure. But by the same token, the reversal of this endothelium breakdown can set the stage for heart-healthy arteries.

How Do You Know If You're Protected?

Antibody Assay Laboratories in Santa Ana, California, has developed an evaluation screening called the Oxidative Protective Screen™, a blood test that measures your antioxidant capability to defend against free radical damage. Your oxidative protection capability is reported as a percentage value called the TOP Index™. Higher values indicate more oxidative protection, while lower values represent a deficiency in oxidative stress protection.

For example, if both your oxidized LDL and lipid peroxides are high but your TOP Index™ is low, then you need to make serious lifestyle changes. You should modify your diet to include more fresh fruits and vegetables, fewer saturated fats, and more phytonutrient sources such as carotenoids, flavonoids, vitamins C and E, and coenzyme Q10. And don't forget the impact that emotional stress has in oxidizing LDL. In my experience of assessing multiple blood analyses, *I have seen the highest oxidized LDL in patients with excessive stress and tension.* It is also important to reduce environmental exposure to free radicals by staying away from drugs, toxic chemicals, rancid fats and oils, and smoking, as well as excessive radiation, sunlight, infections, strenuous exercise, and over-exposure to heavy metals such as mercury, iron, and copper, which can enhance oxidative stress.

In addition, Metametrix in Atlanta, Georgia, and Great Smoky Laboratories in North Carolina are performing sophisticated blood analyses to detect lipid toxins, oxidized LDL, and antioxidant levels (see Resources page 407).

The Fibrinogen Factor: Too Much of a Good Thing?

I recently treated a forty-seven-year-old perimenopausal woman admitted to a major urban hospital with a heart attack and subsequent angioplasty. She was treated by a well-trained, highly competent cardiology team which accurately assessed her traditional risk factors. But when I saw her in a follow-up appointment, her risk assessment revealed very high fibrinogen in her blood that no one had considered.

In younger women, heart attacks are often triggered by a clotting event precipitated by high fibrinogen levels. Too much fibrinogen, an inflammatory product of blood coagulation, can make the blood clot even faster—too fast. Arteriosclerosis—narrowing of the arteries—is the most common cause of heart disease, but in women younger than forty-five, we see more heart attacks caused by improper blood clotting.

But high fibrinogen levels aren't solely the province of younger women. Consider Anna, a fifty-seven-year-old woman who went to her doctor with signs of unstable angina. She had bypass surgery and angioplasty to treat severe coronary disease, followed up with cholesterol-lowering drugs, and other conventional treatments.

But nine years later, Anna had a second heart attack. Now in her mid-sixties and depressed about the recurrence of her heart disease, she came to see me seeking alternative ways to heal her heart. I did a new millennium panel on her and found these three red flags:

ELEVATED FIBRINOGEN   521 mg/dl   normal range <185 to 360 mg/dl

ELEVATED INSULIN   87 uu/ml   normal range 4 to 20 uu/ml

ELEVATED TRIGLYCERIDES 402 mg/dl   normal range 35 to 135 mg/dl

Her HDL "good" cholesterol was also low at 31. I prescribed a fish oil (EPA-DHA) supplement to help give her "slippery" blood platelets and lower her triglyceride levels. I also put her on a Mediterranean-type diet featuring lots of fresh fruits and vegetables and much lower levels of carbohydrates to combat her insulin resistance, plus healthy fats and garlic. I also suggested exercise to help her lose weight (you'd be amazed how many conventional physicians fail to mention the obvious!). Then I added coenzyme Q10, L-carnitine, and pantethine, vital nutrients for cardiovascular health that will assist in helping to pick up her dangerously low HDL. She agreed to go on natural estrogen therapy if these measures failed to improve her blood profile within the next three to six months.

Why is estrogen so important? Fibrinogen levels rise with falling estrogen. Recent research suggests that estrogen replacement therapy can significantly reduce plasma fibrinogen levels.

Although blood levels of fibrinogen are also influenced by one's genetic predisposition, the most important contributor to high fibrinogen levels is cigarette smoking. According to the Framingham researchers, *almost half of all cardiovascular risk can be attributed to cigarette smoking.* Smoking is just about the worst thing you can do for your health, and even more so if you are a woman. A young woman who smokes, takes birth control pills, and has a hidden genetic risk factor for heart disease such as high fibrinogen is writing a perfect recipe for a heart attack in early life.

If you are a smoker, ask your physician to run a serum fibrinogen profile for you. An acceptable range for fibrinogen is less than 300 mg/dl; anything over 360 mg/dl is considered undesirable. If your fibrinogen level is elevated, it should be just the motivation you need to quit smoking. If you don't smoke and are peri- or postmenopausal, consider estrogen therapy, especially if you scored high in other risk categories.

Nutritional support including fresh garlic, cold-water fish, or healthy fish oil and bromelain can help to offset the clotting and inflammatory reactions that excessive fibrinogen produces. (We will further discuss these approaches in Section II.)

"L–P–Little A"—What is this
Strange Creature Called Lp(a)?

Yes, it sounds funny. But it's a serious risk factor just the same. Lipoprotein(a), or Lp(a) for short, is a killer component of the low-density lipoprotein (LDL) or "bad" cholesterol. When it's present at high levels in the blood, Lp(a) can increase your risk of heart disease. Anyone with a strong family history for heart disease should know their Lp(a) level.

Patrick Kelley was forty-nine when I first treated him for chest pain in the emergency room at Manchester Memorial Hospital in Connecticut. He had a history of heart attack and had undergone bypass surgery. Recently, his daughter Kathy had a heart attack at the young age of twenty-eight. Mr. Kelley and his wife were understandably quite concerned and asked for my guidance.

Because Mr. Kelley's Lp(a) had been high, I suggested that Kathy ask her physician in Arizona to test her blood to determine her level. And as it turned out, she had high Lp(a), just like her father. There are no drugs that lower Lp(a) except niacin and estrogen, so I recommended that she begin taking nutritional supplements, including coenzyme Q10, niacin, flaxseed oil, fish oil (DHA), and vitamin C.

Shortly thereafter, I was asked to evaluate the Kelleys' thirty-year-old son, Neil, who had experienced an episode of pressure-like pain radiating into his left arm. Because of the family's significant history of premature heart disease, I ordered a battery of tests for Neil, such as a nuclear stress test (see Appendix A), and metabolic blood profile that included homocysteine, fibrinogen, serum ferritin, and Lp(a).

Neil's stress test results were within normal range. That was a good start, and his homocysteine and fibrinogen were also satisfactory. However, Neil's total cholesterol was elevated at 248 and his HDL "good" cholesterol was excessively low, at 25. But add to that the fact that his Lp(a) was 111—nearly double the desirable range of 60, and like his sister Kathy, Neil was at considerable risk for heart disease.

Many factors influence blood levels of Lp(a), with genetics perhaps playing the major role. According to a 1997 *Journal of American Medical Association* article, Lp(a) appears to regulate clot formation (thrombosis) and inhibit blood thinning. This unwelcome blood process increases in unstable diabetics and menopausal women, perhaps due to their concurrently falling estrogen levels. I suspect that Lp(a) may contribute to the big jump in heart disease among menopausal women, especially since it responds favorably and decreases with estrogen replacement therapy. If your Lp(a) level is elevated, you may need to consider some form of estrogen therapy. (See more about estrogen therapy in Section IV.)

You should be aware that standard cholesterol-lowering drugs (such as Zocor and Mevacor) will have *no impact* on your Lp(a) levels. In fact, a study involving these drugs showed an *increase* in Lp(a) levels! And therein lies the dilemma. While cholesterol-lowering drugs can reduce LDL, they are ineffective when it comes to knocking down Lp(a).

If Lp(a) levels run high in your family, you can counteract them with a regimen similar to the one I prescribed for Kathy. Start off with a combination of 240 to 400 mg coenzyme Q10, 500 mg vitamin C, and 100 mg niacin twice a day. You can increase your niacin dose for better protection (up to 500 mg twice daily) or decrease it as needed if you experience side effects such as flushing or an initial bout of diarrhea or headache.

More good allies are cold-water fatty fish such as salmon, sardines, and mackerel, or fish oils, particularly docosahexaenoic acid (DHA), which blocks the inflammatory and blood-clotting capabilities of Lp(a). Fresh fruits, vegetables, and legumes like chick peas and lentils will help to reduce Lp(a) by lowering insulin levels. Choose monounsaturated fats (such as olive oil) and the best polyunsaturated fats (such as alpha linolenic acid found in organic flaxseed and flaxseed oil) and toss out your saturated fats. Also, be sure to exercise and lose weight if necessary.

By the way, the Kelley's other son, Kevin, also decided to be evaluated for heart disease risk. His Lp(a) and other factors were within normal range, so be aware that not everyone in the family will inherit all the biological traits for heart disease. It's important for you and your loved ones to identify your specific risk factors and take action. I feel strongly that Lp(a) levels be tested on all perimenopausal women who have a strong family history of heart disease. Remember, heart disease does *not* have to be a family affair—prevention is always easier than cure!

C-Reactive Protein: The Case for Cardiovascular Infection

One of the most provocative—and controversial—theories to come along suggests that there may be an infectious component to heart disease (and a number of other chronic degenerative conditions as well). It has been hypothesized that infectious organisms such as *chlamydia pneumoniae, herpes virus,* or *cytomegalovirus* could trigger a chronic inflammatory process in the blood vessel walls that sets off a cascade of events leading to the formation of artery-clogging plaque.

As long ago as 1985, one Finnish study found that half of their patients with coronary heart disease had high levels of an antibody known as C-reactive protein (CRP) compared with only 17 percent of healthy controls. In other investigations, CRP levels were elevated in patients with unstable angina as well as those who had suffered heart attacks. But since CRP also increases in response to reduced blood flow to the heart (ischemia), researchers aren't yet certain whether elevated CRP is the cause or the effect of heart disease and heart attacks. However, other studies have demonstrated that C-reactive protein levels are indeed elevated *often years ahead of a coronary event.*

In 1997 data from the well-publicized Physicians' Health Study indicated that CRP could predict future vascular events, such as heart attack, in healthy as well as high risk individuals. Also, a European study involving 3,043 men and women showed positive correlations between elevated CRP and fibrinogen and ongoing inflammatory responses. In patients with arteriosclerotic heart disease, both CRP and fibrinogen levels shot up. Their results suggested a link between inflammation and heart disease. Other major findings of the study, as reported in 1997 in the *Journal of Cardiology Rounds*, included:

❖ Risk estimates for CRP were stable over long periods, implying that the inflammatory effects may be secondary to a chronic inflammatory process associated with atherosclerosis.
❖ The risk of heart attack from CRP was independent of total and HDL cholesterols, triglycerides, Lp(a), homocysteine, fibrinogen, body mass index, diabetes, hypertension, family history, and several other indicators.
❖ Levels of CRP were predictive of future heart attacks—even for a subgroup of patients with "low-risk" lipid profiles.

In high-risk individuals, some researchers believe that antimicrobial therapy may help thwart heart disease by inhibiting the infectious organisms implicated as the source of chronic inflammation. Clearly, a great deal more research is needed before we start prescribing antibiotics as a preventive for heart disease. For now, be aware of this new risk factor, especially if you are a smoker, and follow the research. In addition, a very recent study published in the *Journal of the American Medical Association* found that exercise reduced levels of CRP in women, and described inflammation as a factor in heart disease.

Iron (Ferritin) Overload: Heavy Metal, Heavy Heart?
Most of us have been raised to believe that getting enough iron is critical to health. But we now know that while some people—such as growing children and menstruating women—have to be

mindful of their iron consumption, others of us must be cautious about getting too much of this heavy metal in our systems. And newer research indicates that iron overload (medically called *hemochromatosis*) can actually contribute to heart disease risk.

This information may seem somewhat paradoxical to you because everyone in our culture, especially women, has been told from childhood that iron is good for us, and that we should be sure to get enough of it in our diet to avoid iron deficiency or anemia. It is true that iron is necessary throughout life for stimulating the bone marrow's production of hemoglobin, the red blood cell pigment that carries oxygen to our cells. Without it, we couldn't survive. And growing children and menstruating women do need to maintain the level of iron in their diets to make sure they're getting enough. This is not difficult, though, because our food industry sees to it that we get more than enough by fortifying hundreds of common foods, including cereals, breads, and pastas with iron.

However, iron is necessary only up to a certain point: too much of a good thing is dangerous. Iron levels in the body are cumulative (stored in the muscles and other tissues), and unless iron is lost through menstruation or donating blood, over the years toxic levels can build up in the system. While this danger always exists for men, it becomes a real risk for women after menopause. At that point, excess iron poses a greater risk than deficiency, and can increase a woman's risk of heart disease.

Even though this risk is not widely known, it is very real and has a strong genetic component. It is now believed that 10 percent of American adults may carry the gene for hereditary hemochromatosis. Many people will not discover that iron overload is responsible for their symptoms until years of damage have taken place. Their physicians are often perplexed by their symptoms of fatigue, abdominal pain, organ failure, immune dysfunction, skin bronzing, irritable bowel syndrome, menstrual irregularity, hair loss, and explosive diarrhea. If you suspect you have iron overload, request from your doctor a pair of simple blood tests: the Serum Ferritin Test and the Fasting Transferrin Saturation Test.

Iron overload can directly affect the heart. One study of Africans who drank local beer brewed in large iron pots revealed high levels of iron in their body tissues, from the iron that leached into the beer. They were getting seven to ten times the recommended daily allowance (RDA) for iron of 10 to 18 mg a day, and many showed signs that they had too much iron infiltrating the heart tissues, a condition called *hemosiderosis*, which can cause deterioration of the heart muscle.

A 1992 study by Finnish researchers examined the role of iron in coronary artery disease (Finland has the highest incidence of coronary artery disease in the world, along with an extremely high per-capita consumption of meat). After studying 1,900 Finnish men aged forty-two to sixty for five years, the researchers found that men with excessive levels of a protein-carrying iron called ferritin had an elevated risk of heart attack, and that every 1 percent increase in ferritin translated into a 4 percent increase in heart attack risk. Ferritin, like C-reactive protein, can readily increase with any inflammatory process, but it can also reflect too much iron in the body. If your TIBC (total iron binding capacity) is greater than 40 percent saturation, and your serum iron and ferritin levels are also high, your body probably has too much iron on board. *Those with high levels of ferritin were more than twice as likely to have heart attacks than those with lower levels.* The authors of this study concluded that the level of ferritin may be even a stronger risk factor than high cholesterol, high blood pressure, or diabetes.

Although the subjects of this study were male, the findings are also important for women. Not only do postmenopausal women lose the protection of regular menstrual iron depletion—which can account for the loss of up to 400 to 500 mg ferritin per year (equal to about two pints of blood)—their levels of ferritin begin to rise steadily after menopause, more than doubling between the ages of fifty-five and sixty-five, and increasing even further after that, in all likelihood subjecting them to the same iron-related risks as the men in the Finnish study.

Indeed, in the early 1980s, Jerome Sullivan, MD, a pathologist, following the idea that iron reduction due to menstrual blood loss protected women from heart disease, theorized that men who regularly donated blood would derive similar protection. He conducted a study which indicated that this was true. Sullivan's findings, first published in the British medical journal *Lancet* in 1981, were years ahead of their time, and since then have been supported by research such as the Finnish study.

No one is yet sure exactly how elevated levels of iron contribute to heart disease, but researchers have a number of ideas. Some research has indicated that iron released from ferritin may play a role in causing the formation of free radicals, which oxidize LDL cholesterol in the blood, making it more likely to adhere to artery walls to form plaque. Other research has indicated that iron released from ferritin at the site of the tissue damage from a heart attack may expand the injury to the heart muscle.

While we have yet to collect data on the specifics of iron excess and women, you do need to be aware that high levels of iron are a risk factor for both genders. And, as we shall see, the increased risk for women after menopause may be related to the fact that they lose the protective benefit of iron loss through menstruation as well as the protection of estrogen and progesterone.

We shall now look at some creative ways to make women less vulnerable to heart disease.

SECTION II

How to Prevent and Heal Heart Disease:
The Four Pillars of Health

CHAPTER FOUR

Nutritional Healing: Eat the Heart-Healthy Way

Over the years, I have seen many trendy diets come and go. After a great deal of observation, study, and personal research, I've concluded that the best overall choice is the Mediterranean diet.

Not only does it have well-documented cardioprotective benefits, the Mediterranean diet will also help protect you against breast cancer *and* osteoporosis. And best of all, it's not really a "diet"—we know that diets are doomed to fail—it's a lifestyle choice.

But, what exactly *is* the Mediterranean diet? Is it eating pasta and drinking red wine? Yes, but it's much more than that. I have modified the Mediterranean diet to address the nutritional issues of most Americans. This is a *moderate*-carbohydrate diet with slightly *more* protein than is often recommended. My version of the Mediterranean diet includes 15 to 20 percent protein, especially from cold-water fish such as salmon and halibut; 30 to 35 percent healthy fats such as olive oil; and 45 to 50 percent slow-burning, low-glycemic carbohydrates, such as root vegetables like garlic and onions, fruits, legumes like lentils and chickpeas, and nuts.

With their nutrients balanced within these ranges, my patients feel better, have more energy, are losing (and keeping off) weight, experiencing a better quality of life, and enhancing their survival from coronary heart disease and cancer. You can too!

Dr. Sinatra's Modified Mediterranean Diet

DECREASE YOUR INTAKE OF:

❖ Processed foods containing refined white flour and sugar, such as breads, cereals (Corn Flakes, Frosted Flakes, Puffed Wheat, and sweetened granola), flour-based pastas, bagels, and pastries;

❖ Foods containing hydrogenated or partially hydrogenated oils (which become trans fatty acids in the bloodstream), such as most commercially prepared crackers, chips, cakes, candies, cookies, doughnuts, and processed cheese;

❖ Starchy, high-glycemic* cooked vegetables such as potatoes and corn;

❖ Processed canned vegetables (they are usually very high in sodium);

❖ Processed fruit juices (often loaded with sugars—try juicing your own carrots, celery, and beets instead);

❖ Red meats and organ meats;

❖ Oils such as corn, safflower, sunflower, peanut, and canola;

❖ Dairy products such as whole milk, high-fat cheese, and whole-milk yogurt.

INCREASE YOUR INTAKE OF:

❖ Oatmeal and higher-fiber pastas made with spelt or Jerusalem artichokes instead of semolina flour pasta;

❖ Slow-burning, low-glycemic vegetables such as asparagus, broccoli, kale, spinach, cabbage, brussels sprouts; and legumes such as lentils, soybeans, and chickpeas;

❖ Onions and garlic;

❖ Herbs such as rosemary, basil, oregano;

❖ Fruits such as grapefruits, cherries, peaches, plums, dried apricots, rhubarb, pears and apples; plus cantaloupes, grapes, and kiwi, although they contain more sugar;

❖ Protein such as fish, especially fatty, cold-water fish like salmon, mackerel, sardines; and shellfish. Flavor your sauces with small amounts of lamb, lean beef, chicken, or turkey. Eat up to six eggs a week;

❖ Soy products like tofu, soybeans, tempeh, and soy milk;

❖ Extra-virgin olive oil on salads or veggies;

❖ Nuts and seeds, including walnuts, almonds, and flaxseed;

❖ Low-fat cottage cheese, feta cheese, and small amounts of grated Parmesan.

*The glycemic index is a ranking of foods, mainly carbohydrates, based on how quickly they increase your blood sugar. For many people (especially those who are overweight, insulin resistant, or diabetic), the glycemic index can be a useful tool in managing the risks of blood-sugar fluctuations.

My modified Mediterranean diet encourages a healthy combination of essential fatty acids (EFAs) and monounsaturated fats (olive oil, nuts) while discouraging the intake of saturated fats often found in red meats, poultry, and high-fat cheeses. Foods higher on the food chain are more likely to contain saturated animal fats.

Mediterranean people, in general, flavor their sauces with meat instead of eating large portions of meat as Americans do. At nearly every meal, Mediterraneans consume fiber-rich fruits and vegetables packed with phytonutrients, vitamins, carotenoids, flavonoids, polyphenols, and monounsaturated fats, so precious to well-being and cardiac health. Their diets are naturally rich in omega-3 fatty acids, coenzyme Q10, and potassium, calcium, and magnesium.

Like many cardiologists, I used to recommend low-fat, high-carbohydrate foods to my cardiac patients. I was caught up in the low-fat, high-carbohydrate craze that swept across the country ten years ago. Boy, was I off the mark! Many of my patients did initially lose weight on no-fat, low-fat diets, but over time their HDL "good" cholesterol decreased and their triglycerides shot up, and they often regained the weight.

Two Big Problems With Low-Fat, High-Carb Diets

What was happening with my patients on high-carb diets? Many were developing *insulin resistance*, a common malady that can lead to diabetes, premature aging, and increased risk of heart disease and stroke, among other conditions. As previously mentioned, insulin resistance reflects the body's ineffective use of glucose due to high amounts of carbohydrates (starches) in the diet. Basically, unmetabolized carbohydrates are stored as fat. Over time, this scenario may be expressed in weight gain, low HDL "good" cholesterol, and high triglycerides that could predispose you to coronary heart disease. Some fifty million Americans are afflicted with some level of insulin resistance—reflected in recent research revealing that one in six Americans are overweight.

At the same time, the no- or low-fat diets were creating a *deficiency in essential fatty acid (EFA) intake*. When people avoid all or most fat in the diet, they begin missing out on the "good fats," too. Although some fats can kill, others can heal. Your body needs fat to burn as fuel and for proper heart and brain function. This is

---

Food-Preparation Tips

- Remove all visible fat and skin from chicken, steaks, and chops. Should you choose hamburger on occasion, select top round steak and ask your butcher to trim excess fat before grinding it.

- Use a rack for broiling so the fat falls away from the food.

- Avoid frying. When you must, use a nonstick frying pan and wipe away or blot excess oil with a paper towel.

- Steam vegetables whenever possible.

- Avoid making gravies with butter or margarine. Instead, use the natural juices from meat, skimming off the fat. Fresh herbs and veggie juices make excellent gravies.

- Substitute fresh or dried herbs for salt.

probably why many of my patients on high-carb, low-fat diets also developed depression, lethargy, and irritability.

In one study of essential fatty acids, ingestion of two fatty fish meals a month were associated with a 30 percent reduction in cardiac arrest; four fatty fish meals a month were associated with a 50 percent reduction in cardiac arrest. Compared with no fish intake at all, you can significantly reduce your risk of cardiac death by eating only one fish meal a week!

Trendy no-fat or very low-fat diets are hazardous to your health. It is time for many of the "no-fat/low-fat" diet gurus to redefine their dietary strategies and introduce vital fats back in the diet.

Look at some of the benefits of the Mediterranean diet:

Ten Benefits of the Mediterranean Diet

1. Offers several cold-water fish selections, such as salmon and halibut, that contain an abundance of beneficial essential fatty acids— omega-3 oils that reduce arterial clotting and inflammation. They are also excellent sources of coenzyme Q10, an energy-boosting nutrient.
2. High in low-glycemic legumes such as lentils and chickpeas, which slow the release of sugars into the bloodstream, helping to prevent excess insulin release leading to heart disease, obesity, high blood pressure, and high LDL cholesterol.
3. Offers a cornucopia of fresh fruits and vegetables packed with phytonutrients—carotenoids, flavonoids, and polyphenols— associated with a lower incidence of cardiovascular disease, cancers, eye disease, and more.
4. Lower in dairy and excessive quantities of meat, thus less methionine, an amino acid precursor to homocysteine, which is formed without adequate B-vitamin support.
5. Rich in root vegetables such as garlic and onions, two terrific

heart healers noted for their antioxidant effects and ability to lower blood pressure.

6. High in vitamin C, vitamin E, magnesium, zinc, and L-glutathione—key antioxidants necessary for the control of free-radical–induced diseases and premature aging; vitamin E is especially important for cardiovascular health.

7. Low in saturated fat, creating less arterial plaque, the major precursor to heart disease.

8. High in fiber, further helping to stabilize blood sugar by slowing the absorption of carbohydrates and supporting healthy intestines.

9. High in olive oil; far healthier than margarine—which contains trans fatty acids.

10. May include small amounts of red wine—a rich source of quercetin, which prevents the deposit of arterial plaque.

Eating fewer processed carbohydrates and consuming more complex carbohydrates like chickpeas, lentils, and broccoli, to name a few, will help your insulin levels to drop, thus sparing your vascular system from insulin excess (hyperinsulinemia), which many researchers now believe is a major cause of premature vascular disease and high blood pressure.

Research Confirms Benefits of the Mediterranean Diet

Research has confirmed that heart-attack survivors on a Mediterranean diet had a 76 percent reduction in their risk of future cardiac events, including subsequent heart attacks and even sudden death, compared with those who followed their doctor's diet advice or a typical American Heart Association diet. The Lyon Heart Diet Study followed 605 patients, all of whom had survived their first heart attack. Only fourteen cardiac events occurred in people following the Mediterranean diet, compared to fifty-nine major cardiac events including stroke, heart failure, and heart attack for subjects on the other diets.

Even more compelling, there were *no sudden deaths* among those on the Mediterranean diet, while there were eight sudden deaths among those following the typical American Heart Association diet. Research has also noted that the difference between the two groups was striking even within the first year.

What Makes the Mediterranean Diet so Protective?

Omega-3 fatty acids, antioxidant vitamins (especially vitamin E), and various carotenoids and flavonoids in fresh fruits and vegetables give the Mediterranean diet its unique cardioprotective effects.

For example, alpha-linolenic acid (ALA), which is found in plants and vegetables (and which acts like an omega-3 fatty acid), appears to prevent blood clots. ALA also is a precursor to omega-3 oils like DHA (docosahexaenoic acid) and EPA (eicosapentaenoic acid), which are found in fish and shellfish. Both help to reduce inflammation and blood clotting—dual processes that may block coronary arteries and ultimately result in a heart attack or sudden death.

What? No Bread?

FRANKLY, THE WORST THING MODERN MAN AND WOMAN has introduced into the diet is bread. While a no-bread–diet is preferred, it is probably impractical, so try to limit your intake to two or three pieces of seven-grain bread per week. Why is bread (and bagels, and frozen waffles, and crackers) so bad for you? It's mostly processed white flour and sugar. It ferments in the gut, which can cause overgrowth of *Candida* yeast. These rapidly absorbed, high-glycemic carbohydrates trigger your insulin levels to rapidly rise, then fall even more quickly, encouraging insulin resistance and "rebound hunger." So you keep snacking and gaining weight. If you limit your intake of white flour products, along with most other pastas, white potatoes, and commercial cereals, your triglyceride levels will plummet and you'll lose weight, too.

How Women Can Benefit from Essential Fatty Acids

These good fats, which cannot be manufactured by your body, penetrate the tenacious layers of cholesterol-laden plaque, doing their anti-inflammatory work and preventing blood-clotting deposits from lining the coronary arteries—all within days! Essential fatty acids also can prevent spasm of the coronary vessels as well as rupture of plaque, which can close the heart's life-sustaining blood vessels, resulting in a heart attack.

The Lyon study provided compelling evidence of the benefits of essential fatty acids in the diet. In this study, the profiles of patients on a Mediterranean-type diet demonstrated that their bodies had an increased ability to decrease free radicals and thus were better equipped to offset oxidative stress. The researchers concluded their higher intake of essential fatty acids to be the reason that no sudden deaths occurred among those on the Mediterranean diet. In addition to protecting vulnerable arteries from rupturing, essential fatty acids appeared to rein in oxidized LDL particles—the notorious "bad guys" in coronary artery disease.

These research results underscore the problem with high-carb, low-fat diets: they are often insufficient in omega-3 fatty acids. While such restricted diets will indeed lower LDL "bad" cholesterol levels, they will simultaneously limit healthy sources of HDL "good" cholesterol. And since it is *oxidized* LDL that you need to be protected against—not just the LDL level alone—the trade-off with the low-fat/high-carb diet may be quite risky. There is further evidence to support this theory.

My Top Nutritional Foods for Women

1. Omega-3 fish oils
2. Soy
3. Flaxseed

Population studies show that cultures with diets low in saturated fatty acids but high in essential fatty acids (such as omega-3) have lower coronary risk when their physical energy needs are met with unsaturated fatty acids instead of carbohydrates. If you're concerned that you may not be getting enough essential fatty acids, here's what you can do:

❖ Eat fresh ocean fish like salmon, halibut, or scrod one to two times a week, as well as soy products like tofu and soybeans.

❖ Eat seeds, like flaxseed and nuts, and especially walnuts, which have omega-3s. I especially like ground-up organic flaxseed. Take at least two tablespoons every day mixed with soy milk.

❖ Consider a high-quality fish oil—check your local health food store. In a recent large placebo-controlled trial of eleven thousand patients who had a recent heart attack, those given omega-3 fatty acids had far fewer incidents of recurrent heart attack, stroke, and death over a three-year duration. Sudden cardiac death alone was reduced by an amazing 17 percent.

Beware of Killer Fats

BEWARE OF "NO-SEE-UM" OR HIDDEN FATS IN YOUR DIET. These include the fatty streaks in lean meat, dark poultry meat, pastries, cheese, crackers, margarine, and processed oils such as partially hydrogenated coconut, palm, corn, cottonseed, and soybean oils. These oils, along with margarine, are *killer fats*. They contain trans fatty acids, which increase harmful Lp(a) and enhance blood clotting. They decrease testosterone levels and are associated with an increased risk of cancer. A word to the wise: Read the labels on all food products that you buy. If they contain margarine or any of the oils mentioned above, don't buy them! Stick with healthy fats such as fish oil, flaxseed oil, and olive oil.

"Healthy" Fat Is Your Friend

When we look at the total picture, it is the Mediterranean diet that offers the most scientific and nutritional approach to heart disease. Remember, the more recent population and research studies suggest that health care providers who continue to endorse no-fat, low-fat diets as "heart-healthy"—in spite of evidence to the contrary—are leading others dangerously astray. (I know, I was among them at one time. I gained 10 pounds on the high-carb, low-fat diet myself.) Therefore, I strongly encourage you—as I do my own family and patients—to stay far, far away from high-carb, low-fat diets.

When considering any dietary plan—whether Mediterranean or a variation thereof—please keep in mind that healthy fat is your friend. Although too many saturated animal fats are bad, the real health threat comes from no-fat, low-protein, high-carbohydrate-type diets, which can run up your insulin levels and result in weight gain, lethargy, fatigue, and even high blood pressure.

On the other hand, the Mediterranean diet can even out your blood sugar levels and reduce insulin resistance while giving you more energy and helping you find your ideal weight or body mass. (To get you started, see the "The Sinatra Modified Mediterranean Diet Seven-Day Meal Plan" in Appendix C.)

Heart-Healthy Foods

By choosing foods off the following list, you will get much of the potassium, magnesium, and calcium you need each day to lower your blood pressure and maintain heart health. These foods are an integral part of my modified Mediterranean diet.

Recommended Foods High in Potassium

Dried Fruits	Meats and Poultry	Vegetables	Fish and Shellfish
dates	beef eye round	avocado*	salmon
prunes*	wild goose	beet greens	mackerel
raisins*	range-fed chickens	chickpeas	halibut
figs*	deer	garlic	snapper
	buffalo	baked potato	sole
	antelope	w/skin	trout
	elk	sea vegetables	mussels
		sweet potato	bass
		swiss chard	bluefish
			anchovies
			lobster
			haddock
			clams, blue
			flounder

Beans	Nuts and Seeds	Milk/Yogurt	Fresh Fruit
adzuki*	soybean nuts*	yogurt, nonfat	apricots
pinto		natto (soy	bananas
white*		product)	cantaloupe
lima			nectarines
turtle			
black			
kidney			
lentils			

* Foods highest in this mineral.

Recommended Foods High in Calcium

Cereals and Grains	Fruits	Milk/Yogurt	Nuts and Seeds
oatmeal	figs*	skim milk*	sesame seeds
	dates	yogurt, non	
	prunes	fat/lowfat	
	raisins	1 percent	

Cheeses	Vegetables	Other Foods	
milk*	asparagus	molasses	
feta	collards	turtle beans	
ricotta, part	broccoli	white beans	
skim*	kale*	tofu*	
	cabbage		
	kelp		
	parsley		
	daikon*		

* Foods highest in this mineral.

Recommended Foods High in Magnesium

Cereals and Grains	Fish	Fruits	Nuts and Seeds
All-Bran	all seafood	figs, dried*	pumpkin
brown rice		apricots*	seeds*
		bananas	sesame seeds
			sunflower
			seeds

Vegetables			
adzuki beans			
black beans			
kelp*			
spinach			
wakame			

* Foods highest in this mineral.

CHAPTER FIVE

Vital Supplements: Unleash a World of Prevention

When I first tell my patients that it is critical for them to take vitamins, minerals, and other nutrients—what I call nutritionals—many of them challenge me to know why. There are five good reasons.

First, very few adults—less than one in ten—eat a truly *healthy* diet, such as a Mediterranean-style diet. Such a diet contains at least five to nine servings of fresh fruits and vegetables per day—the recommendation of the National Institutes of Health.

Second, even if you are eating a balanced diet, you are probably not getting the higher, more therapeutic levels of certain antioxidant vitamins and minerals—such as coenzyme Q10, folic acid, selenium, and vitamins C and E—which may be effective in preventing heart disease, cancer, and other degenerative diseases.

Third, no matter how pure your intentions, it's likely that you are eating at least some highly processed, refined foods which have had many of their natural vitamins and minerals stripped away.

Most cereals, chips, crackers, pastas, and breads made with white flour fit this category.

Fourth, our soils have been depleted of key trace minerals through decades of fertilization and intensive farming, which means that many of our foods do not have enough natural nutrients to begin with. Buying organic produce can help a great deal, and I strongly encourage you to begin incorporating organic foods into your diet.

Fifth, our water and air contain environmental toxins ranging from radiation, chemical poisons, and heavy metals to industrial waste, auto and truck emissions, and cigarette smoke. All of these poisons can affect us at the cellular level, causing free radicals to form. Free radicals are implicated in accelerating the aging process and contributing to the development of degenerative diseases. In a process not unlike that of a cut apple turning brown, your cells are exposed to the damaging effects of free-radical–induced oxidation.

Under ideal conditions, your body compensates for this damage and can repair its cells. However, exposure to radiation, chemical pollutants, alcohol, or heavy metals can tip the balance in favor of free radicals. This is where antioxidant nutritional supplements can play a critical role in combating—and even reversing—the process.

Nutritionals to the Rescue

Hundreds of studies have shown that adding antioxidant nutrients to your diet can protect you from free radicals, neutralizing these molecular marauders before they do serious damage. Antioxidants protect your genetic DNA, cellular membranes, and even the enzyme systems that run your cells' metabolism.

Among what I consider "elite" antioxidants are vitamin E, vitamin C, B vitamins, coenzyme Q10, carotenoids (flavonoids—OPCs), and magnesium, to mention a few. Researchers are not only looking at their benefits to inhibit or prevent heart disease, but also to thwart a host of other chronic disorders, including cancer, diabetes, and Alzheimer's. I can tell you from personal experience and from analyzing the blood of many of my patients that high levels of antioxidants in the blood do protect patients from heart disease, stroke, and even cancer. And this is not only *my* opinion. In a randomized poll of cardiologists, *44 percent take vitamin E themselves to prevent heart disease.*

Vitamin and mineral supplements are not substitutes for a proper diet, but even the rare American who eats a balanced diet does not get the amount of nutritionals needed to combat the toxins that bombard us. *This is why it is critical that you take a quality multivitamin/mineral supplement with antioxidants every day with your meals.*

Key Nutritional Allies

While entire books have been written about these nutritional supplements, here, I am going to single out a handful of select nutrients that support a woman's heart and cardiovascular system. I encourage you to expand your horizons when it comes to nutritional supplements, and read and learn all you can in this rapidly evolving field.

Vitamin E: One of Your Heart's Best Friends

If vitamins could win awards, surely vitamin E would be in line for one of the top prizes. Vitamin E is one of the most versatile of all vitamins, and the evidence of its multiple benefits is irrefutable. There's no question that it helps improve immunity, protects you from cancer, and helps prevent heart disease.

And that's just for openers. There is also evidence that this wonder-nutrient improves circulation, may have blood-thinning properties, reduces oxidized LDL, helps prevent cataracts, relaxes leg cramps, and improves skin and hair. It is considered one of the elite corps of anti-aging nutrients, and it easily earns my vote for blue-ribbon antioxidant status.

Study after study has confirmed my long-held belief that this nutrient acts like a loyal bodyguard as it protects your cell membranes from free radicals. Vitamin E, a lipid (fat)-soluble vitamin, can reduce lipid peroxidation (which causes LDL oxidative stress) by as much as 40 percent. Unimpeded, this progression can cause further oxidative damage which ultimately leads to coronary heart disease.

The American Heart Association touted the Cambridge Heart Study on vitamin E as one of the most "noteworthy scientific accomplishments" in 1996. This controlled trial looked at the effect of vitamin E on 2,000 patients with documented heart disease. Those who took between 400 and 800 I.U. vitamin E daily had a 77 percent decrease in cardiovascular disease over a year's time.

The Cambridge Study supports other studies in the United States, Canada, and Europe. Research has even demonstrated that long-term supplementation with large doses of vitamin E alone increases resistance to oxidized LDL, the low-density lipoprotein form of "bad" cholesterol considered a precursor to heart disease.

Another study, sponsored by the National Institute of Aging, followed 11,178 seniors, aged 67 to 105, for a nine-year period. Those who supplemented with 400 I.U. vitamin E daily had a 41

Why Take Vitamins and Nutritional Supplements?

- Boost your overall energy and sense of vitality;
- Increase your resistance to disease and illness, including coronary artery disease, cancer, Alzheimer's, diabetes, and more;
- Offset the effects of physical and emotional stress;
- Support cellular metabolism and repair;
- Delay the aging process by preventing free radical oxidative stress.

percent reduction in heart disease, a 22 percent reduction in death from cancer, and a 27 percent lower risk of mortality overall.

Dr. Marguerite M. B. Kay of the University of Arizona College of Medicine told the National Academy of Sciences that vitamin E "...may play an important role in preventing free radical damage associated with aging by interfering directly in the generation of free radicals or by scavenging them."

In the Nurses' Health Study involving approximately 87,000 women, the research reported a 41 percent reduction in the risk of heart disease for those taking vitamin E for more than two years. Women taking 200 units of vitamin E had the most protection and even more protection than women taking 100 units or less.

Vitamin E and Women

Although there are several lines of evidence to support the relationship of vitamin E and coronary artery disease in both men and women, the dietary intake of vitamin E may have even greater implications for women. This was seen in an epidemiological study involving 5,133 Finnish men and women, initially free from coronary artery disease. After a follow-up period of fourteen years, a total of 244 cases of fatal coronary heart disease had occurred.

The results showed that the relative risk of heart disease mortality was 32 percent lower for men and 65 percent lower for women in those groups having the highest vitamin E intake compared to those groups with the lowest vitamin E consumption. And women with both dietary vitamin E and carotenoid intakes in the highest one-third had a whopping 84 percent lower adjusted relative risk of coronary heart disease mortality than women for whom both vitamin intakes were in the lowest one-third of the study population.

Be aware that vitamin E requirements for men and women are different. The Nurses' Health Study showed that most women need a baseline of 200 I.U. of vitamin E a day. Other research indicates that most men may need 400 to 800 I.U. per day. Although I have found that a dose of 200 I.U. affords most women sufficient cardiac protection, if you can answer "yes" to two or more of these seven risk factors, consider taking 400 I.U. vitamin E:

1. One or more risk factors for heart disease, overweight status, a smoking history, high cholesterol, or high blood pressure.
2. A family history of premature coronary disease under age sixty.
3. Prolonged exposure to environmental toxins, chemicals, or radiation.
4. A diet high in saturated fats or polyunsaturated fats (omega-3s and monounsaturated fats like olive oil are fine).
5. Excessive consumption of alcohol (more than two alcoholic drinks per day).
6. Severe physical or emotional stress of any kind (family, marital, work-related, etc.).
7. Exercise fewer than four times a week.

In addition, if you have menopausal symptoms such as hot flashes or night sweats and 200 I.U. of vitamin E is not sufficient, consider increasing the dose to 400 to 600 I.U. a day. For women with fibrocystic breast disease, even higher doses—800 to 1,200 I.U.—have been useful in alleviating symptoms of breast tenderness, especially when combined with natural progesterone therapy.

Vitamin E is the Key

YOUR FIRST LINE OF DEFENSE AGAINST FREE RADICALS and highly oxidized LDL "bad" cholesterol is to increase your daily dose of vitamin E.

What to Look for When Shopping for Vitamin E

Most vitamin E products contain d-alpha tocopherol, one of several compounds that comprise vitamin E. But don't settle for anything less than one of the newer generation of products that contains, mixed tocopherols including alpha and gamma fractions, and tocotrienols, a recently discovered group of related compounds. These will do an even better job of protecting you from oxidized LDL, lowering your cholesterol, and offer more antioxidant protection than standard vitamin E products. In addition, maintain your intake of foods rich in vitamin E, including fresh fruits, dark green leafy vegetables, almonds, peanuts, and wheat germ.

Note: If you are taking the blood thinner Coumadin, don't take more than 200 I.U. vitamin E per day because an excess combination of the two could potentially cause excess blood thinning and bleeding.

Colorful Carotenoids: Disease-Fighting Phytonutrients

Carotenoids are extremely important phytonutrients that give fresh fruits and vegetables their various bright colors. Consumption of

---

More Vitamin E Benefits

TOCOTRIENOLS ARE COMPOUNDS THAT HAVE DEMONSTRATED vitamin E–like activity, with some added benefits to reduce your risk for coronary heart disease: they help lower cholesterol (which standard d-alpha-tocopherol does not), and there is evidence that tocotrienols provide greater antioxidant protection against lipid peroxidation than standard vitamin E. They have demonstrated superior anti-tumor activity, especially in breast tissue. The data suggests that the effects of vitamin E and related tocotrienols may have even greater health implications for women.

TOCOTRIENOLS CAN BE PURCHASED IN HEALTH FOOD STORES as a stand-alone supplement or purchased as part of a mixed-tocopherol vitamin E product. The usual dosage is 40 to 80 mg/day.

fresh fruits and vegetables has long been associated with a lower incidence of several diseases including cardiovascular disease, cancers, and eye diseases.

When your mother told you to "eat your veggies," she intuitively knew what she was talking about. Research has demonstrated that free radicals are neutralized most effectively by a *diverse* selection of antioxidants rather than by just one or two. In one study of 1,899 men over a period of thirteen years, those with the highest level of carotenoids had 36 percent fewer heart attacks and deaths than those with the lowest levels.

Those of you who consume at least five to nine servings of fresh fruits and vegetables per day will, on average, take in enough carotenoids to meet your body's needs. But many of you—myself included—will find it a challenge to consume this many servings of fresh fruits and vegetables every day. In such instances, it makes sense to take out the additional "insurance" which can be found in supplements. You should still eat as many fruits and veggies as you can, because it's difficult to duplicate the sheer *variety* of carotenoids found in nature. (For example, lycopene—extremely important in preventing cervical cancer in women and prostate cancer in men—is found predominantly in tomatoes.)

Look for a special supplement or read the label to find a *mixed carotenoid complex* within your multivitamin supplement. Strive for a carotenoid complex total of 12,500 I.U. per day, including alpha carotene, beta carotene, gamma carotene, xeaxanthin, cryptoxanthin, lycopene, and lutein.

Beta Carotene: Not the Only Carotenoid That Glitters

A carotenoid that has gotten quite a bit of attention over the last several years is beta carotene. You may recall reports disparaging the value of beta carotene as a nutritional supplement. One of these, the

Harvard Physicians' Health Study, showed no significant benefits—or harm—from high intakes of beta carotene supplements over a thirteen-year period. Another major trial, the Beta Carotene and Retinol Efficiency Trial (CARET), was actually halted after preliminary results indicated possible adverse effects in long-term smokers given beta carotene and retinol palmitate (vitamin A).

These reports generated considerable controversy and confusion, but I believe the results merit closer investigation. Research subjects appeared to be from a high-cancer-risk group of heavy smokers and asbestos workers. In addition, CARET study participants received extremely high doses of both synthetic beta carotene and vitamin A.

It is well known that vitamin A, a fat-soluble vitamin, is absorbed by and stored in body fat; excessive intake can lead to toxicity over time. On the other hand, beta carotene—a precursor to vitamin A—is water soluble and, therefore, a much safer nutrient. The CARET study combined 50,000 I.U. beta carotene with 25,000 I.U. vitamin A for a whopping aggregate dose of 75,000 units daily! This would be overkill for anyone, regardless of their health status.

Another factor that may have skewed the results: in the Harvard Physicians' Study, *synthetic* beta carotene was taken as a supplement in high dosages. Some chemists and researchers have indicated that high-dose beta carotene *in the absence of* other carotenoids (such as lutein, lycopene, alpha-carotene, and zeaxanthin) may actually work *against* you by literally "washing out" your body's natural carotenoids. For example, too much beta carotene may overwhelm your lutein receptors in the gut, binding them, and preventing the absorption of other carotenoids. This backlash may cause a relative lutein deficiency.

A similar situation has been observed with overzealous consumption of vitamin B6. People who take high doses of vitamin B6 for various reasons, such as carpal tunnel syndrome, without taking a multiple B-complex, have created a similar B-vitamin washout, resulting in a relative B-vitamin deficiency.

In fact, some of the doctors in the Harvard Physicians' Study developed signs of macular degeneration—an eye condition that improves with lutein (another important carotenoid) supplementation and so may be caused by low lutein levels. Therefore, I do *not* recommend that you take high-dose supplemental beta carotene alone, but get it in combination with your diet. It is always best to combine a good diet with some supplements.

The fact remains that beta carotene is an extremely important ingredient for cardiovascular health. Over two hundred studies have confirmed that foods rich in flavonoids, carotenoids, and other antioxidants can reduce your risk of cardiovascular disease (as well as cancer) through regular consumption of antioxidants and phytonutrients. In one study, patients who stored high levels of beta carotene from dietary sources alone in their fat tissue had a lower incidence of heart attack. Many other studies have demonstrated the positive impact of dietary beta carotene for heart disease and cancer.

So, what should you do? First, check the label of your multivitamin to be sure it includes *mixed natural carotenoids*. Then eat foods like carrots, spinach, and squash. Three carrots equal 12,000 units of beta carotene; a large serving of spinach will give you 10,000 units. If your diet is rich in these natural sources, keep your supplemental beta carotene to less than 12,500 I.U.

Lutein—The French Paradox Explained

When news broke a few years ago that red wine seemed to protect the French—who eat a diet high in saturated fats—from heart disease, some of you may have stocked up on Cabernet or Beaujolais. But you needn't risk liver disease for the sake of your health. There's a far healthier and less expensive way to protect your heart and your eyes, and that is found in a carotenoid called lutein. This antioxidant nutrient is found in most fruits and vegetables, most abundantly in spinach, kale, and collard greens, and to a lesser degree in broccoli and brussels sprouts.

To tease apart the paradox, Cambridge University researchers compared the level of antioxidants and carotenoids in people of Toulouse, France, with those of residents of Belfast, Ireland, where the incidence of coronary heart disease is much higher—four times greater in men and an alarming *eight* times greater in women. They discovered that the blood levels of lutein and another carotenoid, beta cryptoxanthin, *were twice as high in the French as in the Irish.* It's also interesting to note that the daily intake of lutein for the French was a healthy 3 mg per day (6 mg is the optimal level).

Since the French diet is as high in fresh fruits and green leafy vegetables as it is in saturated fats, the effects of excess saturated fat intake appears to be offset by the fruits and veggies. In Belfast, however, there's a lower intake of these foods, which likely contributes to high rates of coronary artery disease.

Why is lutein so beneficial? Scientists have found that lutein is present in HDL "good" cholesterol, and it may prevent LDL "bad" cholesterol from oxidizing, a key step in the lethal process which initiates the cascade for coronary heart disease.

Because lutein is so important to your health, I recommend that you take in at least 3 to 6 mg a day. To achieve these levels, you could eat spinach or kale once or twice a week, but you can have the best of both worlds by taking a dietary supplement. Lutein supplements are available in health-food stores, pharmacies, and grocery stores.

So before you build that wine cellar in the basement, take a trip to your local grocery or vitamin store. That's a far wiser way to invest in your health.

Magnesium: Unsung Hero of Cardiovascular Health

Did you know that noise pollution in combination with magnesium deficiency can be a harbinger for sudden death? Years ago, when I was a cardiology fellow, I remember reading a paper from the Dutch literature in which a patient wearing a twenty-four–hour Holter monitor experienced ventricular fibrillation and sudden cardiac death at the time her alarm clock went off. Although we didn't know it back then, research now reveals that loud noises or startle situations in the presence of low magnesium states can cause the heart to go out of rhythm or even stop. Magnesium is in a class of essential nutrients that promotes optimum cardiovascular health.

A light metallic element that burns with a brilliant white flame, magnesium (Mg) commands position number twelve in the periodic table of the elements. Dissolved as a salt (electrolyte) in your bloodstream, it shines as a cofactor in over three hundred enzymatic reactions in the human body. Among its unique properties, magnesium acts like a calcium channel blocker to stabilize cardiac conduction, heart muscle, and vascular membranes.

Magnesium is essential for healthy heart function. It is crucial to produce the high–energy bonds that drive the energy machinery of your cells. *Yet low magnesium is one of the most underdiagnosed electrolyte abnormalities in clinical practice today.*

Your cells need a steady supply of magnesium to maintain proper smooth muscle function in your blood vessels. In addition, magnesium helps shuttle potassium and sodium, two other essential electrolytes, in and out of cells, maintaining proper membrane balance (homeostasis). Magnesium deficiencies can lead to muscle weakness and tremors (spasm) and a host of cardiovascular problems ranging from high blood pressure to arrhythmias. Several factors that cause magnesium depletion are:

❖ **CHRONIC EMOTIONAL AND MENTAL STRESS.** Your body responds to various types of stressors by releasing the "fight or flight" hormones adrenaline and cortisol. These hormones are vital, perhaps even life-saving when you are trying to outrun a predator or meet a deadline, but they are only meant to kick in during times of danger. If the stress level in your life is high, especially if you don't get enough exercise, your bloodstream may be flooded with these hormones on a regular basis, causing magnesium to be released from cells and lost in the urine.

❖ **LONG-TERM USE OF DIURETICS.** If you have a history of heart attack, congestive heart failure, or high blood pressure, you may be on diuretics, which can cause magnesium depletion as the mineral is lost through the urine. In a landmark study reported about fifteen years ago, men with high blood pressure on diuretic therapy had a higher death rate than those whose high blood pressure was left untreated.

It was suggested that many of these men suffered sudden cardiac death from heart rhythm disturbances that were the result of a deficiency of magnesium and/or potassium. The study created chaos in the medical establishment, since treating hypertension was thought to reduce cardiovascular complications, including sudden cardiac death. As a result of this study, many physicians now prescribe magnesium, potassium, and zinc to all of their patients who must take diuretics.

❖ **THE TYPICAL AMERICAN DIET.** Most people (including physicians) are not aware that the typical American diet contains food sources that are frequently depleted in magnesium. Approximately one hundred years ago, magnesium and other minerals were widespread in the American diet. But "modern" technology now employs large amounts of inorganic fertilizers that are often low in magnesium. Overuse of phosphates, nitrates, and ammonia drains much-needed magnesium from the soil. This combination of low magnesium soil concentrations and the damaging impact of modern food processing results in decreased availability of magnesium in the typical American diet.

❖ **TOO MANY CHEMICALS.** Consider, too, the age of chemicals in which we live. Our bodies are insulted by multiple pollutants, such as aluminum, lead, and mercury, that interact with magnesium. By binding to and claiming the body's magnesium stores, these elements further increase your magnesium requirements. Magnesium loss is also linked to a host of medical conditions, including alcohol abuse, prolonged use of antibiotics, anorexia nervosa (or any state of starvation or malnourishment), and excessive use of H-2 receptor antagonists such as Tagamet or Zantac.

Does Your Body Have Enough Magnesium?

This can be a difficult question to answer. Although most hospitals and laboratories can measure blood levels of magnesium quite readily, the magnesium level in the blood has a very weak correlation with the level of magnesium in the heart *cells*.

In addition, an insidious problem can occur even if your blood level of magnesium falls within the normal range. You (and your doctor) might think all is well, but a normal magnesium level in the blood does not always guarantee that the heart tissue has normal magnesium levels in its energy-hungry cells. Modern technology has yet to develop an ideal system for measuring magnesium. Although some tests include measuring the blood cell and skeletal muscle magnesium, these tests are technically difficult and very expensive. For now, the best test is a mononuclear blood cell magnesium ($Mg++$) determination.

Because of these pitfalls, I do not routinely order blood level magnesium tests on my patients. I believe that since magnesium is safe, inexpensive, and easy to use, it should be considered a mineral that deserves more respect for chronic and acute cardiological problems.

Magnesium Can Be Life-Saving

Here's when to use it:

- ❖ If you have suffered a heart attack or are at risk for heart attack;
- ❖ If you are prone to ventricular arrhythmia;
- ❖ If you have had or are planning open-heart surgery or a heart transplant;
- ❖ If you have congestive heart failure or cardiomyopathy;
- ❖ If you have high blood pressure;
- ❖ If you have "sticky" blood;
- ❖ If you are taking diuretics long-term;
- ❖ If you suffer from chronic migraine headaches (which in rare instances, can lead to stroke).

There is a great deal of evidence that magnesium, when administered promptly according to specific protocols and in appropriate dosages, can reduce mortality in patients who have suffered a heart attack. For example, when a person comes in with a heart attack, two grams (2,000 mg) intravenously can be given gradually over an hour's time.

Magnesium can prevent or reduce the severity of life-threatening ventricular arrhythmias that often occur after heart surgery, chiefly through its membrane-stabilizing effect and its ability to maintain potassium, another crucial mineral for the heart, in the cells. Some enlightened cardiac surgeons administer magnesium intravenously prior to bypass surgery.

Magnesium also has been shown to be effective in the treatment of patients with congestive heart failure and cardiomyopathy. Research has determined that patients with very diseased hearts, especially those undergoing cardiac transplantation, have low levels of magnesium as well as coenzyme Q10 in their myocardial cells.

Magnesium and High Blood Pressure

One of the best indications for magnesium, with huge implications for large numbers of people, is in the treatment of high blood pressure. There is a direct relationship between low magnesium and high blood pressure. In addition, magnesium deficits are found in insulin-resistant individuals, particularly Type II (adult onset) diabetics. Many diabetics are hypertensive as well.

Researchers have yet to figure out the "chicken-or-egg" relationship between magnesium deficiency and high blood pressure and diabetes—that is, whether low magnesium levels in the body cause or contribute to these disorders, or if the magnesium depletion is the *result* of these conditions. But regardless of "who-done-it," with such a strong association of magnesium deficits and these problems, it makes sense for any woman with diabetes and/or high blood pressure to include supplemental magnesium in her daily supplement regimen as well as her diet.

Magnesium is "endothelial-cell friendly," helping the lining of your arteries stay smooth and elastic. Over time, low magnesium levels may predispose the interior of your vessels to constrict (tightening the opening) or contract (go into spasm); eventually, high blood pressure can result. Magnesium can come to the rescue of contracted blood vessels and even reverse some of the damage.

There is also evidence that magnesium deficiencies may predispose you to migraine headaches (a vascular disorder) and may aggravate the symptoms of mitral valve prolapse.

Foods rich in magnesium include whole grains, fish and seafood, leafy green vegetables, soy products, brown rice, bananas, apricots, seeds, and nuts. The foods highest in magnesium include kelp, tofu, figs, and pumpkin seeds. I also recommend that you take a magnesium supplement, particularly if you are on diuretics or have any of the cardiovascular conditions previously mentioned.

The Calcium–Magnesium Relationship

Calcium is important, too, because of its synergistic relationship with magnesium. Although most women associate calcium deficits with osteoporosis, low calcium levels can also increase your vulnerability to high blood pressure. *But you must be careful about the amount of calcium you take.* More than 2,000 mg of calcium per day can cause your kidneys to *excrete* magnesium.

You may be wondering whether you can get both of these crucial minerals from diet alone. You can eat foods rich in calcium, such as green leafy vegetables, tofu, low-fat cheeses, and skim or 1 percent

---

Women and Kidney Stones

MANY WOMEN WITH A FAMILY HISTORY OF KIDNEY STONES have been told by physicians to avoid calcium in their diet as well as calcium supplements, even though they have a vulnerability toward osteoporosis. There have been large studies involving nurses who looked at the effects of calcium intake on kidney stone formation. In the Nurses' Health Study, a twelve-year-long project, investigators found that calcium-rich diets actually had an inverse relationship to kidney stones. In other words, women generally developed fewer stones as they consumed more dietary calcium. In contrast, women tended to form more stones as they increased their consumption of calcium supplements.

THE SCIENCE BEHIND THE UNDERSTANDING OF DIETARY CALCIUM involves the body's level of oxalate, a salt from oxalic acid. The higher your oxalate level, the higher your risk for kidney stones. The good news is that dietary calcium lowers oxalic levels. If you're a woman with a family history or personal history of kidney stones, there is no reason to avoid high-calcium foods. Although you should use calcium supplements with caution, you may still take them if you exercise a little care.

JUST REMEMBER TO TAKE YOUR SUPPLEMENTS immediately after your meals. Taking calcium supplements on an empty stomach is a "high-risk behavior" when it comes to kidney stone formation. If you are a menopausal woman and you feel you need higher doses of supplemental calcium in addition to what you're getting from your diet, you can avoid the oxalate dilemma by taking your calcium supplement on a full stomach.

milk, but *you still must supplement to be sure you're getting the right ratio and balance of each mineral.* You should take 400 mg "magnesium insurance" every day in conjunction with 1,000 mg calcium. Postmenopausal women are often recommended to take 1,500 mg of calcium, which is fine, but most of you will be able to make up the difference in your diet with 1,000 mg. Remember to take calcium after meals to prevent the development of kidney stones (see "Women and Kidney Stones" on page 101).

I like the calcium or "CalMag" preparation in softgels because of their rapid disintegration time (six minutes or less) and better bioavailability. In people with poor digestion, solid calcium tablets may pass through the digestive tract intact and fail to be utilized by the body. So, choose a calcium formula that contains mixed compounds such as citrate, carbonate, aspartate, and gluconate in combination with a similar magnesium complex. Even though calcium supplementation is frequently given to help prevent osteoporosis in aging women, it also plays a role in easing the symptoms of PMS in premenopausal women. Other recent research also shows that calcium may help to prevent the growth of polyps in the rectum.

B-Vitamins & Folic Acid: Starring Roles for Your Heart

Recently, a national survey on "What We Eat in America" yielded crucial information to scientists and new insights about vitamin nutrition in the United States. One major concern was the fact that only 45 percent of women between the ages of twenty to twenty-nine have a folate intake that achieves 100 percent of the RDA. This means that slightly over half of women in this age group have low intakes of folic acid, which in turn increases their risk of having a child with serious—and fully preventable—birth defects.

Are you aware that folate helps prevent neural tube defects such as spina bifida? Although the USDA has advised all women and teenage girls who are capable of becoming pregnant to consume at least 400 mcg folic acid daily to minimize their risk of having a deformed child, many women have not followed this advice or are unaware that it even exists.

Unfortunately, in 1989 the RDA for folic acid was cut in half for both men and women. The revised RDA dropped to 200 mcg per day for men and 180 mcg per day for women. At that time, scientists failed to realize the extreme importance of adequate folic acid intake to both prevent neural tube defects and modify elevated homocysteine levels.

What to Look for in a Multivitamin

WHEN SHOPPING FOR A MULTIVITAMIN, here are the overall ranges of "the basics" I'd like to see included. As you will see, I am not a proponent of "mega-dosing."

12,500 I.U. mixed carotenoids (beta carotene, lycopene, lutein, zeaxanthin, beta-cryptoxanthin, and alpha-carotene)
200–400 I.U. vitamin E, mixed tocopherols, gamma tocopherol, tocotrienols
500 mg vitamin C
400 I.U. vitamin D
125–250 mg calcium
200–280 mg magnesium
50–100 mg potassium
100–200 mcg selenium
400–800 mcg folic acid
10–20 mg vitamin B-1 (thiamine)
10–20 mg vitamin B2 (riboflavin)
10–20 mg vitamin B3 (niacin)

20–40 mg vitamin B-6
20–40 mcg vitamin B-12
25–50 mg vitamin B5 (pantothenic acid)
10–15 mg zinc
100–200 mcg chromium picolinate
10–40 mg quercetin
200–500 mcg vanadium
25–50 mg bromelain
1 mg manganese
200–500 mcg boron
150–250 mcg copper
75–150 mg iodine (kelp)
75–150 mg molybdenum
50 mg inositol
25–150 mcg biotin

But research coming in within the last few years has convinced many experts that the RDA should be returned to its older, higher levels, especially for women. A major fourteen-year study, which appeared in the February 4, 1998 issue of the *Journal of the American Medical Association*, drove the point home in terms so clear that even the mainstream media began to encourage women to voluntarily increase their intake of folic acid. Here's what researchers at the Harvard School of Public Health in Boston found:

❖ An intake of folic acid and B6 above the current RDA (180 mcg folic acid; 1.6 mg B6) could significantly lower a woman's risk of heart disease and heart attack.

❖ Women who typically consumed 400 mcg folic acid and 3 mg of B6 daily—significantly above the current RDA—were half as likely to suffer a heart attack than those who consumed the lower levels.

Most of the women in the study received the bulk of their folic acid and B6 from multivitamins and fortified cereals. Researchers examined the amount of folic acid and B6 in the diets of 658 women who had survived heart attacks and compared them to women who had never suffered a heart attack. They found that the more of each vitamin the women consumed, the less likely they were to have suffered an acute cardiac event.

Although you can get folic acid and B6 from food, including green leafy vegetables, beans, legumes, oranges, and orange juice, your diet alone may not give you all that you need to protect you against heart disease or a heart attack. I've always believed that a higher dose of folic acid, as well as other B vitamins, is the antidote for high homocysteine, a harmful amino acid that causes free radical stress to the cells that make up your blood vessel linings.

Homocysteine, as we discussed in Chapter 3, is one of the more recently recognized risk factors for heart disease, along with oxidized LDL and Lp(a), a lipoprotein that can cause premature heart disease in women. Researchers believe that excess levels of homocysteine may set the stage for cholesterol to penetrate blood vessel walls and start plaque formation.

I believe that every woman over the age of fifteen should take folic acid supplements or at least fortified cereals and/or green leafy vegetables every day. And it's never too soon to start heart disease prevention. Even young women who take B vitamin supplements can reduce their risk of heart disease and stroke. In fact, any woman with a history of high blood pressure and high homocysteine faces an alarming twenty-five times normal risk for stroke.

And here is more to motivate you. B vitamin supplementation has also reduced the risk of cervical cancer. Any woman who has a family or personal history of cancer of the female reproductive organs should be aware of the basic protection she can have just by making sure her B vitamin intake is on the mark. Think of it: 400 mcg of folic acid and 3 mg of B6 can cut your risk of heart attack in half. It is time to pay attention to the tremendous impact B vitamins can have on your health.

Vitamin C: Still the All-Around Antioxidant Champ

Vitamin C, also known as ascorbic acid, is one of our best-known antioxidants, first made famous by the work of Linus Pauling, the two-time Nobel laureate who pioneered much of the research into its benefits. It's likely that more research has been done on vitamin C than any other single nutrient, precisely because of its proven benefits in preventing and treating chronic diseases.

In addition to its wide-ranging antioxidant talents, vitamin C aids in the absorption of calcium and magnesium, two key minerals for heart and bone health as previously discussed. It lowers your risk of depression by perking up levels of serotonin and dopamine, two neurotransmitters that keep you on an even keel. It stimulates your adrenal glands, helping to protect you from fatigue and stress. Essential for the development of healthy connective tissue, it speeds healing of wounds and surgical incisions and stimulates the immune system for faster recovery from burns, infections, and disease. It's also essential for maintaining healthy joints and can be crucial in the treatment of arthritis. Last but not least, vitamin C also helps protect blood-vessel linings and will help lower levels of Lp(a), a recently recognized type of cholesterol that is a major cardiac risk factor.

There is near-universal agreement that you need a minimum of 200 mg of vitamin C daily—more than three times the RDA (60 mg). Even higher amounts may be beneficial. For instance, we know that 180 mg daily has been shown to reduce colon cancer by 50 percent and bladder cancer by 60 percent. Cancers of the breast, stomach, esophagus, and lung have also been improved at higher doses.

There is often debate about dosage level for vitamin C. I am quite comfortable recommending a daily maintenance dose of 500 mg. In fact, short-term use of higher doses (up to 5,000 mg, or 5 grams, taken in one-gram increments every few hours throughout the day) can reduce the duration of a cold and combat seasonal allergies, especially when combined with quercetin. In addition, you should eat foods rich in vitamin C, such as broccoli, tomatoes, strawberries, and citrus fruits like pink grapefruits and oranges.

Look for vitamin C in 500 mg ascorbic acid capsules; if you have a sensitive stomach, consider an esterified source, such as Ester C. Stay away from chewable types of vitamin C, which are usually loaded with sugars and binders.

Note: If you have high iron (ferritin) levels, be careful about megadosing with vitamin C. Vitamin C enhances the absorption of iron, and too much iron (which can be determined by a blood test) is a risk factor for heart disease.

The New Breed of Supernutrients for Your Heart

I would be committing nutritional malpractice if I didn't tell you about a number of other heart-healthy nutrients that can safeguard the health of both women and men. Consider making these cutting-edge nutritionals part of your nutritional profile.

Coenzyme Q10: Energy on Call for Your Heart

There have been more than one hundred clinical studies at major universities and hospitals documenting the benefits of coenzyme Q10. It has demonstrated ability to improve congestive heart failure (CHF) and angina and reduce high blood pressure. The research also shows that CoQ10 helps patients get through—and recover more quickly from—bypass surgery. It also helps offset the toxic effects of statin drugs used for lowering cholesterol as well as chemotherapy. I have long considered CoQ10 a wonder-nutrient, because this energizing nutrient essentially improves the heart's ability to pump more effectively.

My Top Ten Nutritional Supplements for Women

1. Coenzyme Q10
2. L-carnitine
3. B-Vitamins (folic acid, B12, B6)
4. Carotenoids (lutein)
5. Magnesium/calcium
6. Vitamin E
7. Vitamin C
8. OPCs (grape seed, pycnogenol)
9. Alpha lipoic acid (ALA)
10. NAC (N-acetylcysteine)

Some Heart Drugs Could Deplete Coenzyme Q10 and Cause Breast Cancer

WOMEN WHO TAKE CERTAIN "STATIN" DRUGS to lower cholesterol (often prescribed for those with a history of coronary heart disease) are dangerously depleting their CoQ10 stores and could be making themselves vulnerable to breast cancer. Low levels of CoQ10 have been found in people with various cancers, particularly women with breast and cervical cancer. Two studies in Europe have reported that women with levels of CoQ10 under 0.6 ug/ml are more vulnerable to breast cancer. In one study of 200 women with documented breast cancer, 40 percent had low Q10 levels. The lower-than-normal levels of CoQ10 have been associated with women taking statin drugs, also called HMG-CoA-reductase inhibitors, such as Lipitor, Mevacor, Zocor, Pravachol, and others. The problem with these drugs is that they interrupt approximately twenty biochemical pathways in the body. The result is not only do they lower cholesterol, but they also interrupt the synthesis of CoQ10 (and squalene as well). It is important that women at high risk for breast cancer understand this association between statin drugs, low CoQ10, and cancer, and strongly consider taking CoQ10 supplements if they must be on a statin drug.

WHO ARE HIGH RISK WOMEN FOR BREAST CANCER? Certainly, any aging post-menopausal woman is more likely to get breast cancer than a younger woman. Also, increased body fat, family history of breast cancer, and an increased exposure to insecticides or pesticides place women at additional risk for developing breast cancer. Another important factor is vegetarianism. Vegetarian women are at risk if they don't get sufficient doses of CoQ10, as well as L-carnitine, in their usual diet. Both CoQ10 and carnitine come predominantly from animal flesh.

ANY WOMAN TAKING A STATIN DRUG, especially those at high risk for breast cancer, should take at least 100 mg of CoQ10 a day.

ONE OF THE MOST IMPORTANT CHOLESTEROL-LOWERING STUDIES evaluating statin-like drugs was the CARE Study. In this study of approximately 500 post-menopausal women with heart disease, 250 were placed on a placebo while another 250 took Pravachol, a statin drug. Although the incidence of subsequent heart events (i.e., heart attack, repeat angioplasty, repeat bypass surgery) were all markedly lower in the Pravachol group, their incidence of breast cancer was significantly higher. In fact, only one woman in the control group developed breast cancer compared to twelve in the group receiving the statin drug.

THERE NEEDS TO BE MORE RESEARCH into the potential risk of breast cancer for women taking HMG-Co-A-reductase inhibitors to lower their cholesterol. Doctors owe it to their patients to look further into this issue before routinely prescribing what may have the potential to be a dangerous medication for some women.

TO KEEP OUT OF HARM'S WAY, consider many of the other creative cholesterol-lowering options. For women who are still unable to decrease cholesterol levels and have a history of moderate to severe coronary heart disease, then a statin drug is a suitable choice, but only if she protects herself with supplemental CoQ10 as well.

Every cell must have a way of obtaining energy. In cardiac cells as well as throughout the body, oxygen-based production occurs within the cellular power plants called mitochondria. Here, CoQ10 provides essential energy in its most basic form—adenosine triphosphate (ATP)—the energy of life. Without adequate CoQ10 as a cofactor, ATP synthesis slows down, eventually leaving the cell in a vulnerable state.

As oxygen-based production takes place within the cellular mitochrondria, CoQ10 concentrations in heart cells can be ten times greater than in any other body tissues including the brain and colon.

The heart is one of the few organs in the body to function continuously without resting; therefore, the heart muscle (myocardium) requires the highest level of energetic support. Thus, any condition that causes a decrease in CoQ10 could impair the energetic capacity of the heart, thus leaving the tissues more susceptible to free radical attack.

Since free radical stress is more pronounced in advancing stages of heart failure, the heart becomes even more vulnerable in these situations. Higher doses of CoQ10 will be required for severe heart failure. I recommend at least 300 to 400 mg per day in such instances.

Dietary sources of CoQ10 come mainly from beef heart, pork, chicken livers, fish (especially salmon, mackerel, and sardines). Vegetarians typically will not get enough CoQ10 unless they eat large quantities of peanuts and/or broccoli. The average person only gets 5 to 10 mg

CoQ10 each day from diet alone. As you can see, most people would benefit from far more CoQ10 than can be gleaned from the daily diet.

Although CoQ10 can be synthesized by the body, I see many patients who are very deficient in this vitamin. Illness depletes the body's stores even further. Taking cholesterol-lowering drugs such as HMG-CoA reductase inhibitors can literally "kill" CoQ10 synthesis. Other drugs, such as beta blockers and some of the older antidepressants, also interfere with CoQ10–dependent enzymes, lowering its concentration in the body.

I recommend CoQ10 according to the following tiered dosage schedule:

300 TO 400 MG/DAY—advanced congestive heart failure

120 TO 240 MG/DAY—high blood pressure, angina, arrhythmia, mitral valve prolapse, and periodontal disease.

90 TO 150 MG/DAY—diabetes type II, insulin resistance, or family history of diabetes

60 TO 90 MG/DAY—preventive maintenance for healthy hearts and anti-aging of mitochondria

For Added Nutrition

HERE ARE A NUMBER OF OTHER EXTREMELY BENEFICIAL NUTRITIONALS that are not likely to be included in your multivitamin that can further protect your heart and overall health. Stay on the lookout for some high-quality multivitamin and multimineral supplements that contain most, if not all, of these ingredients:

10–20 mg coenzyme Q10
12.5–25 mg L-carnitine
3–6 mg lutein
25–50 mg alpha lipoic acid
10–25 mg proanthocyanidins (such as grapeseed extract)
75–100 mg N-acetylcysteine (NAC)
100–150 mg L-arginine

If your initial response to lower doses is poor, increase the dosage and maintain it over time. High levels may be required to achieve a therapeutic effect, and bioavailability among products varies greatly.

Side effects are rare, but I have had a few patients report feeling "too much energy" and a few describe it as a feeling comparable to consuming too much caffeine. For these people, I simply adjusted their dose until a more comfortable level was found. Like most nutritional supplements, for best results take it in divided doses with meals. CoQ10 also works synergistically with its "sister" L-carnitine in anti-aging medicine (more of which we will discuss later).

Alpha Lipoic Acid: Antioxidant With a Twist

Alpha lipoic acid (also called lipoic acid) is considered a universal antioxidant because of its talent for neutralizing free radicals. It also has a unique ability to conserve and rejuvenate other important antioxidants such as vitamins C and E. When oxidative stress wears down your stores of front-line antioxidants, lipoic acid comes to the rescue.

And because it's fat *and* water soluble, alpha lipoic acid (ALA) is readily dissolved and carried in your blood for distribution throughout all the tissues and cells of your body, including the brain, where it readily crosses the blood/brain barrier to protect neural tissues from free radical attack. Recent theories suggest that some mental illnesses and neurological disorders may be aggravated by free radical damage at the nerve synapses in the brain. At the very least, ALA may support memory function, an important consideration as we age. Topical ALA is also popular to help rejuvenate the skin, protecting it from the damaging effects of environmental toxins and rendering the skin more firm with prolonged usage.

Some researchers believe lipoic acid's greatest asset is its ability to regenerate *L-glutathione*, an essential nutrient that helps deter atherosclerosis. But this versatile antioxidant also plays a role in preventing cataracts, improving sugar metabolism and insulin release (critical for those with diabetes), and enhancing the liver's ability to detoxify heavy metals. In Germany, lipoic acid has been approved for the treatment of diabetic nerve damage. It also has been shown to improve blood flow to nerves and to stimulate the regeneration of new nerve fibers.

As you age, your stores of lipoic acid decline. Sure, you can get some of what you need from food, but, unfortunately, the best dietary source of lipoic acid is red meat, which often contains high levels of saturated fats, hormones, insecticides, pesticides, and radiation. As a result, it's far better and safer to get this antioxidant in supplement form.

The usual recommended dose is 50 to 100 mg daily. For patients with severe diabetic neuropathy with a highly compromised quality of life, I recommend up to 500 mg lipoic acid per day without fear of side effects. ALA, even in modest doses, will protect you from heart disease, diabetes, heavy metal intoxication, and even aging itself.

N-acetylcysteine (NAC): Tireless Free Radical Fighter

N-acetylcysteine (NAC) also helps raise levels of L-glutathione, one of the most potent free radical scavengers around and one, unfortunately, that decreases in those with heart disease. You may be wondering, "Why not just take glutathione supplements instead?" But I discourage this because glutathione is difficult to absorb.

NAC, on the other hand, breaks down into natural glutathione and, in combination with vitamin C and selenium, forms glutathione peroxidase, one of the best defenses against atherosclerosis. Glutathione also supports red blood cell function and helps to eliminate heavy metals such as arsenic from your bloodstream.

I believe you're going to hear a lot more about NAC in the future, as it's showing promise in research against certain types of cancer as well as chronic bronchitis and many other conditions. It is one of the best nutrients to take during a flu-like illness. Research has shown an improvement in flu-like symptoms, mucus production, and well-being through taking 1,200 mg of NAC per day. This sulfur-containing compound has been shown to improve the endothelial cells lining your coronary arteries and keep blood flowing smoothly by producing various chemical substances which cause blood vessels to relax.

When damaged—whether by free radicals, oxidized LDL, or other factors—endothelial cells can lose their protective ability, setting the stage for conditions ranging from atherosclerosis to coronary artery spasm. Because we are all at risk for developing atherosclerosis, we need to safeguard these cells. You should take at least 100 mg of NAC daily and 600 to 1,200 mg for upper respiratory infections.

Oligomeric Proanthocyanidins (OPCs): Bioflavonoids With Clout

Oligomeric proanthocyanidins (OPCs) may be a mouthful to pronounce, but once in your system, they get right to work doing wonderful things. In addition to their many heart-friendly effects, they help control allergies, fight off disease, slow down aging, and may even put a little extra zing in your step. For me, they have earned rights to the elite status of universal antioxidant.

You may have heard of polyphenols, flavonoids, flavones, Pycnogenol (pinebark), grapeseed, catechins, tannins, quercetin, and flavonol. You've also probably heard about the benefits of red wine, green tea, and grape juice. All are in the family of OPCs, which are really the cream of the crop.

It absolutely amazes me how nature gives us so many opportunities to nurture our bodies and improve our health. OPCs, which were discovered about fifty years ago, are particularly abundant in nature: there are approximately six thousand flavonoids in the plants around us! These free radical scavengers not only help prevent the oxidation of LDL, they also boost your body's overall resistance to disease. OPCs enhance collagen's ability to repair itself, thereby protecting your collagenous tissues from age-related degenerative processes.

Because they are highly bioavailable, OPCs are quickly absorbed into the bloodstream, where they also cross the blood/brain barrier to protect the brain from free radical stress. As a class, the proanthocyanidins also have a "lipoic acid effect" by regenerating oxidized vitamin E back to its reduced form. Although OPCs belong to the larger class of polyphenols, their subclassification is further broken down into flavonols, which have been found to have extraordinary health benefits. Here are a few:

❖ as efficient free radical scavengers, they prevent the oxidation of LDL "bad" cholesterol, thereby lowering your risk of cardiovascular disease;

❖ may reduce cholesterol plaque buildup on blood vessel walls;

❖ prevent blood stickiness and thus excessive blood clotting;

❖ increase strength and elasticity of capillaries, improving vascular function;

❖ reduce swelling, edema, inflammation and degeneration of veins, helping to prevent circulation problems, especially varicose veins;

❖ reduce discomfort associated with menopause and premenstrual syndrome;

❖ protect against diabetic retinopathy, the most common cause of blindness in diabetics;

❖ improve blood vessel elasticity and may lower blood pressure by having an "ACE-inhibiting effect."

Consider the "Far East Paradox." China and Japan have traditionally had lower rates of cancer and heart disease than the West. Studies show that the Chinese and Japanese also have lower LDL "bad" cholesterol concentrations in their blood. In a small but significant study, fourteen healthy subjects taking in flavonoids and polyphenolic antioxidants via their daily tea had less oxidation of their LDL cholesterol. It was suggested that tea flavonoids taken on a daily basis may lower the risk of atherosclerosis.

Flavonols, a subcategory of flavonoids, inhibit oxidation and reduce toxicity of low density lipoproteins (LDL) as well as inhibit blood clotting in the laboratory. In population studies, a higher intake of flavonols reduced the risk of coronary heart disease mortality as well as a first heart attack.

Animal studies have also demonstrated that OPCs lower cholesterol as well as reduce the amount of cholesterol plaque on blood vessel walls. And the research continues to show that even grape juice can be as effective as red wine in protecting you from atherosclerosis. *Grape juice*, like wine, contains flavonols that have been shown to inhibit blood platelets, thus making your blood less prone to clotting, which can help prevent heart attack and stroke.

If you're not already convinced that OPCs are a combination healer and fountain of youth, consider that OPCs have also been linked to fighting chronic fatigue, arthritis, allergies, cataracts, and Alzheimer's disease as well as other degenerative diseases. And they've also been connected to resveratrol, commonly found in grapes and other plants. Resveratrol helps prevent the initiation of cancer and possesses potent antioxidant and cardio-protecting properties.

You can find grapeseed extract and pinebark extract (under the patented brand name Pycnogenol™) in your local health food store. I recommend 30 to 60 mg daily.

Flavonoid-rich *green tea* is an easy way to further protect yourself from heart disease and cancer. One Japanese study showed that people who drank five cups of green or black tea containing 24 mg of tea flavonoids had fewer free radical indicators in their blood compared to a control group. As little as one cup of green tea per day may provide adequate polyphenols to inhibit LDL "bad" cholesterol, the cornerstone of cholesterol damage to the blood vessels. Furthermore, green tea inhibits blood clotting that promotes arteriosclerosis, strokes, and heart attacks.

The British medical journal *Lancet* reported that the antioxidant effect of green tea was greater than vitamin C, and equal to vitamin E, two premier antioxidants. As a bonus, green tea can help prevent skin cancer and gingivitis, and it has a mild diuretic effect.

While plain green tea itself has a delicate flavor, try it in one of the many formulas that combine it with lemongrass and other herbs. Add a little honey and lemon and I think you will find that this healthy brew is quite delicious. My wife Jan is not fond of the green tea flavor but finds that if she brews it with another flavored

Should You Have an Aspirin a Day?

IF YOU HAVE DOCUMENTED CORONARY ARTERY DISEASE (CAD) or have had a heart attack, angioplasty, or bypass surgery, it's fine to take a baby aspirin a day if you can tolerate it. However, if you don't have a documented history of heart disease, I do not recommend aspirin therapy. In women over the age of seventy-five, aspirin can increase the risk of stroke. And there are strong data to show that aspirin is poorly tolerated by a lot of people, with gastrointestinal bleeding being a major adverse side effect.

HERE'S AN ALTERNATIVE: drink a cup or two of ginger tea a day. Ginger inhibits platelets and makes blood less sticky, reduces inflammation, and also has some cholesterol-lowering ability. I drink ginger tea every day; you should, too. It's a way of improving or assuaging any subtle inflammation while reducing your risk of CAD.

tea it has much more appeal. If you can, in the process, break the coffee habit, you'll be doubly rewarded as you'll also be reducing the amount of caffeine. Black teas also contain less caffeine than coffee and have medicinal effects similar to green tea, but to a lesser degree.

CHAPTER SIX

Get Moving! Exercise Can Save Your Life

How do you sidestep osteoporosis, lift your spirits, and protect your heart all at the same time?

Exercise.

There is no other lifestyle modification with such immediate and long-lasting benefits on your health and well-being, both mentally and physically. The benefits of regular exercise to maintain body weight, improve your mood, curb food cravings, and lower your blood pressure cannot be emphasized enough. Here are my top ten reasons to exercise:

1. Your heart will love you for it. Your blood pressure will go down, and so will your resting heart rate. Your heart will become more efficient, maintaining the same level of output with fewer beats per minute.
2. It will reduce your risk of cancer (a recent study revealed that women who exercise an hour a day reduced their risk of breast cancer by 30 percent).

3. You'll minimize your risk for stroke.

4. You'll increase your muscle strength and restore your range of motion (flexibility), thereby reducing painful signs of arthritis.

5. You'll rev up your metabolism and burn calories, thereby losing weight.

6. You'll beat depression. Exercise releases endorphins and triggers release of the neurotransmitter serotonin, which will lift your mood.

7. Your blood sugar will go down, improving your body's regulation of insulin and preventing insulin resistance and diabetes.

8. You'll age more gracefully and look and act younger than your years.

9. You'll sleep like a baby. Not only will you fall asleep more quickly and sleep more deeply, your concentration and memory will improve.

10. You'll feel more amorous. Exercise not only increases your growth hormones, it improves your self-image, making you feel better about yourself.

Inactivity is the single most prevalent risk factor for heart disease. And a report by the Centers for Disease Control and Prevention found that nearly 30 percent of adults aged eighteen and older reported being inactive. If you're obese (20 percent more than your ideal body weight), you are at greater risk of dying prematurely from a heart attack as well as developing hypertension, which can predispose you to heart attack or stroke.

The reason is simple: The more weight you carry, the harder your heart has to work. When you are overweight, your heart actually has to push your blood through fat that lines and narrows your blood vessels. It's like trying to battle your way through a subway station at rush hour.

Aerobic Movement: The Foundation

Did you know that thirty minutes of exercise will keep your metabolic rate up for another hour? So, the longer you exercise, the greater the benefits. JoAnn E. Manson, professor of medicine at Brigham and Women's Hospital and Harvard Medical School, analyzed the histories of over 72,000 women enrolled in the Nurses' Health Study. She found that women who walked briskly five or more hours a week cut their risk of heart attack by 50 percent. She also found that brisk walking three hours per week cut the risk of cardiovascular disease by 40 percent.

You don't need a lot of fancy equipment. Nor do you need to join a health club. Just put on a pair of comfortable lace-up shoes

---

What About Running?

MANY OF MY PATIENTS ASK ME ABOUT RUNNING as a way of healing the heart and lowering blood pressure. Although running is considered an aerobic activity, it is a more strenuous one and should be avoided for heart patients, especially if you're just embarking on an exercise program. Studies have shown a connection between heart attacks and sudden exertion. At the same time, moderate exercise has been shown to reduce the long-term risk of coronary artery disease. But you can gain the benefits of exercise without the added strain to the heart. The Nurses' Health Study found that women who walked briskly at least three hours per week achieved results equivalent to jogging or aerobic dancing. Those who walked five times or more a week over time had substantially lower rates of heart attacks triggered by strenuous exertion. Still, you should be alert to any of the warning signs that may indicate you are exercising too strenuously. If you experience any of the following, stop immediately. If they persist, consult your physician.

- Lightheadedness or dizziness
- Palpitations
- Shortness of breath (unable to carry on a conversation)
- Jaw pain
- Arm tingling or numbness
- Tight feeling in the lungs

and start walking. If you haven't been active for a while, start out easy—try ten minutes a day. (Please consult with your doctor before you initiate any exercise program.) Add five minutes a week to your walking regimen, building up to thirty minutes total, five days a week. If you can devote more time to exercise, forty-five to sixty minutes a day is even better. Walk with friends to make it fun. If the weather is bad, head over to your local mall and get moving!

Dancing is also great aerobic exercise and reduces stress at the same time. You don't have to work up a sweat or push yourself until you're out of breath. Find your own rhythm and "go with the flow."

Aerobic exercise enhances well-being and puts a spring in your step—it also strengthens your heart and cardiovascular system. Add a bit of stretching and yoga and spice it up with a bit of weight training to create a great exercise session. Put on your favorite music, warm up with a good stretch and some deep-breathing, then walk for ten to fifteen minutes. Mix it up with some free weights, finish with a little yoga, stretching, and cool-down.

Weight Training: Tone and Strengthen

Many of my patients have asked me if using hand-held weights will benefit their heart muscle. In other words, can resistance exercises be used to strengthen your muscles *and* your heart? The answer is yes. Studies suggest that there is considerable benefit to be gained from strength training in both healthy women and cardiac patients, especially for lowering your heart disease risk and preventing osteoporosis. But a strength-training program can also help protect you in everyday situations that require muscle strength such as lifting, pushing, or pulling.

Many activities of daily life include lifting objects, pushing, and even straining. Without the ability to maintain daily activity, women are at greater risk for heart problems. A recent study revealed that an elderly woman's inability to perform daily activities, such as making the bed and vacuuming, correlate with her risk of heart disease.

Consider also the phenomenon called "airport angina." This term describes a scenario for many people, some of whom don't even know they have heart disease. Victims develop a chest cramp—shortness of breath or some other symptom of angina—while rushing to catch a plane, and weaving quickly through the airport lugging carry-on bags. The combined effects of lifting and squeezing the suitcase, along with brisk walking and maneuvering between people, can place quite a stress on the cardiovascular system. Add in the vigilance and psychological stress involved with air travel, and you have a great recipe for a heart attack.

We all find ourselves lifting at one time or another, whether under stress situations or as a part of normal daily living. We move furniture, lift children or grandchildren, change an occasional tire, bag wet leaves, shovel snow, carry wet laundry upstairs, bring firewood into the house, and so on, any one of which may place considerable demands on our cardiovascular system.

Research has indicated that not only does strength training have a positive impact on cardiovascular endurance, it can also lower your blood pressure, decrease your lipids (fats), and enhance your sense of well-being. In fact, some researchers believe that in addition to improving your cardiovascular health, strength training may also reduce subsequent cardiac events and even the risk of sudden death.

And for those who are frustrated with the limitations heart disease has imposed upon their active lifestyle, strength training is a way to fight back. Many of my cardiac patients have learned how to be maximally active within the restrictions of having some form of heart condition.

In 1994 Miriam E. Nelson, PhD, researcher at the Jean Mayer USDA Human Nutrition Research Center on Aging at Tufts University, made headlines with her report in the *Journal of the American Medical Association (JAMA)*. Her research described the effects of a strength training program on postmenopausal women. After one year, the women's bodies were "15 to 20 years more youthful." As they increased their muscle mass and lost fat, their scores on strength tests soared. They actually gained bone and in some instances reversed osteoporosis at an age when women are typically losing bone. Their balance and flexibility improved. As their bodies changed, their lives became more active and the women felt happier and more confident. All this from lifting weights just twice a week!

The resulting outpouring of interest prompted Nelson to write *Strong Women Stay Young*. Now a classic in its field, she followed up with a companion book, *Strong Women Stay Slim*. I highly recommend both of these books to any woman concerned about her bones, health, and longevity.

Yoga and Stretching for Flexibility

As we age and exercise less, we lose muscle tone and balance. This is significant, as a loss of the ability to balance can predispose you to falls, which can be a life-threatening event, especially if you have osteoporosis.

One of the best ways to maintain balance is with yoga, stretching, tai chi, or qi gong. These gentle exercises have their roots in Asian medicine and can have a positive impact not only on your balance but even on your strength.

A few of my patients' favorite ways to exercise is to tune in every morning to the Denise Austin "Fit & Lite" show on cable television's Lifetime Channel (check your local listings). They report that in just three weeks of daily half-hour sessions, their aerobic capacity, strength, and flexibility are all noticeably improved. They've shared with me that exercising this way is just like having a personal trainer come to their home—and it works no matter the weather. Although the show is aired early in the morning in most locales, you can tape it in order to exercise any time of day, although most found it a terrific way to start the day.

Austin, an exercise physiologist and former gymnast, opens each session with deep breathing and stretching to warm up, then heads into low-impact aerobics (what she calls "cardio-lite"), followed by strength training with light hand-held weights. The half-hour sessions warm down with a bit of yoga or tai chi. Following such a program three to five times per week, then remaining active on weekends ("recreating") can improve the exercise profile of any woman, no matter what her age or level of fitness.

If You Are a Cardiac Patient...

Where and how do you get properly evaluated for strength training? Although some of my patients have taken it upon themselves to go to gyms and work out with three- to five-pound weights to improve their muscular strength, this, in my view, is not the best approach. Just as a cardiologist uses a stress test to prescribe an exercise prescription for you, you can and should be evaluated for your muscular strength. A certified exercise specialist or exercise physiologist (usually an MS or PhD) can prescribe an individual program for you to build muscle strength and endurance.

Once you get a baseline muscular strength capability, a prescription can be written that specifies the amount of weight to use, the numbers of repetitions to do, and an appropriate time duration and intensity level. There are experienced clinicians, especially in various cardiovascular rehabilitative programs, who can test you, write you a prescription, and follow your progress.

Although testing your maximal strength capacity may not be accomplished in one session, once your "threshold strength" is determined, an exercise prescription can be developed to enhance that strength. Once you gain some self-confidence and body strength, you will be better able to perform most everyday lifting activities at a lower cardiovascular workload, i.e., lower heart rate and lower blood pressure.

When, after training, the heart can do the same work at a lower level of exertion, the oxygen demand on the heart to perform at that intensity of workload is reduced, thereby decreasing the stress on the heart. Once you know your own muscular strength, you will know which activities are safe for you. You will also better understand how to adjust your daily workload to one that you can handle, such as lightening a ten-pound bag to your comfort level of five or seven pounds, or resting mid-task before you become short of breath. Muscle strength training is a great way to learn your own limitations, extend them when possible, and have an overall better sense of freedom and independence.

Ask your doctor about centers that include muscular strength training for cardiac patients. Your local hospital-based cardiac rehabilitation program is a great place to start. They have experts to teach those who already have heart disease how to exercise safely and to their maximum capacity. If you have recently had a heart attack, bypass surgery, or angioplasty, your insurance will probably pay for cardiac rehabilitation for a few sessions or even a few months.

Most rehabilitation centers also have state-of-the-art cardiac monitoring equipment along with exercise equipment so you can have instant feedback on what your heart rate and blood pressure are doing while you exercise. I know my hospital even has special classes for those who are at risk for coronary artery disease. Patients pay only a small out-of-pocket fee for as many sessions as they feel they need. It's a great place to get started.

Remember, exercise is *the key* to a healthy heart—it can be safe and fun, too.

CHAPTER SEVEN

Emotional Healing, Stress Management, and Spiritual Healing

The word "stress" is used so often these days that it has become a badge of sorts for the age in which we live. In years to come, ours may well be viewed not so much as the "High-Tech Age" but the "Stress Age." In fact, stress has spawned its own industry, one rife with quick-fix cure-alls and personality quizzes that promise a better quality of life in no time at all—and with very little effort on your part!

I wish it were so easy. While stress can be a time bomb, manifesting itself in a host of illnesses, those most in need of help will not find it by taking a pop magazine quiz. In fact, the reality of the grip that stress has on people's lives and their health usually isn't apparent until they end up in a doctor's office seeking treatment for anything from skin rashes and headaches to heart disease and cancer.

While stress has always been a factor in disease, it appears to be an even greater one now. Surveys indicate that stress today accounts for about *80 percent of all visits to doctors' offices.* While this figure may be relatively new, the premise certainly is not. For centuries, we have known of the role that psychosocial and behavioral factors play in disease. Over one thousand years ago Hippocrates and Maimonides both concluded that emotional disturbances cause marked changes in the body.

Stress—Connecting the Heart–Brain Hotline

Why does everyone appear to be so stressed out these days? It is difficult to escape the fact that we live in a high-tech society poised to compete on demand—one where business is highly structured and ultra-demanding, and where the word "leisure" no longer accurately describes how most folks spend their precious spare time. "Leisure" activities are more likely to be active, even competitive. Little time, if any, is devoted to relaxation or even to casual conversation. Our cultural motto has become "work hard, play hard."

We live in a society that rewards left-brain activities like analysis, counting, scheduling, and planning. Intuition and creativity, which stem from our right brain, are perceived as having less value.

Indeed, there can no longer be any doubt about the relationship between stress and disease. What we think and how we feel can affect the very workings and intricacies of the heart. I am always impressed by the way in which our underlying emotions, often masked by stress, can inhibit our ability to heal ourselves. I have seen many heart attacks and even unexpected sudden death brought on by severe stress.

Tragically, such was the case for Mary Ann, a forty-two-year-old mother of three teenagers. Her father had a heart attack at age fifty-eight and fortunately recovered. One afternoon, Mary Ann found herself in the emergency room with her fifteen-year-old son, Rob, who was having an acute asthma attack. On this particular day, the hospital's interventions were not working as quickly as they had in the past. Rob was struggling for air, his lips and nails turning blue. He was becoming more and more frightened, and so was Mary Ann.

Fearing for her son's life, Mary Ann suddenly collapsed on the floor, in full cardiac arrest. The ER staff responded quickly, working hard and long to bring her back, but they failed to save her life. Her death had a devastating effect on her family, her friends, and all the medical personnel who rallied to save her. But the effects of intense fear and impending doom had stolen her away.

Most physicians and cardiologists who have been practicing on a day-to-day basis know that emotions have a direct and definite effect on the heart. Although it is difficult to measure the impact of stress, research over the years has consistently demonstrated that blood pressure and blood lipids, particularly cholesterol and triglycerides, become elevated as a result of severe stress. For example, researchers have found a connection between stress and blood cholesterol levels in certified public accountants evaluated from January 1 to April 15. Extremely high cholesterol elevations were found during this intensely time-urgent period without a change in the diet. Other acute stressors, such as racecar driving, have demonstrated massive elevations in free fatty acids and triglycerides when drivers risk their lives negotiating high speeds and threatening turns.

Coronary heart disease may be lurking in the background for years, partially blocking an artery, but not enough to create any symptoms, and then *wham!*—something happens to tip the balance, like the loss of a job, an argument with a teenager, a divorce, the death of a child or a spouse—and the heart literally breaks down or goes into full cardiac arrest. The cascade of events that lead to the clotting of a critical vessel in the heart is oftentimes initiated by

Get in Touch with Your Emotions

EMOTIONAL RELEASE AND FEELING VULNERABLE have as much to do with recovering from heart disease as eating a healthy diet, exercising, and taking supplements.

hormones resulting from strong emotions such as intense disappointment, loss, grief, sadness, anger, depression, and especially fear which was tragically seen in the case of Mary Ann.

After the storm of an acute cardiac event has passed, I often ask my patients what was going on in their lives just before, the day of, or even prior to the day that their heart literally attacked them.

For some folks, there was no apparent emotional connection to the event; for them it seemed to be a matter of chance, or a sudden physical exertion was the cause. More often, my heart patients, especially women, make the connection right away. Some even respond, "I knew I would have a heart attack over it" or "I have been so sad, I am not surprised."

Others take some time to reflect on their lives, and later report that certain psychological stresses had been taking a toll on their body. In the process, they often come to understand to what extent they have been disconnected from their feelings. For such people, a cardiac event or early warning sign can be a gift in disguise—the messenger that they needed to reevaluate their lives. A heart attack offers some patients a way to reconnect with themselves and set new priorities for the way they choose to live in the world.

Emotional Risk Factors: The Missing Link

We've touched on the common risk factors that have been reported in the popular press and medical journals, such as older age, unfavorable family history, poor diet, elevated blood cholesterol, obesity, sedentary lifestyle, diabetes, high blood pressure, and cigarette smoking as well as some of the newer cardiovascular risk factors like homocysteine, fibrinogen, and C-reactive protein. Although these risk factors must be considered in anyone with heart disease, 50 percent of all cases of heart disease are *not* related to the conventional risk profile. The missing link is often *emotional risk factors*—behaviors and conditions, often hidden or ignored by conventional medicine, that can make you vulnerable to developing heart disease.

It would not surprise me to learn that you haven't heard much about the connection between heartbreak and heart disease. Heartbreak is not considered a "medical condition" because "love" is not recognized as a physiological function. Until recently, physiology has limited itself to the mechanics and chemistry of how organs work and has ignored the impact of various emotional states on those functions. Science has been necessarily confined to phenomena that can be measured and quantified. But how can you measure love, or heartbreak?

Although the more subjective "feelings" lie outside the realm of science, I think it is a big mistake to exclude them from our understanding of how disease affects the human body. Feelings such as love, faith, and hope are tremendously vital forces in human behavior, and I firmly believe that we must try to understand their nature and the role they play in our emotional and physical health.

While love, faith, and hope alone may not "cure" heart disease, these emotional states can certainly lift up your spirits and encourage what I call *dispositional optimism*. When you learn to cope with heartbreak, anger, or resentment, rather than suppressing these emotions, you can harness their power to help heal your heart.

Indeed, research has documented that our emotions are intimately connected to our immune systems, manifesting themselves as behaviors and physiology that can place us at higher risk for heart disease. One such devastating factor can be the impact that internalized anger can have on your heart.

Anger and Your Heart: Claiming the "Shadow Side"

Cynicism, alienation, and hostility are perhaps the most devastating personality traits that can hurt the heart. The origin of this unholy trinity resides in the common emotion we define as anger, a major psychological risk factor for the heart. Anger, and to a greater degree, hostility and rage, are components of everyone's personality, but most of us are hesitant to claim this "shadow" or "dark side" of ourselves. But getting in touch with these hidden emotions and becoming aware of their contribution to heart disease is crucial not only to healing the heart, but to survival itself.

This is reflected in the case of Jean, a woman in her early sixties, who had been married for approximately thirty-eight years. Jean had no children or siblings, and her parents were both deceased. Bob, her husband, was her only vital connection. After Jean discovered that her husband had become involved with another woman, she experienced the full gamut of angry emotions: rage, heartbreak, humiliation, resentment.

After four days of intense panic, disbelief, "mental torture," and heightened physiological arousal (the "fight-or-flight" state), Jean wound up in the emergency room in full cardiac arrest. Fortunately, she was resuscitated, and when I performed a cardiac catheterization on her several days later, she had normal coronary arteries. Did Jean's intense heartbreak, anger, and rage set up her heart to go out of rhythm, making her vulnerable to sudden death? She certainly had a very healthy heart with a well-functioning muscle, free of disease. Although Jean did not experience a full-blown heart attack, she had a life-threatening cardiac arrest stemming from her body's reaction to deep, intense heartbreak. Research has shown that women like Jean who experience hopelessness or a sense of doom face tremendous cardiac vulnerability. In fact, women who rated highest on hopelessness measures had two times the incidence of a fatal cardiac

Find a Friend

RESEARCH HAS SHOWN THAT WOMEN with the least number of social connections have the highest mortality compared with women with varied social support networks.

event within an eight-year period. And this statistical risk can be compounded by a lack of vital connections.

So what made Jean so vulnerable to cardiac arrest? Was it the shock of the affair? The impending fear of isolation and loneliness? The intense shame? The lack of other vital supports? Or was it the anger and rage she was experiencing? Although it was most likely a combination of all of the above, I believe that internalized anger and rage were mainly responsible for her acute cardiac episode.

Anger, whether repressed or festering, creates an undesirable burden on the cardiovascular system by increasing resistance in blood vessels with high constriction. It's like driving your car with the brakes on—something has to give. The problem for many people is that we don't really want to acknowledge that we possess a "dark side" in our personality. Most of us are not in touch with—we even deny—our anger, hostility, and rage.

Several years ago I gave a lecture on stress and the heart to a group of psychiatrists in Massachusetts. As I spoke about anger and how it impacts the cardiovascular system, I clearly struck a nerve in a member of the audience. As I referred to the mind-body interaction between anger and cardiac disease, one psychiatrist became extremely agitated and upset. He interrupted the lecture, clenched his jaw, made a fist, and shouted, "Why is a cardiologist talking about anger when that is *not* your domain?" I tried to diffuse the situation by calmly responding, "I see that you are angry." He immediately shouted at the top of his lungs, "I am *not* angry!"

Needless to say, this person was completely out of touch with his own hostility and anger. The reason I relate this story to you is to demonstrate how anyone can be in denial of these emotions. The truth of the matter is that each and every one of us has anger at some time, whether it be chronic or situational. Over time, chronic anger becomes part of your biology, structured in the body's muscular tissues as well as the blood vessel walls, where it is often an unrecognized contributor to high blood pressure.

What to Do with Anger?

There has been much written on the subject of anger; many authors suggest interventions from stress-management to relaxation techniques to deal with it. Some say that the best way to deal with anger is to stay cool and calm, forgetting your problems and stresses. Others advise you to "have your anger outward," experiencing the feelings and discharging the emotion.

But as damaging as anger can be, it does not have to be an "ugly" emotion. There is energy in anger that, when channeled correctly, can be utilized as a powerful healing force. When you are in touch with your anger and can identify what is happening in your body, you will be able to release the body sensation of anger and move on, whether it's to "reframe" that anger into some constructive action or to simply let go of the situation completely. Even people with cancer, heart disease, or any life-threatening illness can learn to direct their emotions in a way that gives them strength, clarity, and purpose. How do you know if you have anger that you need to address? Ask yourself the following questions:

❖ Do I ever give a "look that could kill?"
❖ Do I ever strike out verbally or physically?
❖ Do I sometimes flare my nostrils or hold my breath when I am upset?
❖ Do I ever become hostile and impatient to the point of interrupting others?
❖ Do I feel that it would not be feminine to show my anger?
❖ Do I "stuff" my negative feelings, blame myself, or become depressed?

Some of my patients need to express their anger in a physical way and have asked me for guidance in how to do this.
Learning how to say "no" with real feeling behind it is a crucial
step in the right direction. Sometimes, even letting yourself go
with a temper tantrum in the privacy of your own home will
release withheld emotions, resulting in a general relaxation of the
body. Using the voice and expressing negativity, jutting out the jaw
and making a fist, and even using upper arm motions such as striking out or hitting pillows can offer your body and psyche considerable relief, loosening up the tension of the upper back and neck,
throat, and chest.

Although one or two exercises are not going to release you
completely, performing these maneuvers over time will assist the
body to discharge chronic tension. Sometimes I work psychothera-
peutically with my patients individually or in groups employing these
techniques to work out not only anger and hostility, but also rage.

Rage: The Most Damaging Emotion

Rage is uncontrolled, suppressed anger. Uncontrolled rage can be
hazardous to you and others. Most of us are reluctant to give in to
our rage out of fear that we may lose control and hurt someone.
This is where one-on-one supportive psychotherapy is not only
helpful but also therapeutic. Unfortunately, many people are reluctant to see a therapist, social worker, or counselor. If this is your
case, follow these simple suggestions to work with your anger.

First, be aware that anger is inherent. You have it. Your next
challenge is to own it. Next, know that this insight in itself is cur-
ative. If you are in a situation which evokes a negative feeling,
acknowledge that feeling. You may simply tell yourself "I am
angry." Then you have to ask yourself this question: "Is this event
worth my emotional investment?" And if it is, ask yourself: "If I

have or resist my feeling, is it worth getting tense, raising my blood pressure, or having a heart attack?" Or, "Is it worth dying for?" Or, "If I get so upset and angry, is it going to make a difference anyway?" Take a few deep breaths, listen to what is happening in your body, make your decision, and then go with the flow.

An occasional flash of temper or angry feelings is perfectly reasonable, perhaps even cathartic. When you are in touch with your anger and have access to it, you "own" it. When you give up hostile, angry feelings, you become more vulnerable and less defensive. You are now more open and living in your heart.

Chronic hostility, grimaces, and resentments will make you anxious and tense, eventually isolating you from others. Remember, when angry emotions implode or explode, the result can raise havoc with your blood pressure, your heart, and even your life. When anger is turned against the self instead of out onto others, depression can occur, and research shows that this affects women to a much greater degree than men.

How to Overcome Anger and Attend to Your Spirit

Take time to reflect on your own relationship with your "dark" or "shadow side." Do you have an unresolved conflict that makes your blood boil every time you think about it? Do you often become angry or upset with your spouse, children, colleagues, or even a driver who cuts you off? You may be thinking, "Of course I do. Doesn't everybody? That's life." But each of these incidents triggers a basic physiological survival mechanism known as the fight-or-flight response, which dumps stress hormones such as cortisol and norepinephrine into your bloodstream. Over the short term, there is no problem—we're designed to outrun (or outthink) danger, and blood values return to normal. But as you can see, when you get "stuck" in emotional states such as anger, grief, sadness, shame, or fear, the same stress hormones continuously flood your body, constricting your blood flow, making your platelets sticky, and perhaps even causing heart palpitations or chest pain. Chronic negative thinking can actually lead to high blood pressure, clogged arteries, and even a heart attack.

Building walls around your emotions—whether you are seething silently or being a "good soldier," enduring your fate stoically—is decidedly *not* healthy. I have found, over the last ten years, that men and women who have trouble expressing their emotions have the highest cortisol rates and are, therefore, at higher risk of developing high blood pressure and heart disease.

You have a choice about how you express your anger. But first, you must recognize that you cannot be effective when you are possessed by anger, and indeed you may be harming your heart. So begin searching within; quiet your heart, and, if necessary, quench your unresolved anger. Here are some ways to get started on the road to relaxation.

Eight Steps to Relaxation and Spiritual Healing

1. INCLUDE SOME "SPIRITUAL EXERCISE" IN YOUR DAY. Take up yoga, tai chi, qi gong, dancing, or deep-breathing. Spend at least part of every day outdoors doing something that *you* enjoy, such as browsing outdoor flea markets, walking your dog, or bird-watching. Exercise opens and expands the chest, lifts your mood, curbs food cravings, and lowers your blood pressure. It will also help you sleep better—an often overlooked aspect of health.

2. TREAT YOURSELF TO A MASSAGE OR OTHER TYPE OF BODYWORK, such as Reiki, Feldenkrais, or Alexander Technique. In addition to lowering your resting heart rate and blood pressure, massage and bodywork promotes muscle relaxation, helps break up scar tissue, relieves certain types of pain, promotes circulation, and more. Most importantly for the heart, many types of bodywork can facilitate emotional release. Expert bodywork can access old traumas, release stored emotions, and free blocked energy that is literally stored in cellular memory.

It's not uncommon for the release of long-held sadness to occur as a result of bodywork. Once freed, these energies and emotions can be redirected toward health and healing. Remember that touch is crucial to growth, healing, and well-being. It's like a nonchemical tranquilizer with no side effects. Many studies have documented the benefits of massage therapy for the treatment of pain, muscle spasm, anxiety, depression, and psychoemotional stress, which can aggravate heart conditions.

3. CRY IT OUT. There is often sadness just beneath the anger. Explore this with a trusted friend and don't be afraid to let the tears flow. The discharge of sadness, grieving, and hurt through crying is one of the most cleansing experiences you can go through. Deep sobs originating in the pelvis and belly open the chest, allowing energy bound up by stress to be released. Crying frees your heart of muscular tension that might otherwise strain it. A good cry also enhances oxygen delivery to the cells while stimulating release of biochemicals in the brain that help you to relax. That's why you always feel better after a good cry.

When you relieve emotional tension with tears, you also lower circulating levels of cortisol and adrenaline—two hormones implicated in coronary artery disease. When these hormones are elevated, blood surges more forcefully through your arteries, potentially weakening their walls, and making them vulnerable to forming pits and scars, which act as nets for fatty deposits of cholesterol.

If possible, do your crying in the company of an empathetic "witness"—a friend, loved one, trusted therapist, or clergyman. Such a person can not only help you keep the process going, but can also offer understanding, comfort, and unconditional support as you access and work through your heartbreak.

4. VISUALIZE A NEW REALITY. Your imagination is one of your most powerful healing resources, and you can harness and channel it with a process called guided imagery or visualization. The relationship among mental imagery, relaxation, physiological responses, and behavior has been documented in many studies to decrease anxiety, reduce stress and depression, increase a sense of well-being, and even influence the outcome of serious illness. One of the most powerful ways to visualize is through prayer or meditation.

5. TAP INTO THE POWER OF PRAYER AND MEDITATION. Whether you pray, meditate, or simply sit quietly for ten to fifteen minutes every day, cultivating your spiritual side is an important part of releasing your anger and lowering your blood pressure. Such activities quiet your sympathetic nervous system, which is biologically encoded to "kick in" during high-stress activities.

Herbert Benson, MD, author of *The Relaxation Response* and *Timeless Healing*, cites scientific evidence that faith, religion, and/or belief in God lowers mortality rates and improves health by reducing anxiety, depression, anger, and blood pressure. According to Dr. Benson, "Faith quiets the mind like no other form of belief." Prayer creates peace and positive images that foster healing.

To induce the relaxation response, repeat a simple, neutral word such as "one" for several minutes. Benson and his colleagues noted even more profound physiological changes when patients incorporated what he terms the "faith factor" into repeating a simple prayer or statement reflecting one's spiritual roots. For example, you could use the word "shalom" or "om." Or, "The Lord is my shepherd" or "Hail Mary, full of grace." After you have chosen your phrase, close your eyes, relax your body and mind and breathe in through your nose and out through your mouth. Say your word or phrase silently as you exhale. When stray thoughts come by, gently release them, and continue your mantra. To achieve relaxation, use this technique for at least ten to fifteen minutes each day.

Following your session, simply be still and be by yourself for another few minutes. Do not jump right up and do things. Rather, give yourself time to acknowledge whatever comes up. You may get an urge to call an old friend or have an intuitive flash about your health or emotional well-being. You may wish to reach out to a friend, or record your thoughts and insights in a journal.

When you include prayer in your daily life, you will begin to notice some changes. You may become more open to life, less inflexible in your outlook, and more centered. You may find it easier to resolve your problems and cope with stressful situations. Your relationships with others will deepen.

Rosemary Ellen Guiley, author of *The Miracle of Prayer*, has written of seven essentials to enrich your prayer life. I wholeheartedly endorse her approach, which includes the following:

❖ Be honest with yourself and God;
❖ Make every thought a prayer—your thoughts create your reality;
❖ Make your life your prayer—in other words, "walk your talk;"
❖ Pray regularly—not just when you have a crisis or special need;
❖ Pray in a group—it's comforting and powerful;
❖ Be willing to trust and surrender completely, turning the matter over to God. Realize that it is an act of courage to place your life in God's hands rather than to think you have all the answers. It may be difficult to surrender, especially in the middle of a crisis, but the more you pray that God's will—not yours—be done, and the more you are willing to surrender, the more you can trust in your faith that all will be well;

❖ Give thanks—every time you pray, be grateful that you are blessed with your life and the continued opportunities that you have to connect with others. When you experience feelings of appreciation, your heartbeat becomes more rhythmic, skipping fewer beats. Keep a "gratitude journal," in which you regularly write down all the things for which you are grateful.

6. SPEND TIME IN SILENCE EVERY DAY. In today's high-tech world of the Internet, fax machines, cell phones, and voice mail, it is increasingly difficult to access a space of silence. Yet reconnecting with stillness and silence is a necessary step in our quest for health and balance. When you can quiet the internal chatter enough to not be obsessed with the "busyness" of life, you begin to approach your spiritual self. This sacred space often opens you to an untapped healing response.

Each day, take a little time to release from your mind all thoughts, images, and concerns. Learning to quiet yourself will help to lower your blood pressure (as do most of these relaxation activities), stimulate the release of endorphins, and perhaps most importantly, bring you closer to what's in your heart, which never lies.

Sit down and block out all outside stimulation by closing your eyes and not touching, listening, smelling, tasting, or thinking about things. During this quieting time, focus on something involuntary, like your breathing. When thoughts come along, picture them floating downstream like a log going down a river.

7. FORGIVE. Simply stated, forgiveness means letting go of the past. Insidiously, the negative energy you hold from past events not only

Don't Overlook the Emotional Factor

REPRESSED EMOTIONS are often overlooked, hidden risk factors in heart disease and hypertension.

erodes your spirit but also takes a toll on your physical body. In order to heal and stay healthy, you must give up your grudges and resentments; believe me, you are the only one who is suffering from them. Often, sharing your story with an impartial counselor, clergyman, or friend can help you see things in a new light. Chances are, they'll help you to see how futile it is to hold on to your resentments.

Granting forgiveness to someone who has injured you is just as important as seeking forgiveness from another. In the process of asking for forgiveness, you may need to ask God to give you courage.

8. CONNECT WITH AN ANIMAL FRIEND. If you've had bouts of "the blues," either short- or long-term due to social isolation, I highly recommend that you consider bringing an animal into your life.

Research shows that the survival rate of people who suffered a heart attack is five times greater for those who come home from the hospital to a loving pet than for people who come home to a lonely house. In other words, that dog you have—whose biggest moment of the day is your homecoming—could be saving your life with that wet kiss!

Animals have much to teach us, and I am among those who believe they can be guides for our souls. Here are some of the lessons that we can learn from our animal friends:

❖ **APPRECIATION**—pets bring a tranquil and playful energy into a space, and they can teach us to be more relaxed and in tune with our bodies. For pets, every day is a new adventure.

❖ **RELAXATION**—have you ever watched a cat stretch and arch her back as she wakes up? Some yoga postures mimic this stretch, which involves deep breathing. Take a hint, and start your day with some "cat stretches." Notice, too, how your cat never seems to be in a hurry.

❖ SILENCE—animals can teach us a great deal about being present in the moment and silent at the same time. They know how to "be" and how to sit in silence for long periods of time. Animals can hold a space as sacred, whether it's their favorite sunning spot or the mat by the front door. Observe your pets at these times and allow yourself to absorb their peace. Watch as they tune out the world and practice the "art" of silence.

❖ STRESS REDUCTION—animals can be a lot smarter than people when it comes to stress. They often simply walk away from a potentially futile or hopeless situation that threatens their well-being. Cats especially have an innate ability to tune out the environment and become aloof in difficult situations. How many of us get "hooked" by a stressful situation that has the potential to harm our heart? How often do we sacrifice our needs until we're exhausted, with nothing left for ourselves? Animals have a keen sense of self-preservation, one that we humans should emulate more often.

❖ PLAY—Pets reinforce the value of play. Many of us mix up "play" with "compete" or turn something that started out to be fun into a serious competition. True recreational play is spontaneous. When physical activity doesn't involve any preconceived agenda, it can be one of the most healing things we can do. In true play there is a feeling of lightheartedness that usually leads to laughter and surrendering to the experience.

A dog, cat, or even a songbird will lift your spirits and give you something outside of yourself to cherish and care for. And, something that relies upon *you* for its physical and emotional well-being will give you one of the greatest gifts of all—unconditional love. Studies have shown that simply stroking an animal's fur can lower your blood pressure. Animals help us release pent-up emotions and put us in touch with memories. I often bring my Chow Chow Chewie, my Elkhound Charlie, and my new Chow puppy Kuma into my office. My patients adore them. If you don't have one, I urge you to take a trip down to your local animal shelter to adopt a pet. You won't regret it!

The Four Pillars of Healing: Putting It All Together

When my patients combine my modified Mediterranean diet with a low-level exercise program, targeted nutritional supplements, stress reduction, and relaxation exercises, they come into my office, show me their diary of blood-pressure readings, and, with a smile on their face, ask me: "Dr. Sinatra, what drug can we take away now?" It's a gratifying experience for both of us as we go about the process of eliminating traditionally prescribed drugs with all their negative side effects and enhancing prevention and natural healing, one by one. Sometimes we can cut dosages in half; other times we can eliminate them entirely. What really touches my heart the most is how empowered my patients become. They love it, and it makes my job a lot easier, too. Instead of me telling my patients what to do, they become my partners. Together, we do the dance of healing. You have the power to join in the dance—the information is at your fingertips!

SECTION III

Common Cardiac Conditions Women Encounter

CHAPTER EIGHT

The Great Pretenders: Conditions That Disguise Themselves as Heart Attacks

It often starts in the middle of the night. You may be sleeping comfortably when you are suddenly awakened by a tightening sensation in your chest, followed by shortness of breath, chest pressure, and paralyzing fear. You may think you're having a heart attack. The next morning, you go directly to your doctor's office, certain that you are headed for "the big one." Your doctor runs a stress test or electrocardiogram (EKG) and assures you that all is well... your heart is fine. You breathe a big sigh of relief.

This is an example of what cardiologists call "atypical" or "noncardiac" chest pain (NCP). More common in women, chest pain can be the harbinger of many things that are *not* overt heart disease. For example, chest symptoms can be triggered by indigestion, anxiety, or panic attacks. Sometimes becoming preoccupied with the thought that your heart is at risk can set off an episode of chest pain. But more often than not, chest discomfort is masquerading as coronary artery disease... it's a pretender.

At least three cardiac conditions—among them coronary artery spasm, mitral valve prolapse (MVP), and a type of cardiomyopathy or heart muscle disease called *idiopathic hypertrophic subaortic stenosis* (IHSS)—share a common physiological feature: a stiffening of the heart muscle that prevents it from stretching and filling with blood normally. It's called *diastolic dysfunction*. In some instances, it's considered a very early sign of heart disease. In some cases, diastolic dysfuntion is well tolerated and the patient may not even experience any symptoms at all.

Over many years, diastolic dysfunction may not cause you any harm, but having it may increase your risk of future congestive heart failure. Diastolic dysfunction is often seen in women with a long history of high blood pressure as well.

Coronary Artery Spasm:
That Frightening, Tightening Feeling
What is happening in your heart when you're awakened in the

How Does the Heart Beat?

WITH EVERY BEAT OF YOUR HEART, there are three basic components: During (1) *systolic function,* the lower chambers of the heart muscle contract, squeezing blood out to the arteries. This stage requires adequate energy in the cells of the heart muscle and a competent muscle to respond and contract effectively. The systolic contraction (which correlates with systolic blood pressure) empties about 50 to 70 percent of the blood out of the heart chambers. Next, there is a (2) *brief rest*—usually less than one-third of a second—before the heart refills with blood in preparation for the next contraction. During the (3) *diastolic stage,* the heart's lower chambers refill with blood. This phase is dependent upon the energy and the ability of the heart muscle to s-t-r-e-t-c-h without sagging, fill, and accommodate adequate blood volume—about 200 to 400 ml, or about one cup. This entire cycle—your heart beat—occurs approximately 50 to 80 times a minute on average, depending on the activity or energy demand.

middle of the night with chest pain? Most likely a condition called *coronary artery spasm*. Your blood vessels actually contract quickly over a period of seconds to minutes, producing that tight feeling. Most of the patients I have seen with this affliction are younger or middle-aged women. After thorough investigations of these patients, including stress tests, echocardiograms, and even cardiac catheterizations, I've found normal coronary arteries that simply went into spasm. (See cardiac diagnosis and testing in Appendix A.)

The good news is that coronary artery spasm, despite its scary symptoms of chest pain and perhaps even diminished blood flow to the heart (*transient ischemia*), is usually a harmless condition. Rarely have I seen women develop heart attacks as the result of coronary artery spasm or mitral valve prolapse (MVP), another condition that is often overrated as a health threat. Even more rare are situations where coronary artery spasm is associated with some degree of diastolic dysfunction.

Compared with coronary artery *disease*, these conditions are clowns playing a cruel joke—messing with your mind, as I like to put it. There are times when they can make your life exceedingly uncomfortable, and occasionally they can progress to something more serious. But most of the time, they are quality of life issues rather than matters of life and death.

What Brings on Such Alarming Episodes?

Researchers have concluded that emotional and/or physical stress can provoke the vessels in your heart to contract. (So can smoking.) An awareness of the contribution of psychological factors to chest pain has been known as far back as two centuries ago. During the Civil War, Dr. J. M. DaCosta noticed soldiers were falling out of the ranks, dizzy, lightheaded, and complaining of chest discomfort. Unsure of the cause of what has come to be known as DaCosta's Syndrome or "Soldier's Heart," the concerned physician suggested that it was due to "disordered innervation" as a result of intense emotional stress.

Yet he documented that, with few exceptions, his patients were found to be essentially normal. We can speculate that the mega-stressors of war and combat brought on the symptoms. But there would later be similar observations in nonmilitary populations. Many of the symptoms Dr. DaCosta described are probably related to either coronary artery spasm or mitral valve prolapse. Modern-day stressors can come from many sources.

Today, we know much more about what's happening inside the blood vessels. In one European study, patients prone to coronary artery spasm were found to have high levels of free radicals in their bloodstreams. The researchers proposed that the treatment of this syndrome might include antioxidants to scavenge and neutralize free radicals. I have long seen good results with supplemental vitamins C, E, carotenoids, and flavonoids, as well as coenzyme Q10 to help eradicate free radicals.

The Super-Amino L-arginine

Recently, the amino acid *L-arginine* has earned high marks from both researchers and consumers as an excellent natural treatment for coronary artery spasm.

I have been recommending L-arginine to my patients for chest pain due to coronary artery spasm as well as the chest symptoms caused by congestive heart failure. Here's why: There is convincing evidence that regular supplementation with L-arginine induces smooth muscle relaxation within the arterial wall, preventing episodes of coronary artery spasm. This nutrient also inhibits the accumulation of plaque. Also, L-arginine is thought to be the primary agent responsible for the production of nitric oxide (NO) which maintains blood vessel elasticity. Research has also shown that L-arginine improves circulation, particularly for those with high cholesterol.

Good natural sources of L-arginine include nuts, especially almonds and peanuts. You can also find L-arginine in meat, and to a lesser degree, in dairy products, though I'd rather you limit your intake of these foods. L-arginine capsules can be purchased in health food stores as an amino acid supplement. I recommend 2 to 3 grams daily in divided doses, which can be taken at bedtime by those who are awakened regularly in the middle of the night with symptoms such as tightness in the chest and shortness of breath due to coronary artery spasm.

In addition to reducing cholesterol and retarding plaque development, L-arginine has been reported to improve the immune system, accelerate wound healing, and—in megadoses team up with conventional chemotherapy to treat breast cancer. The versatility and potential of L-arginine continues to grow!

Mitral Valve Prolapse—"You Have a Heart Murmur"

Coronary artery spasm isn't the only "pretender" when it comes to cardiac conditions that women commonly encounter. Mitral valve prolapse (MVP) is an ominous-sounding condition that is a source of

---

Congestive Heart Failure (CHF)...

IS THE MOST SERIOUS OF ALL cardiovascular conditions that usually afflict women in their seventies and eighties. In fact, CHF's five-year survival rate is worse than breast cancer, and is often an end-stage symptom of coronary artery disease, high blood pressure, ischemia, myocardial infarction, chronic alcohol abuse, or acute viral infection. One-third of cases have no known cause. It is highly probable that these unknown cases spring from a nutritional cause, as aging women (and men) have low blood levels of CoQ10 and other vital nutrients.

great confusion among cardiologists and their patients. More likely, you may have heard your doctor say, "You have a heart murmur." If your physician has confirmed that your particular heart murmur is due to MVP, then there are some things you should know.

In many cases, MVP is detected during a routine examination with no other signs. Its distinctive murmur or "click" can be heard with a stethoscope as the blood flows through the chambers of the heart, momentarily caught in the mitral valve as it opens and closes. MVP is diagnosed most frequently in adolescents and premenopausal women. It can be congenital (present at birth) or acquired later in life (only occasionally is MVP associated with diastolic dysfunction).

The mitral valve has two cusps or flaps and is so named because its appearance resembles that of the dual-peaked miter (hat) of a bishop. The mitral valve sits between the left atrium and the left ventricle, where its major job is to open freely and far enough to allow blood to enter the left ventricle, and shut tightly enough so that blood does not backwash into the left atrium.

If the valve prolapses, or falls backward into the left atrium, the blood leaking or "sloshing" in reverse mode creates the trademark clicking sound we call the cardiac murmur. Usually, a thickening of one or two of its specialized, cartilage-like tissue flaps (called leaflets) causes the flopping back of the valve's cusps. Most often, the mitral valve prolapses intermittently, and so it can be missed during an exam.

Most people with MVP have no symptoms. But if you are one of the few women who does experience symptoms, you know how alarming they can be because they often mimic the signs of heart attack: chest pain, shortness of breath, palpitations, weakness. And even if you *know* that you have MVP, and *not* coronary artery disease, the symptoms can be distressing. They can come on abruptly and without warning, interfering with your daily activities, making you feel anxious or depressed.

Unfortunately, the causes underlying MVP's symptoms have yet to be fully explained (research suggests that there is gradual degeneration of the connective tissues that make up the valve), so treatment options have targeted the few sources we can identify. Increased adrenaline-like activity and, more recently discovered, magnesium deficiency have been suggested as causing many of the symptoms of MVP. So medications that block adrenaline response—such as beta blockers—have been helpful in assuaging some of the distress for women who suffer symptoms. Medical therapy has not been effective for specific symptoms, such as the quick jabs of knife-like chest pain and/or the skipped heart beats that may be experienced during episodes of prolapse.

While some women respond well to a class of drugs called beta blockers—Inderal (propranolol), Corgard (nadolol), Lopressor (metoprolol)—many do not. But though we may not completely

---

Carotid Artery Disease Can Affect Women

CAROTID ARTERY DISEASE is essentially caused by the same process as heart disease, except the arteries affected are the carotids, those large arteries that run up each side of your neck to your brain. Because they deliver blood flow from the neck up, so to speak, the symptoms of blockage that manifest are *visual* and *neurological*.

SYMPTOMS OF CAROTID ARTERY DISEASE INCLUDE *weakness* and/or *tingling of the hand*, *loss of part of your field of vision*, or even transient ischemic attacks (TIAs) or "mini-strokes." The symptoms of a mini-stroke are similar to those of a stroke (see page 160), such as *slurred speech* and *extremity numbness*, but with a mini-stroke, the symptoms resolve without permanent damage. But that does not mean that a mini-stroke is harmless; it is a warning sign to seek medical evaluation. In much the same way that angina is a harbinger of heart attack, a mini-stroke can be a precursor to a stroke or cerebral vascular accident (CVA) in which permanent damage may result.

understand the causes of MVP, we do understand its physiology and factors that can aggravate or precipitate episodes.

First, stress is a major player, most probably because the hormonal response to psychological stress is to dump out the excess adrenaline that can overtax the heart muscle. Several chemical stimu-

---

It's Not a Heart Attack But You Still Have Pain

NONCARDIAC OR ATYPICAL CHEST PAIN (NCP OR ATP) is an expensive and disconcerting phenomenon in medicine. Not only does it cost individuals and insurance companies millions of dollars each year, it causes an intolerable amount of human anguish, suffering, and disability. The causes of NCP range from acid reflux, to disorders of the esophagus, to mitral valve prolapse (MVP), to abnormal visceral proprioception—a perception of pain that is an inappropriate attribution to a physical source from your gut. A few other individuals will have what we call *microangina*, pain from diffuse and widespread blockages in the smallest blood vessels in the heart, or they may have coronary artery spasm where the walls on the coronaries contract so forcefully that the blood flow to the heart is compromised.

IN MY CARDIOLOGY PRACTICE, many individuals come to me for assessment of some type of chest pain or chest discomfort. In fact, *about 50 percent of the patients who consult any cardiologist are experiencing chest pain.* Half of these individuals will find out that their pain is not cardiac in origin and that their prognosis is excellent. Still, it is estimated that 34 to 70 percent of these patients will continue to suffer multiple painful attacks, repeatedly consulting physicians for ongoing symptoms.

OVER A DECADE AGO, it was calculated that the costs of managing noncardiac chest pain were in the range of $4,000 a year per person. That figure included 1986 costs for an average of 1.2 prescriptions per month as well as 2.2 emergency room visits and one hospitalization per year for cardiac work-ups. I'm sure that those costs have skyrocketed since then. In 1992 it was reported that of the 2 million angiographies (at a present cost of about $10,000 a piece) performed each year in the United States, most of them for chest pain, 10 to 30 percent were negative. While a negative report is always great news for the patient and family, it means that a huge chunk of those undergoing this invasive procedure still have to explore other causes for their chest pain.

lants also trigger prolapsing of the mitral valve in vulnerable women. Those include caffeine; cocoa and chocolate; food additives such as MSG (monosodium glutamate), which are hidden in many foods, especially Chinese food; and preservatives such as sodium benzoate, potassium sorbate, and coloring agents. Over-the-counter cold remedies with ingredients such as ephedrine often increase heart rate and can also provoke MVP. Alcohol, simple sugars, and flour are other dietary culprits. Food allergies can even precipitate increased heart rate, chest pain, and shortness of breath. If you suffer from MVP, your first step is to try to eliminate as many of the above triggers as possible, and then look at targeted nutritional supplements that can help.

Coenzyme Q10—A New Approach

For years, I experienced tremendous frustration treating mitral valve prolapse. While only a small proportion of women with MVP syndrome had symptoms distressing enough to require drugs to improve their quality of life, I found myself in a bind when many failed to respond to conventional beta blocker therapy. And for the few who did, many complained of troublesome side effects such as fatigue, mental confusion, hair loss, insomnia, and even nightmares. Then there were the women who had very infrequent symptoms, and so took their medication only when needed. Yet they had to struggle for thirty to sixty minutes waiting for the drug to kick in, less than an optimal plan of action. Then I tried a new approach, so simple that I was amazed: a vitamin and mineral combination that was virtually free of side-effects.

I discovered that about 25 to 50 percent of my MVP patients responded quite favorably to coenzyme Q10 (CoQ10). They reported a decrease in chest discomfort and shortness of breath on 90 to 180 mg of CoQ10 daily. In fact, episodes of irregular heartbeat responded exceptionally well to CoQ10 in this dose range.

CoQ10 is a naturally occurring, vitamin-like substance found in small quantities in many foods and synthesized in all cells of the body. CoQ10 has many functions, including antioxidant activity, membrane stabilizing capacity, and energy enhancing activity. The energy enhancing activity of CoQ10 is probably its most important function.

CoQ10 supports each cell's power plant, or mitochondria, by helping to produce ATP (*adenosine triphosphate*), the most fundamental form of energy. Its membrane-stabilizing ability can help reduce irregular heartbeat. There's research documenting that MVP symptoms may be related to a CoQ10 deficiency, so supplementing with this nutrient makes sense for anyone with MVP. Syndromes of diastolic dysfunction and decreased energy production in the heart also respond well to the ATP-stimulating properties of CoQ10.

Magnesium and MVP

New research findings have been reported that demonstrate the effectiveness of *magnesium* in alleviating symptoms of MVP, so I've added it to my natural treatment protocol. Consider this two-phase study on MVP and magnesium:

A double-blind study was performed with 181 subjects. Magnesium blood cell levels were assessed in 141 patients with MVP and compared to that of forty healthy control patients. Lower-than-normal magnesium levels were found in 60 percent of the patients with MVP; only 5 percent of the controls showed similar deficiencies.

The second leg of the study investigated response to treatment. Participants with magnesium deficits were randomly assigned to two groups: magnesium supplement versus placebo. The results in the magnesium-supplemented patients were dramatic:

❖ the average number of symptoms per patient was significantly decreased;

❖ there was a significant reduction in weakness, chest discomfort, shortness of breath, palpitations, and anxiety-related symptoms;

❖ there was a decrease in the amount of adrenaline-like substances in the urine.

The researchers made two conclusions: First, many patients who are severely symptomatic with MVP have low serum magnesium levels. And secondly, supplementation of this crucial mineral leads to an improvement in symptoms as well as a decrease in adrenaline-like hormones. For these patients, magnesium supplementation may be just the solution to reduce their symptoms and improve their quality of life.

Certainly, magnesium is not a drug, and its administration is safe and simple. For my patients with MVP who have healthy kidney function, I recommend a combination of CoQ10 (usually 120 mg per day) along with 400 to 800 mg magnesium in divided doses after meals. I am no longer frustrated with MVP treatment, because this nutrient combination offers many women relief from its troublesome symptoms.

IHSS: Too Much Muscle

A third manifestation of diastolic dysfunction has the tongue-twisting name of *Idiopathic Hypertrophic Subaortic Stenosis*, or IHSS.

Symptoms of a Mini-stroke or Impending Stroke

Inability to speak or slurring of speech
Inability to swallow
Facial droop
Visual disturbances like blurring or loss of part of visual field
Weakness, numbness, or paralysis of extremity
Dizziness or vertigo
Fainting or loss of consciousness

To break that down:

IDIOPATHIC—indicates that the cause is unknown.
HYPERTROPHIC—means increased muscle mass of the muscular wall dividing the right and left ventricle, right down the center of the heart.
SUBAORTIC—refers to the area right below the aortic valve.
STENOSIS—means blockage of normal flow.

It sounds complicated, but basically with IHSS (a type of cardiomyopathy), too much of the heart muscle blocks the left ventricular cavity, causing obstruction of blood flow out of the heart and into the aorta. This impediment to blood flow often results in symptoms of lightheadedness, dizziness, passing out, and, rarely, sudden cardiac death.

Medical therapy such as calcium channel blockers and beta blocking drugs has long been used to reduce symptoms of IHSS. More recent research has shown that CoQ10, with its positive effect on cardiac energy, can also assuage the symptoms of IHSS and improve quality of life as well as chance of survival.

Anxiety—Tricky to Diagnose, Slippery to Treat

About one-third of the people who seek advice from any cardiologist are actually having symptoms as a result of anxiety or even panic disorder, one of its more extreme manifestations. To complicate matters even further, the chicken-egg phenomenon of non-cardiac chest pain (NCP) is that it can be hard to tell which comes first. Anxiety about having a heart condition can precipitate cardiac-like symptoms, even when the heart appears to be uninvolved.

And what about the other group of individuals who battle unexplained chest pain? What about those with a known history of cardiac disease—a heart attack, angioplasty, or bypass surgery—

who continue to experience chest discomfort despite medications and procedures?

What's Behind Disabling Anxiety?

Many of the people I see with NCP are actually exhibiting symptoms of panic disorder (PD). PD is defined as a specific, disabling anxiety disorder that is characterized by recurrent unexpected episodes of intense fear or discomfort associated with several specific somatic and cognitive complaints. Its cause is the imbalance of several brain chemicals.

PD patients have a well-documented tendency to catastrophically misinterpret their anxiety symptoms as physiological in origin, creating a negative feedback loop that accelerates their already high anxiety level, raising it to the point of sheer panic. Researchers know more about how to treat PD than its exact physiology.

Why is Panic Disorder So Commonly Seen in Cardiology?

Most manifestations of PD—ten out of thirteen diagnostic symptoms—are known as somatic (body symptoms), rather than psychological or cognitive (involving mental/thinking states), as you might expect. So most PD patients will initially seek treatment

---

Panic Disorder: Another Great Mimicker of Heart Disease

INDIVIDUALS WITH PANIC DISORDER (PD) suffer with panic symptoms on a chronic basis. They react disproportionately to stressful triggers. But at other times, anxiety attacks may hit without any real warning. Some individuals with anxiety get so tense that they dump out enormous amounts of adrenaline, giving them palpitations, sweats, tremors, and even chest pain and tightness, or general uneasiness. Research supports the fact that such anxiety disorders are one of the major noncardiac causes of chest pain syndromes.

from a doctor. And because seven of those ten body symptoms are so cardiac-like—chest pain, shortness of breath, palpitations, sweating, feeling of choking, numbness or tingling of the extremities, and hot flashing—a majority of patients will rush to a cardiologist.

The Story of Elaine

Elaine came to me for disturbing episodes of chest pain and discomfort that were associated with a lot of other physical symptoms. On physical exam, she was healthy. The results of her echocardiogram and exercise stress tests were within normal limits. Nonetheless, Elaine was convinced that there was something wrong with her heart. She insisted on an angiogram, which came back negative for heart disease. She was evaluated for other noncardiac sources for her symptoms, which, again, ended without a diagnosis. Like many people with PD, Elaine was *not* reassured; she continued to seek a diagnosis and treatment. She sought a second cardiac opinion and another series of diagnostic tests, which again indicated no problem with her heart.

I appreciate the dilemma for women like Elaine. Often, their symptoms are dismissed as emotional, and they have to be savvy enough to insist on a thorough cardiological evaluation. But when an intensive workup has been done, as it had in Elaine's case, then

Therapeutic Approaches and Healing

WOMEN ARE NOT ONLY MORE VULNERABLE to the physical risk factors of coronary artery disease than men, they are also more prone to subsequent cardiac events, such as recurrent heart attack, bypass surgery, recurrent angioplasty, and even sudden cardiac death. Since recurrent morbidity as well as mortality is more common in women, aggressive emotional and psychological interactions will have a more profound impact. For women, understanding the delicate balance between the emotional and physical must be acknowledged in the overall scheme of healing. That is why an awareness of therapeutic approaches to heart disease is so important.

consideration must be given to the possible psychological component for her distress.

If you asked about my concern that someone like Elaine
could eventually create a self-fulfilling prophecy and develop heart
disease because of her overinvestment and preoccupation, I have
to admit that yes, that does concern me. And, if you challenged me
that perhaps Elaine is a victim of heartbreak and intuitively knows
she is at risk, I would again have to agree that her symptoms
should not be dismissed out of hand.

In any case, whatever the emotional root and potential physical
outcome of Elaine's distressing symptoms, the optimum course for her,
when everything physical is ruled out, is to consider deeper self-explo-
ration through psychotherapy. That's my ideal treatment scenario for her.
At the very least, a good psychological assessment should identify the
possible source of her symptoms and can guide her treatment options.

I recognize that psychotherapy may not be the most comfortable or reasonable course of action for everyone, but there are
possibilities that can be opened to you through this work (see
Chapter 14). You may want to consider relaxation, breathing techniques, and other cognitive-behavioral therapies such as gradual
exposure to anxiety-provoking cues. These approaches, used in
combination with lifestyle changes (outlined in Section II), have
been helpful for more than 80 percent of my patients.

Inositol: New Hope for Panic Disorder

One of the best nutritional supplements that I've found for panic
attacks (not to mention anxiety and depression), is inositol, a key
ingredient in the central nervous system. Inositol helps regulate
serotonin, the "happy hormonal" neurotransmitter. Inositol is beneficial for treating panic disorder as well as the insomnia that may
come with anxiety. Anxiety is often the flip-side of depression (see

Chapter 13). Although it seems that the two are energetically very different, people with depression often have a strong anxiety component and vice versa.

Many of my patients report that they feel calmer when they take inositol, which is natural and a perfectly safe alternative to prescription drugs (and it's virtually free of side effects). If you suffer with symptoms of anxiety and panic, I recommend 12 grams a day of inositol, which can be found in most health food or vitamin stores.

If you want to try inositol, you should do so for at least four weeks. Research shows that's the minimum amount of time required to experience its therapeutic benefits. I expect we will see more research on this compound in the future. In the meantime, don't take inositol if you are on an antidepressant or medication for anxiety or depression. Always talk to your doctor first.

CHAPTER NINE

Congestive Heart Failure and the Power of Coenzyme Q10: A Miracle in the Making

In October 1996 I was on my way home from a conference when I took a call from a man nearly frantic with concern for his mother. Mary was seventy-nine years old, laying unconscious, on a respirator, in a community hospital in Connecticut. She was in congestive heart failure complicated by pneumonia. With the exception of giving birth to her children, she'd never been in a hospital in her life and had always been a vibrant, healthy woman.

Her son, Bob, quickly filled me in on the details: Mary had been on a ventilator for three-and-a-half weeks, receiving powerful steroids to reduce inflammation in her lungs and tissues, along with high concentrations of pure oxygen. Bob happened to be a biochemist with a doctorate degree and was familiar with nutritionals such as coenzyme Q10 (CoQ10). He had asked the doctors to place his mother on CoQ10, but they had refused. He then brought in a two-foot-thick stack of references, attesting to the efficacy of this agent, but still they refused to cooperate with his wishes, and instead told him that his mother was "terminal." In fact, on two separate occasions the doctors tried to convince the family to pull the plug. They even accused him of "interfering" with his mother's care!

But when Bob called me on the phone even I thought he was asking for the impossible. He wanted me to take Mary in transfer to my hospital in Connecticut so that I could take over her care. I had to be very direct with Bob: "I can't take your mother in transfer. She is dependent upon life support and probably would not survive the forty-minute ambulance trip to my hospital."

Bob didn't miss a beat: "At least she will have a fighting chance. Where she is now she will certainly die." He and his sister were willing to accept responsibility for the outcome, so the arrangements were made for their mother's transfer.

When I first saw Mary in the intensive care unit at Manchester Memorial Hospital, she was semi-comatose, respiratory-dependent, and had minimal response to stimulation. I continued her conventional pulmonary care, making just one change in her therapy: 450 mg CoQ10 was given through her feeding tube daily, 150 mg every eight hours. She also received a multivitamin/mineral preparation, crushed and delivered via feeding tube, plus 1 gram of magnesium delivered intravenously each day.

Although I held out some hope for Mary, my colleagues—both doctors and nurses—were quite skeptical of using CoQ10 in this case, despite the fact that it had been on formulary at our hospital for years.

But what we were all about to observe was truly a miracle.

On the third day of the program, Mary began to "wake up." And after ten days of steady improvement in her condition, we were able to wean her off the ventilator. Four days later, she was discharged to an extended care facility, and was sitting up in a wheelchair with only supplemental oxygen to accompany her.

I have had the good fortune to continue to see Mary in my office on several occasions over the last four years. She is now completely asymptomatic for congestive heart failure (CHF) and enjoys a good quality of life on her combination therapy: conventional medicine plus 360 mg CoQ10 in divided doses every day. When I last spoke with her family, she was reorganizing a library of three thousand books and still reading many of them.

Mary's story is not an isolated case. I have treated dozens of cases (and have heard of many more from colleagues) of people literally "left for dead" who have been similarly resurrected by the remarkable compound called coenzymeQ10.

Remember coenzymeQ10 is an antioxidant compound similar to vitamin K and is naturally manufactured in the liver as well as every cell in the body. But even though CoQ10 is produced in the body, many people have deficiencies, especially those suffering from cardiovascular disease and heart failure. The best dietary sources of CoQ10 are organ meats, beef, fish, nuts, spinach, and broccoli. Supplemental CoQ10 can be found in health food stores.

Clinical research has demonstrated that significant CoQ10 deficiencies exist in our population due to a multitude of factors, including the fact that production of this key energy nutrient declines in the body with aging. Women are more vulnerable to this fall-off than men. Because the heart is so metabolically active and requires a constant supply of adenosine triphosphate (ATP) to continue beating, it is especially vulnerable to CoQ10 deficiencies. Fortunately, however, the heart can be very responsive to CoQ10 supplementation.

It is unthinkable for me to practice good cardiology without the help of this nutritional agent. Hundreds of scientific studies and thousands of clinical applications have documented that this substance has proven benefits for treating a wide variety of cardiac conditions including congestive heart failure, coronary artery disease, high blood pressure, angina, and more. Despite the large body of research, a therapeutic description in 1997 in a mainstream textbook, and the fact that CoQ10 is used by many board-certified cardiologists throughout the United States, Europe, and Japan, this vitamin-like substance is still virtually ignored by the majority of clinical cardiologists and most of the conventional medical establishment.

The ongoing resistance of the medical community to employ this essential nutrient represents one of the greatest missed opportunities in modern medicine. I find it tragic that many patients who are not helped by conventional treatments alone could be supported, and perhaps saved, by the simple addition of CoQ10.

As with many potent nutritional agents, CoQ10 is not patentable, since it is a widely occurring substance in nature. Therefore, there is little or no economic incentive for major pharmaceutical companies to develop and market CoQ10 as a proprietary product. The education and marketing is just too costly for any company to take on when it cannot expect to have an exclusive patent on the market.

I have been using CoQ10 since 1986, when I first prescribed just 10 mg three times a day to one of my patients undergoing bypass surgery. Since that time, my comfort level—and dosage level—have risen considerably. Now I have thousands of patients in my practice and across the country taking CoQ10 at various dosage levels, based on their conditions. I have learned that if individuals fail to respond to low-dose CoQ10 therapy, we need to increase the dosage, and maintain it over time. Up to 500 mg per day or more, given in divided doses, may be necessary to achieve a therapeutic effect. A significant blood level of CoQ10, usually greater than 3.5 ug/ml, is necessary to obtain a therapeutic effect, especially in cases of congestive heart failure.

What is Congestive Heart Failure?

With congestive heart failure (CHF), the heart becomes so weak that it can no longer effectively pump blood throughout your body. During an acute episode of CHF, the percentage of blood pumped out of the left ventricle may drop well below the normal level of 50 to 70 percent. Anyone with an ejection fraction of 30 to 35 percent or less is probably fighting to get enough air into their lungs as fluid backs up into the lungs, the extremities (puffy ankles and fingers), and the liver (congested). At times some will need hospitalization and aggressive treatment with diuretics.

Others with an ejection fraction of 10 to 15 percent may be so compromised that they can barely sustain everyday activities. Just moving from a bed to a chair may be exhausting. At this point, a heart transplant may be the only option.

With CHF, the heart is not strong enough to pump blood effectively out of the left ventricle, and it begins to flow back into the lungs. There, it blocks the life-giving exchange of oxygen-for-carbon dioxide. People with early stage CHF usually experience fatigue and shortness of breath with minimal exertion.

This creates "air hunger"—that sense of gasping for breath—and will eventually lead to a state in which the extremities of the afflicted individual begin turning blue. Supplemental oxygen is needed at this point, and many people with chronic low-level CHF must remain attached to a portable oxygen unit in order to remain active.

As the lungs become more congested, blood backs up further, collecting in the body's various tissue "compartments." At this point, swelling occurs where gravity tends to settle the blood: feet, ankles, lower legs, fingers, or the small of the back when one is lying down. Eventually, the congestion backs up to the liver and can be detected by a professional during a physical exam.

When CHF strikes abruptly, as it can during a heart attack, it can be cataclysmic and life-threatening. Within minutes, the body can go into full-blown *pulmonary edema*—a rapid-fire, flash-flood type of CHF in which time is critical, and only emergency medicine can save the day.

The most common cause of CHF is coronary artery disease and large areas of stiff, scarred mucle tissue from earlier heart attacks. Long-standing high blood pressure, toxic drugs, chronic alcohol abuse, valvular diseases, and viral illness can also contribute to congestive heart failure.

Congestive Heart Failure and Women

The April 1998 issue of *Internal Medicine News* reported some shocking and disconcerting statistics based on findings of a national study involving nearly one hundred thousand women. The average duration of survival for women aged sixty-seven and older who survived their first hospitalization for congestive heart failure (CHF) was only 2.5 years. The study further reported:

❖ Medicare claims identified 99,135 women sixty-seven and older discharged in 1986 following what was probably their first hospitalization for CHF;

❖ During six years of follow-up, 82 percent of these women had died—about 30 percent in their first year of discharge;

❖ There were no racial differences in mortality rates after adjusting for age; and

❖ Women with diabetes in conjunction with CHF were significantly more likely to die during follow-up.

As you can see from this research, congestive heart failure is a major cardiac problem affecting women with a very high mortality rate. Thus, both prevention and treatment are concerns for any woman.

Most cases of heart failure in men can be traced to a specific cause. In women, heart failure is often "idiopathic"—that is, it has no discernible cause. Based on research and the female patients I've treated, I believe that most of the idiopathic heart failure I've observed among women is due to a dangerous decline in their bodies' production of CoQ10, which leads to a critical loss of energy in the heart muscle cells. This could be accounted for by the tendency for a woman's liver to lose its ability to produce CoQ10 as she ages, and may be why the use of high levels of CoQ10 have resulted in dramatic recoveries.

Laura: a Case of High Blood Pressure Leading to CHF

Laura, a seventy-nine-year-old woman with a long-standing history of hypertension, had developed her first episode of congestive heart failure in 1977 at the age of sixty. By 1984 she had experienced her first episode of pulmonary edema, which had been treated with traditional therapy (digoxin, diuretic therapy, and ACE inhibitors).

Laura's heart was pumping blood out at 35 percent, still well below the normal ejection fraction of 50 to 70 percent, and placing her at risk for acute CHF. Following a second episode of pulmonary edema in 1992, Laura underwent a procedure called cardiac catheterization, which confirmed that she had an enlarged and weakened left ventricle. Her coronary arteries were normal. Laura continued to be treated with standard medical care, including ACE inhibitors, and increasing doses of diuretics. Although her quality of life continued to be satisfactory for a number of years, she continued to suffer intermittent bouts of CHF, and her condition gradually deteriorated.

By October 1994 Laura was failing. She weighed only seventy-seven pounds and was suffering from advanced congestive heart failure. Her heart was pumping just 10 to 15 percent, barely enough to support a bed-to-chair lifestyle. I felt desperate for her, and decided to start her on coenzyme Q10 therapy at 30 mg three times per day, a level I was comfortable with in 1994. (Now we know that side effects associated with CoQ10 are extremely rare and, when they do occur, mild—less than 1 percent may have slight nausea or diarrhea.)

From October through February 1995 Laura continued to remain homebound. I shared her disappointment. Despite the addition of CoQ10 therapy, her quality of life had become completely unsatisfactory. Laura developed marked edema (fluid-filled tissues)—her belly was swollen, and she was severely fatigued from the lack of oxygen. Her respiratory status became so compromised that she required tubes to withdraw the excess fluid from around her lung cavities.

But in March 1995 a miracle happened. Laura was "accidentally" started on a higher dosage of 300 mg CoQ10 daily. Inadvertently, her son had purchased 100 mg capsules instead of the usual 30 mg—more than tripling her dose. About four weeks later, Laura experienced a steady and marked improvement in her functional status. Clinically, I observed improvement in both the right and left sides of her heart. We decided to maintain the 300 mg daily dose which seemed to be responsible for her dramatic turnaround.

By June 1995 Laura was becoming more active and mobile. A repeat echocardiogram demonstrated that her ejection fraction was exceeding 20 percent. By October 1995 Laura was shopping and visiting relatives. In fact, she became so active that, unfortunately, in January 1996 she fell and fractured her hip. Previously considered a high surgical risk, Laura tolerated a total hip replacement with flying colors.

When I last saw her in September 1996, Laura was continuing to enjoy a good quality of life and was walking with the assistance of a cane. She was active with symptoms of CHF occurring only with exertion.

Unfortunately, I must report that in 1998, Laura did succumb to CHF. Following an acute gastrointestinal illness, she had run out of CoQ10 supplement and deteriorated rapidly. (It is dangerous for people with CHF who take CoQ10 to stop taking it suddenly.) She was admitted to the hospital, where her daughter rushed in with a fresh supply of the nutrient, but it could not pull her back from the edge as it had before. However, I firmly believe that CoQ10 gave her four active years of life that she enjoyed with her family and friends.

Battling CHF

The management of CHF and dilated cardiomyopathy (often end-stage CHF) are perhaps the most difficult challenges faced by cardiologists today. Over my last twenty-five years of practice, I have often found the medication juggling act needed to treat recurring bouts of CHF to be among my worst clinical nightmares. Although there are excellent conventional approaches in the battle against CHF, the fact remains that many patients do not fully respond to even the most high-powered drugs, and some cannot tolerate the many side effects that often occur as a result of taking them on a regular basis. Despite modern medicine and technology, the quality of life for those with a weakened heart muscle and chronic CHF is compromised, and their very survival remains guarded.

Although approximately 85 percent of patients respond to CoQ10 alone, 15 percent do not. Something else is needed to enhance the energy of the heart. I have found that many "Q10 resistant" individuals improve when I team CoQ10 with L-carnitine, an amino acid made in the body and taken in the diet. I call this dynamic duo my "Twin Pillars of Healing."

Coenzyme Q10 and L-Carnitine: The Twin Pillars of Healing

One of CoQ10's most important tasks is to shuttle electrons between enzyme systems in order to generate energy—adenosine triphosphate (ATP), the basic building block of all energy—in the power plants of the cells (mitochondria). In fact, each heart muscle cell can have five thousand mitochondria to support energy reserves. Heart disease, including heart attacks and CHF, reduces the effective number of mitochondria due to scar tissue and other damage.

The heart is so active that it requires a constant supply of ATP. Cardiac muscle cells burn fats for fuel. But the heart demands such a constant and high level of energy resources to pump—60 to 100 times a minute, 24 hours a day, year after year—that it's especially vulnerable to even subtle deficiencies in the factors that contribute to ATP production: CoQ10 and L-carnitine.

While CoQ10 sparks the energy in the cells, L-cartinine is like a shuttle, bringing fatty acids into the mitochondria so they can be used for energy, then carting away toxic byproducts. Think of mitochondria as the furnace, CoQ10 as the generator, and L-carnitine as the delivery service. The heart burns fat as the predominant source of fuel, and L-carnitine is necessary to bring the fuel into the heart cells to be burned for energy.

Researchers at the University of Milan in Italy have done a great deal of experimental work with these two nutrients. They have demonstrated a protective and synergistic effect between CoQ10 and L-carnitine in a number of advanced heart conditions. While the research is persuasive, my personal experience is even more heartening. I've had former treatment "nightmares" walk in breathing easier and with better color, walking about the office with minimal difficulty. It was as if L-carnitine provided the "powerpack" to work synergistically with CoQ10. Interestingly, I have observed the most dramatic effects in my most seriously ill patients. That's why I call these two nutritionals my "twin pillars of healing." They have changed the way I treat heart failures and heart disease.

Like CoQ10, L-carnitine can be safely and effectively taken in combination with beta blockers, calcium channel blockers, nitrates, and ACE inhibitors for a more full-spectrum approach to symptom relief. Keep in mind that the primary mechanism of both L-carnitine and CoQ10 is to enhance energy on a cellular level. This property is natural and selective, unlike the pharmacological actions of drugs that indirectly improve the heart's pumping ability by slowing heart rate and increasing contractility of the heart.

Please note also that you do not have to have a medical condition to benefit from L-carnitine and CoQ10 supplementation. Normal, healthy individuals can also derive benefit from the use of these nutrients, minimizing the risk of future health problems. This is prevention at its best, keeping you one step ahead of the game when it comes to your health.

Classifying Heart Failure

Physicians use the following classification system to document the severity of CHF:

Class I—*No limitations.* Ordinary physical activity does not cause undue fatigue, shortness of breath (dyspnea), or palpitations.

Class II—*Slight limitation of physical activity.* Such patients are comfortable at rest. Ordinary physical activity results in fatigue, palpitations, shortness of breath or angina (heart cramps).

Class III—*Marked limitation of physical activity.* Although patients are comfortable at rest, less than ordinary activity will lead to symptoms.

Class IV—*Inability to carry on any physical activity without discomfort.* Symptoms of CHF are present even at rest. With any physical activity, increased discomfort is experienced.

There are other situations in which a combination of these nutrients can be very helpful, such as athletic activities involving strenuous muscular work. L-carnitine and CoQ10 taken together can help your body meet the greater demand for energy. This health-promoting combo can counter the increase in oxidative stress associated with such exertion and reduce accumulation of harmful byproducts such as lactate, helping to reduce muscular fatigue.

Determining Your Optimal Dosage

This dosage conundrum of CoQ10 prompted researchers to design and carry out a preliminary study to evaluate the effectiveness of different preparations of CoQ10. We observed that most preparations with 120 mg may raise the blood concentration to only 1.5 ug/ml. Although this level may help some patients, the therapeutic level for sick patients is at least 2.5 and preferably over 3.5 ug/ml. For this reason, I recommend that those of you who are not appreciating any symptom relief on lower doses get yourselves a blood level. If this is not feasible for you, then treat your symptoms clinically by doubling or even tripling your usual dose of CoQ10, according to how you feel. It's not unusual for cardiologists, including myself, to recommend the same kind of step ladder dosing approach, even with traditional drugs such as diuretics and ACE inhibitors.

Because L-carnitine, like CoQ10, is a substance made by the body, taking it as a supplement causes few side effects. I've been using L-carnitine for several years and have yet to see any significant side effects other than some fleeting gastrointestinal complaints. If that should happen, I usually tell my patients to take a lower dosage and be mindful to take this nutrient with a small amount of food. Although L-carnitine is absorbed better on an empty stomach, improved delivery systems are being developed, especially softgel formulas.

I usually recommend doses of 250 to 500 mg of L-carnitine fumarate three to four times daily. It's often best to start at the lower end of the dose range and then double or even quadruple the dose to get the therapeutic effect desired. L-carnitine, CoQ10, and some drugs may require individual dose adjustments: there's no "automatic" best dose of these agents that's one-size-fits-all for everyone. Both may require adjustment to obtain an optimum therapeutic blood level and symptom relief.

For example, for CoQ10 to be effective in compromised cardiac patients, oftentimes the blood level needs to be greater than five or six times normal. And many people will fail to have a therapeutic effect with coenzyme Q10 even if their blood level is two or three times above normal. The same may be true for L-carnitine. In some of my patients 500 to 1,500 mg L-carnitine, although a suitable dose, may not be an effective *therapeutic* dose. Occasionally, doses need to be increased as high as 3 to 4 grams daily.

In my experience, as well as based on a review of the medical literature, L-carnitine appears to be safe even at these higher doses. There have been some drug interactions related to L-carnitine. For example, anticonvulsant drugs including phenobarbital, phenytoin (Dilantin), and carbamazepine (Tegretol) have had a significant effect on lowering L-carnitine blood levels. As always, please consult your physician before beginning a program of any nutritional supplement.

CHAPTER TEN

High Blood Pressure: Overcome a Silent Killer

It's no wonder that so many of you are concerned about your blood pressure. Some 50 million people are afflicted with hypertension, making it the No. 1 cardiac condition that doctors treat today. There is a strong association between elevated blood pressure and coronary heart disease in both women and men. High blood pressure is *the* most common cause of stroke, and high blood pressure increases your risk of dying from a heart attack three-fold—from heart failure, four-fold. High blood pressure is one of my patients' most pressing concerns. This does not surprise me, since I have lost all too many patients to this disorder that's justly named the "silent killer."

While hypertension can strike at any age, it is estimated to affect approximately 30 percent of all women over age sixty-five. Several studies have linked this late-onset type of high blood pressure with an elevated risk of death from stroke as well as coronary heart disease. African American women are even more vulnerable to high blood pressure, especially since they most often fail to respond to conventional drugs. Although medications have reduced the incidence of both stroke and heart attack, *thousands* of people die each year from *correctly-prescribed* prescription drugs. This startling finding confirms that prescription drugs are much more potent and potentially dangerous than is widely believed. Obviously a more natural approach is warranted!

Consider this statistic from the *Journal of the American Medical Association:* 78 percent of high blood pressure in men and 65 percent in women can be directly attributed to obesity. Research has shown that control of blood pressure using dietary intervention and weight loss has been moderately successful for women. Some other findings in the *Journal* regarding the prevalence and treatment of high blood pressure in the United States revealed that current approaches to treatment are less than optimal. Here are some of their findings:

❖ One in four adults is hypertensive, and one-third of them don't know it;

❖ Despite several decades of improved detection and treatment, we have failed to reduce the incidence of high blood pressure;

❖ There has been a substantial increase in hypertension in the thirty-five–to–sixty age groups;

❖ Of those who are being treated for their high blood pressure, only 21 percent are adequately controlled;

❖ Hypertension usually coexists with other risk factors, such as diabetes, smoking, and obesity; and high blood pressure is found in conjunction with *three or more* metabolic risk factors at an occurrence rate that is four to five times higher than statistical chance.

But What Is High Blood Pressure?

As previously mentioned, high blood pressure or hypertension is a reflection of overly high systolic and diastolic blood pressure readings. Every time your heart beats, blood is squeezed through your blood vessels. The highest reading of the pressure exerted by the contraction of the heart is called systolic pressure. Between beats the heart relaxes and the blood pressure falls. The lowest reading is called diastolic pressure.

The average normal blood pressure for an adult is usually 120 (systolic) over 80 (diastolic). Systolic pressures in ranges of 140 to 150 mm/Hg or higher, and diastolic pressures greater than 95 mm/Hg, are generally regarded as harmful to the heart and vascular system.

Remember, systolic pressure is the amount of pressure necessary to open the aortic valve for each contraction of the heart; diastolic pressure is the amount of tone in the vascular walls as they "milk" the blood through the arteries. Both pressure levels must be balanced—high enough for optimal circulation and energy requirements, but not so high that excess wear and tear on the cardiovascular system occurs.

When the pressure is too great, the blood vessels can weaken, leading to a breakdown in the wall's protective surface. When this happens, toxic blood components such as heavy metals, cigarette smoke, oxidized LDL, and excess homocysteine start to stick to the roughened sidewalls, setting the stage for plaque formation—and ultimately heart disease.

Should You Take Drugs that Lower Blood Pressure?

Despite my preference for natural, complementary approaches, I frequently need to prescribe drugs that lower blood pressure. While medications like Vasotec, Monopril, Norvasc, Lozol, and Toprol can be lifesavers, they can also have serious—even lethal—side effects.

But no matter what your age, current health condition, or blood-pressure lowering drugs you're taking, you can participate in your own healing, lower your blood pressure, *and* improve the health of your heart. Although this major health risk can be treated with prescription drugs, it's far *safer and easier* to revamp your lifestyle before you hit the high road to danger. It's also your ticket to a better quality of life—free from the unpleasant side effects of potent blood-pressure drugs and the uncertainty of complications associated with long-standing hypertension.

While medication can certainly be an important part of a program to lower blood pressure, every drug has its price. As you know, drugs have side effects, ranging from mildly annoying to outright dangerous. For example, ACE inhibitors (such as Vasotec and Monopril) lower blood pressure by inhibiting specific enzymes that cause blood vessels to constrict. But they can also cause severe coughing, dizziness, headaches, and fatigue.

There are at least sixty to seventy different antihypertensive drugs on the market today. But, *I have yet to find a single antihypertensive drug for high blood pressure control that has no undesirable side effects.* It's because of serious compromises such as loss of sexual desire, fatigue, and constipation that I have never been completely satisfied with the health gains from these medications.

If you have a family history of hypertension or have for years been on drugs that lower blood pressure, my advice is to combine the best of both worlds—conventional medicine and alternative methods.

Monitor Your Blood Pressure Accurately— In Your Own Home

You know the drill: you're sitting in your doctor's office. The nurse walks in and straps the blood-pressure cuff around your arm. *Pfff, pfff, pfff,* it tightens, and you feel your heart pounding faster and harder with each squeeze. In fact, just thinking about that cuff squeezing your arm is enough to send your blood pressure soaring. In some cases, blood pressure rises as soon as the doctor enters the room.

It's all because of a medically documented phenomenon known as "White-Coat Syndrome." In a study published in the *American Journal of Hypertension*, French researchers measured the blood pressure of fifty hypertensive patients. They found that blood pressure rose sharply when a patient talked to the doctor, especially when the conversation focused on the patient's medical history of blood pressure and other stressful factors in the patient's life. But measurements dropped when patients read or sat quietly during the exam.

Anticipation coupled with fear initiates the release of key stress hormones such as cortisol and adrenaline. These "fight or flight" hormones constrict the blood vessels, which in turn elevates blood pressure. When you measure your blood pressure at home, you're much more likely to get a more reliable and accurate reading.

That's exactly why I encourage my patients to do home monitoring. The last thing I want them to do is experience that kind of stress and anxiety when they're talking to me about something as important as their health. You can bypass this syndrome by taking your blood pressure at a rehabilitation center, pharmacy, health food store, or even your local gym. Better yet, get your own blood-pressure unit, and have the flexibility of taking your own readings whenever you want, as often as you want.

Another benefit: when my patients conduct home blood-pressure monitoring, they become directly involved with their health in

---

IMPORTANT MEDICAL NOTE: I don't recommend discontinuing *any* prescription drugs you are currently taking without the advice of your physician. Although all the methods presented here are safe, going "cold turkey" on your medication can be quite risky. So, please work with your doctor!

a hands-on way, which promotes a very proactive attitude about their own blood-pressure lowering program. *They* become, in essence, their own doctor. Then all I need to do is nurse them along, giving them suggestions about natural ways to lower their blood pressure so they can reduce their dependence on blood-pressure lowering drugs. I've tried out a lot of blood-pressure monitors over the years and have found the ones that I trust most and are the easiest to use are computer-driven, some of which the American Heart Association has approved. I most prefer the types that quickly and accurately measure your pulse as well.

My only caution is that you don't become so preoccupied with taking your blood pressure that it becomes an obsession. Once you know your own patterns, try to relax about it. Your home kit is always there if you feel the need to check your blood pressure for some reason, like experiencing a little stress or getting more salt intake than usual. Don't make checking your pressure another stressor, or you will end up pouring out stress hormones and elevating the very numbers that you are trying to bring down.

The Story of Peg: A Blood Pressure Dilemma Resolved

I gave a home blood pressure monitor to my mother-in-law, Peg, who suffers from White-Coat Syndrome. When Peg first came to see me for a formal office visit, her blood pressure was up around 170/92. Her blood pressure had been well controlled on medications for years, enough so that she was able to wean down to lower doses. But lately her stress level was rising and her blood pressure was creeping up along with it. She was concerned that she found herself back to juggling her blood pressure, her medications, and their side effects, which were interfering with her quality of life.

For Peg, the continual, dry hacking cough from her ACE inhibitor was creating as much stress as it was trying to relieve.

Overall, she felt fine, but did admit to a little extra fatigue. She tried to disregard her symptoms as "old age" (she's 78, but looks a decade younger), but fear started creeping in. By the time she decided to share her concerns with her daughter, she was losing sleep. And with good reason.

There's a strong history of heart disease in her family. She is one of nine children. Back in the tumultuous sixties, both Peg's father and older brother had suffered sudden cardiac deaths from heart attacks. Although both were on blood-pressure medication, they had felt just fine right up to the moment their heart attacks struck them. Peg's younger brother had recently been admitted to the hospital in congestive heart failure—and he, too, had a long history of high blood pressure, but felt "just fine"—until the morning he couldn't get enough air. Although he pulled through, it took us a while to get his symptoms, medications, and supplements in the right combination so that he felt more like his old self.

Her only sister is also being treated for high blood pressure. But most importantly, Peg thought of her mother who felt fine right up until the day she suffered a stroke. She was younger than Peg is now, yet she did not survive. So it was no wonder that knowing her blood pressure was bouncing around was not reassuring to Peg. And she still had that irritating cough.

I'm sure Peg thought of her own now-distant introduction to cardiology, that day twenty years ago when I first met her. As a young cardiologist in a busy urban hospital practice, I had resuscitated Peg during a cardiac arrest that we speculate was caused by a combination of a heart conduction problem and some cardiac medications. I'm also sure that Peg also recalled her intermittent bouts of heart palpitations, which slightly increased her risk of forming a blood clot.

Her intuition—mixed with good sense and a push from her concerned daughter—now brought her to my office. After a his-

Targeted Nutrients that Lower Blood Pressure

COENZYME Q10: ALL IN A DAY'S WORK. IS THERE ANYTHING THAT COQ10 CAN'T DO? The precise way coQ10 brings down blood pressure is not fully understood. However, research has demonstrated that the membrane stabilizing and antioxidant properties of CoQ10 may help to normalize cell chemistry in blood vessels. Dr. Peter Langsjoen and his colleagues in Tyler, Texas, in 1993 conducted a study of 109 patients with known hypertension treated with 225 mg CoQ10 daily. They found a significant decrease in systolic and diastolic blood pressure. In a 1999 study in India, 120 mg of a water soluble CoQ10 showed substantial blood pressure reduction similar to Dr. Langsjoen's investigation. In Dr. Langsjoen's study, the researchers were able to wean at least 50 percent of their subjects off at least one or two of their anti-hypertensive medications. My clinical experience is similar. Over the last decade, I have been able to slowly reduce at least half the cardiac medications for my patients who were taking the equivalent of 180 to 240 mg CoQ10. And the good news is that when we can reduce some of these drugs, not only do I reduce the cost of medications, but also limit the everyday problems with side effects.

MAGNESIUM, CALCIUM, POTASSIUM: TRIPLE CROWN OF MINERALS. Although I believe that potassium is perhaps the most important mineral in the treatment of high blood pressure, magnesium and calcium are two essential sister minerals. Magnesium depletion has correlated not only with hypertension, but also with diabetes, migraine headaches, and cases of advanced cardiovascular disease. Most researchers believe that maintaining adequate magnesium intake is like taking a medication to lower your blood pressure. Magnesium acts like a calcium channel blocker, preventing blood-vessel spasm that can jack up your blood pressure. As we know that people who take diuretics lose both potassium and magnesium through increased urination, it is absolutely essential that these minerals be replaced if you're taking a "water pill" of some kind. Including magnesium in your diet will usually give you more energy, less muscle cramping, and a better sense of well-being, but the increase in magnesium alone will also nudge those blood pressure numbers on a downward course. It's known that people with low calcium are more prone to increased blood pressure. Researchers have suggested that supplemental calcium can support blood pressure because of its synergistic relationship with potassium and magnesium.

OMEGA-3 FATTY ACIDS. Another vital nutrient complex for lowering blood pressure (both systolic and diastolic) are the omega-3 fatty acids found in certain fish, fish oils, and flaxseed. In addition to easing hypertension, these "good fats" help lower LDL "bad" cholesterol and triglycerides and reduce platelet stickiness and fibrinogen levels. Preventing blood clotting is a key preventive strategy in preventing coronary artery disease and heart attack. Eating one or two 4-ounce cold-water fish servings a week will have a favorable impact on your blood pressure. Keep in mind, though, that some fish and even fish oils can be toxic with PCBs or heavy metals such as mercury. The healthiest fish include migratory Atlantic or Pacific salmon, deep water halibut, and Atlantic cod. I do not recommend eating tuna or swordfish more than once every three months because of the risk of high mercury content in these bigger fish. I also recommend that you stay away from farm-raised fish, if possible.

Another option is flaxseed oil, which is also rich in alpha linolenic acid. Try drizzling a teaspoon over your salad each day. Look for organic, cold expeller-pressed brands in the refrigerated section of your health food store.

The Phytoestrogen Shake also has enough alpha linolenic acid to have a favorable effect on your blood pressure. Grind up two tablespoons of organic flaxseed and mix with 8 ounces of soy milk. Both can be purchased in any health food store.

HAWTHORN BERRY ROUNDS OUT YOUR LINEUP OF BLOOD PRESSURE-lowering supplements. This herb has been used medicinally for centuries and has become increasingly popular as a preventive tool and remedy for cardiac conditions over the last one hundred years. Studies show that hawthorn increases blood flow in smaller vessels. It acts much like an ACE inhibitor, preventing production of angiotensin 2, a powerful blood vessel constrictor responsible for increasing blood pressure. Hawthorn also helps to ease chest pain, and relieve symptoms of congestive heart failure. I usually recommend 500 mg two to three times a day.

GARLIC. IT'S AMAZING HOW MANY NUTRIENTS ARE packed into a single clove of garlic: 33 sulfur compounds, 17 amino acids, antioxidants such as germanium and selenium, and multiple vitamins and minerals. These beneficial chemical compounds, including a substance called *allicin*, give garlic its unmistakable odor as well as a pharmacological edge in cardiovascular prevention. Think of this herb as a virtual multivitamin—not only is it full of nutrients, it's useful for a host of ailments. Garlic's medicinal benefits include enhancing blood thinning (to prevent blood clots), lowering blood pressure, and reducing cholesterol and triglyceride levels.

Since this herb's chemistry is so complex, researchers aren't sure how it helps lower blood pressure, but my patients and I have been pleased with the results. Garlic's antihypertensive effect may be related to its antioxidant and sulfur content. But some very recent studies suggest that garlic lowers blood pressure by increasing the dilation of blood vessels via an ACE-inhibiting effect similar to the action of hawthorn and grapeseed. Although evidence to date indicates that raw, cold-aged garlic offers the greatest medicinal value, studies have demonstrated that lightly cooked garlic also is effective. The highest quality is grown organically (check the organic food section of your grocery store or health food stores). If you choose to take supplements instead, I recommend those with high allicin content. Rarely, some people are allergic to garlic and others may experience some stomach or intestinal upset. If garlic breath is a problem, try chewing fresh parsley, rosemary, or fennel. Freshly squeezed lemon, a piece of grapefruit, or orange peel may also assuage garlic's pungent odor. Don't worry, these minor drawbacks are worth the results you'll get.

VITAMIN C. IN A 1999 ISSUE OF *LANCET*, a small study showed that 500 mg of vitamin C daily showed mild blood pressure lowering.

L-ARGININE HELPS TO PRODUCE NITRIC OXIDE in blood vessels, resulting in increased blood flow and lowering of blood pressure.

---

tory and physical, we agreed to an echocardiogram. Peg's heart was not enlarged from her blood pressure, and her chambers all contracted evenly and with great energy. Her heart was pumping as one of a healthy adult, one who could be much younger. Luckily, I was able to reassure her that her heart checked out fine.

I advised Peg to follow my combination plan to lower her blood pressure: 400 mg magnesium and 1,000 mg calcium in divided doses after meals, and 60 mg CoQ10 three times daily. In addition, I asked her to monitor her blood pressure two to three times a day (the best times are before breakfast and dinner) for the first week to give her a sense of her own patterns. I also had her discontinue her ACE inhibitor medication because of her cough. Her weight was perfect for her age, but we did encourage her to use relaxation tapes and attend to her prayer life to help assuage her psychological stressors.

When I checked in with Peg two weeks later, her blood pressure readings were back in the normal range, around 138/88. She is now comforted by the fact that she can accurately monitor her own blood pressure at home. She no longer feels that she has to run to a doctor's office every time she gets worried about her blood pressure. That's one major life stressor gone!

If her blood pressure pops up with the anxiety of an office visit, Peg can pull out a record of her home readings to give her doctor a more accurate profile of her blood pressure in her usual routine, and how it responds to her medication. She can also recheck it anytime she is having a little stress. Peg can track those activities that tend to elevate her blood pressure—like going to the dentist or having her car repaired. If she finds that doubling up on appointments tends to bump up her blood pressure, she can schedule herself so that she is not doing both on the same day. That's what I mean about really becoming your own doctor.

Like many of my patients, Peg has had excellent success with a natural blood-pressure-lowering/heart health program that includes the four pillars: (1) a modified Mediterranean diet, (2) daily exercise, (3) targeted nutritional supplements, and (4) reduction of stress and tension.

Controllable Risk Factors for High Blood Pressure

Lower your blood pressure, and you'll put a huge dent in your overall risk for major heart attack or stroke. Even so-called uncontrollable factors, such as age, genetics, and poor general health can be overcome by following my guidelines for diet and lifestyle. Despite your age or current health condition, I can help you lower your blood pressure and improve your heart health by addressing the following issues:

POOR DIET—high in animal protein and animal saturated fats (i.e., cholesterol). Such a diet contributes to clogged or hardened arteries, forcing your heart to pump harder to push blood through. Of all the diets out there, I prefer a modified Mediterranean diet, which is high in fiber and rich in calcium, magnesium, and potassium—three crucial minerals for heart health and blood pressure—and cold-water fish, tofu, soy, and nuts.

TOO MUCH SALT—High sodium levels are hidden in processed foods, canned vegetables, powdered soups and dips, diet soft drinks, and preserved meats such as bacon and sausage. A single dill pickle can contain as much as 1,000 mg of salt! Keep your daily intake within the range of 2,000 to 3,000 mg. For optimal health, use trace-mineral-rich sea salt rather than plain overprocessed table salt.

EXCESS WEIGHT AND SEDENTARY LIFESTYLE—In one study, three out of four patients with hypertension achieved normal blood pressure with no drug therapy after losing a specific amount of weight. Losing even 10 percent of your body weight can have a significant effect on lowering your blood pressure. An easy way to achieve this is to walk between one and two miles every day. A study by the National Institutes of Health revealed that moderate physical activity such as this could save the lives of more than 150,000 people each year.

UNRESOLVED ANGER, HIGH-STRESS LIFESTYLE, AND "WORKAHOLISM"—all can contribute to high blood pressure. I have helped many of my patients lower their blood pressure and heal their hearts by developing an emotional support system. There are many techniques to achieve this, including mental imagery, meditation, prayer, and biofeedback.

SMOKING—is one of the most devastating risk factors. Hypertensive smokers are three times more likely than nonsmokers to suffer strokes, and twice as likely to suffer a heart attack. Smoking constricts your blood vessels. Please stop.

HEAVY DRINKING—Consuming more than one or two alcoholic

beverages per day increases blood pressure by an average of 10 mm/Hg. I recommend no more than one drink or one 6-ounce glass of wine per day for women.

INSULIN RESISTANCE—as discussed in Chapter 3, insulin resistance is a complex of factors resulting from eating too many refined sugars and starches (carbohydrates), which leads to excess insulin production. Eventually, your cellular receptors shut down, preventing glucose—your body's chief energy source—from entering the cells. This is why I do not recommend popular diets that promote low fat and high carbohydrates—they are simply adding fuel to the fire!

OVERRELIANCE ON ANTI-INFLAMMATORY MEDICATIONS—such as ibuprofen (Motrin, Advil, etc.) and naproxen (Aleve), which are widely taken for mild-to-moderate pain of all types, from headaches to arthritis. Check the label—most include a warning that patients with hypertension should consult their physicians before taking such medications. Even if your blood pressure is normal, overuse of these medications can contribute to a kidney problem, especially in those over the age of sixty.

Studies suggest that ibuprofen and naproxen push up blood pressure by an average of 3.5 mm/Hg to 10 mm/Hg. Fortunately, aspirin appears to have little or no effect on blood pressure or salt retention. Antihistamines and other over-the-counter cold remedies can also contribute to high blood pressure. Stay away from them if you can.

Take the Fast Track to Lower Blood Pressure

Now it's time to put it all together into your own personalized plan. To help you take things step by step, I've developed a Four-Week Plan to get you started. At the end of four weeks, you should be well on your way to lowering your blood pressure, experiencing more energy, and feeling really good about your health.

Keep in mind that the National Heart, Lung and Blood Institute's guidelines for lowering blood pressure now recommend eliminating the above risk factors and adding lifestyle changes such as these for a period of six months to one year before turning to medication. If your blood pressure is higher than 160/100, or if you have cardiovascular disease or signs of organ damage, you must see your physician and go on blood pressure medication immediately.

WEEK 1: There's no better time to get acquainted with my modified Mediterranean diet, and start eating some of these foods. (See Chapter 4, "Nutritional Healing: Eat the Heart-Healthy Way.") It's especially important to eat foods rich in potassium, calcium, and magnesium, three key minerals for keeping your blood pressure in the normal range. Try to pick at least five foods each day from the chart (see page 83). And be sure to crush a clove or two of garlic into your dinner every day. Fresh is best, as cooking rapidly destroys the active ingredients. You can also take garlic in tablet form.

You needn't starve yourself on a diet of brown rice, fruits, and vegetables. For example, one morning you may have All-Bran cereal and figs, which are high in potassium. For lunch, you may choose to eat an herb omelet. For dinner, have some salmon and soy or lima beans, which are also high in potassium.

By following my straightforward eating plan, you'll not only have a variety of tasty, nutritious foods from which to choose, you'll also get the foods you need to regulate your blood pressure and start those numbers on a downward course.

WEEK 2: Once you're on my eating plan, take it a step further and make some lifestyle changes. Start walking fifteen to thirty minutes every day. Exercise is critical to lowering your blood pressure and keeping it low (see Chapter 6, "Get Moving! Exercise Can Save Your

Life"). The more weight you carry, the harder your heart has to work. If you stick with exercise you will lose weight and, better yet, your lean body mass—an even better gauge of healthy weight—will improve. At the same time take a good hard look at the high blood pressure risk factors. Pick out one or two at a time and make a change. For example, reduce your intake of alcohol. Minimal to no alcohol is best during this period. If you must have a drink, limit it to one a day. And by all means quit smoking if you haven't already!

WEEK 3: You'll notice how much better you're already feeling this week now that you're "cleaning up your act." This week, it's time to step up the program a bit more by including some targeted nutritional supplements.

Here is my optimal daily nutrient program for blood-pressure lowering:

coenzyme Q10—180 to 240 mg

vitamin C—500 mg

calcium—1,000 mg

magnesium—400 mg

L-arginine—1 to 2 grams

hawthorn berry—up to 1,500 mg

grapeseed extract—300 mg

garlic—one small clove of garlic or one capsule

omega-3 essential fatty acids (fish oil)—1 to 2 grams daily or eat fresh fish two times a week

Generous amounts of potassium in the diet—fresh fruits such as bananas, oranges, and raisins are best.

WEEK 4: By this week, your blood pressure numbers should be heading down. So focus on relaxing this week—literally. Turn off the phone and TV. Sit quietly and listen to some classical music, meditate, read an inspirational text, do yoga or tai chi, pray, write in your journal, walk the dog, or do some deep-breathing exercises. Or, you can just sit silently for several minutes each day. Relaxation is an often overlooked tool that, when combined with the other three steps of my program, can have as potent an effect on your blood pressure as some drugs. Many of my patients have lowered their blood pressure by doing one or several of these activities. They also have found that they begin to sleep better, experience less anxiety and stress, and have more joy in their lives.

Oftentimes insomnia, excess anxiety, and fear of heart disease resulting from palpatations or heart rate increases with hot flashes, may cause your blood pressure to soar. We will now look into how a change in a women's hormonal status may affect her quality of life.

Solving the Riddle of Hypertension in African American Women

HIGH BLOOD PRESSURE PLAYS A SIGNIFICANT ROLE in approximately 750,000 deaths per year in the United States. And when it comes to African American women, the risk is even greater. A November 1, 1999 issue of the *Journal of the American College of Cardiology* attributed hypertension in minorities primarily to women having increased body mass and African American ethnicity. And, in women with this profile, high blood pressure was linked with a higher incidence of hypertensive heart failure.

RESEARCH STATISTICS ESTIMATE THAT approximately one-third of both black women and men suffer from high blood pressure, and about 20 percent of deaths in the black population occur as a result of complications of high blood pressure. This is *double* the risk that Caucasians face. Why is there such a disparity between those of African descent and their Caucasian counterparts?

LOOKING AT THE INCIDENCE OF HIGH BLOOD PRESSURE in Africans as well as people of African descent in the Caribbean and the United States, one is struck by the difference between those living in city environments and those residing on their native continent. There's a much higher prevalence of hypertension among U.S. urban blacks and a much lower one among rural Nigerians. In general, urban groups face more risk factors as part of the environment: stress and tension from overcrowding, noise and air pollutants, a high-salt diet, and more physical inactivity leading to obesity. Average body mass index (BMI), a measure of weight relative to height, has increased for Caribbean people as well as urban blacks. So has the average salt intake. Urban African Americans also get less exercise than, for example, the Intuits of Africa, a primarily nomadic group. (See Appendix D for an illustration.)

OTHERS SUGGEST THAT THE MYSTERY OF HIGH BLOOD PRESSURE in African Americans can be solved by examining the amount of a key blood protein called *albumin*. Manufactured by the liver, albumin helps regulate water distribution in the bloodstream and prevents fluid from leaking out of the cells into the tissues. Kenneth Seaton, PhD, DSc, has studied the impact of albumin on health and longevity for many years. In his research, he notes that albumin is less concentrated in black people. According to Seaton, healthy natives in the rural West African nation of Nigeria have average albumin levels of 48 grams per liter (g/L), and they have low blood pressure. The mean albumin level for Americans is 43 g/L, and it is even lower for African Americans at 39.7 g/L.

ALBUMIN HAS A RECIPROCAL RELATIONSHIP WITH *SERUM GLOBULIN*, a blood protein that increases with any inflammatory condition, such as infection, parasites, or allergies. The lower the albumin concentration, the higher the globulins in blood plasma. Low albumin levels mean higher inflammation, stickier platelets, and a loss of elasticity in blood vessel walls. Dr. Seaton suggests that this blood profile can lead to hypertension by rendering arteries "stiffer" and blood "thicker." These alterations also can cause a shift in the kidney's hormonal cascade that mediates blood pressure. Seaton believes this imbalance is a major contributing factor to disproportionate rates of African American hypertension. Low albumin levels have also been associated with respiratory problems, allergies, and poor hygiene. But once reestablished at higher levels, albumin diffuses through the kidneys, regulating its hormonal response and bringing blood pressure back down to safe levels.

LIVING UNDER NATURAL, RURAL CONDITIONS, NATIVE TRIBES like the Intuits of Africa have excellent hygiene; they get full body exposure to healthy sunlight and clean air as well as spending ample time swimming in unpolluted rivers and ponds. They also use natural "plant soaps." The health-promoting aspects of this lifestyle are exemplified by their high albumin profiles and low blood pressure throughout life. Many Intuits also participate in more "regular exercise" than their American counterparts.

ALL TOO OFTEN, STANDARD PHARMACOLOGICAL DRUGS (with the exception of diuretics, which help reduce blood volume) alone fail to do the job. Treating high blood pressure in African American women requires a multidisciplinary approach that considers risk factors such as stress, immune response, body configuration, salt intake, and serum albumin levels. As do women of all ethnic backgrounds, African American women need to carefully assess their risk profile for high blood pressure and act accordingly. Much research suggests that weight control, minimizing salt intake and lowering body mass index (BMI) are very important. High-risk women of all ethnic groups should also be mindful of raising their albumin levels by reducing stress on the immune system.

ONE WAY TO INCREASE LEVELS OF ALBUMIN IS TO USE A VIGILANT standard of personal hygiene. Seaton's premise is that we can all increase our albumin levels by cleaning the fingernails (the cuticles and under the nail), hands, front of the nasal passageway, nose, and eyes. He also recommends dipping the face in salty water containing special solutions to cleanse the mucous membranes.

KEEPING THE FINGERNAILS, FACE, EYES, EARS, AND NOSE CLEANER will results in less "self-inoculation" from bacteria present on and in our own bodies. This often leads to fewer respiratory infections, less inflammation, and a major reduction in asthma symptoms. All this helps to limit stress on the immune system, which then rebounds to boost albumin and lower globulin reserves. My family uses Seaton's "high performance" hygiene system to boost our own immune systems and intercept those miserable asthma attacks.

WHATEVER YOUR ETHNIC ROOTS, REMEMBER: The higher your albumin levels, the lower your blood pressure. And if you're a woman or man, of any cultural background, who suffers a lot of upper respiratory problems along with high blood pressure, then this approach can help you, too.

SECTION IV

Hormones, Menopause, and Your Heart

CHAPTER ELEVEN

The HRT Dilemma: Should You Take Hormone Replacement Therapy?

"Should I take hormone replacement therapy?" Few women approaching menopause have not asked themselves that question—or had it suggested to them by their physician. You've probably heard about the "upside" of estrogen: how it can protect you from osteoporosis, slash your risk of heart disease, and even stave off Alzheimer's; how it can restore your libido and wipe out hot flashes; turn your "fuzzy" brain into clear-thinking; eliminate night sweats; and make you feel like "you" again.

You've probably also heard about the downside: the increased risk of endometrial cancer from taking estrogen alone; the increasing risk of breast cancer from taking estrogen and progesterone for more than five years; and more recently, studies showing that the addition of progesterone to estrogen therapy does *not* reduce the risk of breast cancer and that the risk may actually *increase* over time. Also, new research is revealing that synthetic progesterone alone may increase the risk of breast cancer.

What's a woman to do?

First, know that every woman is a unique blend of risk factors when it comes to cardiac, bone, and breast health—all tempered by your individual response to perimenopause. So, what works for your sister, friend, or coworker may *not* work for you. In this "Hormones, Menopause, and Your Heart" section, I will lay out the risks and benefits of various approaches, give you real-world case studies of women who have grappled with these issues, and show you some of the pitfalls along the way.

Second, you must *educate yourself.* Don't rely on the daily news, the morning TV shows, or even your physician to have all the answers. Hormone replacement therapy (HRT) is too complex, and each woman's risk profile so distinctive, that no doctor can possibly sort it all out for you in the space of a fifteen-minute office visit. In addition, there is no standardized algorithm—a reliable clinical model for determining the best approach—available for HRT.

Finally, know that ultimately, the HRT decision will be *your choice.* I want you to make it wisely. As you will see, the decision whether to take HRT has implications not only for your heart but also for your bones, brain, and quality of life during the time surrounding menopause. Despite estrogen's many salutary effects, I have grown increasingly conservative on this subject as the evidence against many forms of synthetic HRT continues to mount. As new studies come out, recommendations for HRT must be continuously reevaluated and fine-tuned. The whole thing is like one of those "I've got good news and bad news" games we used to play when we were kids:

GOOD NEWS: High circulating levels of estrogen protect women from heart disease and osteoporosis for the first two-thirds of life.

BAD NEWS: When the estrogen levels fall off around menopause, the incidence of heart disease increases fourfold.

GOOD NEWS: Taking supplemental estrogen can restore the benefits of natural estrogen, protecting your heart and bones and reducing menopausal symptoms.

BAD NEWS: Taking supplemental estrogen can increase your risk of endometrial cancer.

GOOD NEWS: Adding progesterone to your estrogen can prevent endometrial cancer.

BAD NEWS: The added progesterone dampens the beneficial effects of estrogen on your cardiovascular system. Of even greater concern, when given in synthetic form, progesterone also increases your risk of breast cancer. And the longer you take it, the more estrogen alone increases your risk of breast cancer.

GOOD NEWS: There are alternatives to these potent synthetic hormones.

Walking the HRT Tightrope:
Balancing Out Your Risks and Needs

No doubt about it: HRT is a controversial topic. Physicians, women's health advocates, alternative health practitioners, and women of all ages are bombarded with information, much of it contradictory or confusing. The essential question can be stated simply: Should most women take estrogen replacement therapy (ERT) or hormone replacement therapy (HRT) at menopause as a matter of course, the same way they might take vitamin supplements, watch their weight, and do regular exercise? Or, because of the risks of ERT/HRT and because menopause is a natural phase of life, should women avoid hormone therapy unless they have a strong family history of heart disease or osteoporosis?

I wish I could give you a simple answer, but in practice, the pros and cons are not clear cut. While much research to date indicates that the cardioprotective benefits of ERT and HRT may outweigh the risks of cancer for many women, the wholesale prescription of hormone replacement therapy—especially potent prescription medications such as Premarin and Provera—does *not,* in my view, constitute a prudent or safe approach. The risks of such hormones were well-delineated in a large study from the National Cancer Institute (NCI) and published in the *Journal of the American Medical Association* in January 2000. The study of 48,355 women from 1980 through 1995 showed a 40 percent increase in breast cancer in those women on both estrogen and progestin compared with those who were not on hormone replacement. (Interestingly, overweight women did not appear to be at higher risk.)

Millions of prescriptions are written every year for Premarin, one of the most prescribed hormones in America. Such hormone replacement drugs have become so widely used that their use is becoming casually accepted by doctors and patients alike, seen by many as necessary and benign, a remedy that should obviously be used.

Why, in light of evidence that estrogen can promote breast cancer, have doctors continued to prescribe it and women continued to demand it? Well, since ERT and HRT began, more than thirty major research studies have assessed the effectiveness of various regimens and monitored their attendant risks. By 1980 these studies began to consistently suggest some unexpected results: *The incidence of heart disease in postmenopausal women who received ERT and HRT appeared to be lower than in women who did not receive hormones.* It is now generally agreed that estrogens can assuage menopausal symptoms, reduce bone fractures, and probably reduce the risk of heart disease, most likely by restoring the beneficial effects of naturally produced estrogen.

Before we go any further, I want to make it clear that cardioprotection is *not* the medical use for which ERT/HRT was developed. In fact, the cardiovascular protective benefits of hormone replacement therapy were discovered by accident.

Even though there is also strong evidence that HRT protects women against heart disease, it is important to understand that the Food and Drug Administration (FDA) has *not* approved hormone replacement therapy for this use. The agency has approved ERT/HRT *only for the relief of menopausal symptoms*, such as hot flashes, fuzzy thinking, heart palpitations, and insomnia. No clear data exists proving that conventional ERT/HRT saves lives overall. And there is no clinical model which convincingly demonstrates that hormone therapy is effective for preventing heart disease in all or even the majority of women.

As a result, the FDA has not viewed the studies on ERT/HRT's reduction of heart disease as compelling enough to approve the therapy for that purpose. This does not mean that the treatment should not, or cannot, be used to reduce your heart disease risk. Drugs are frequently prescribed without FDA approval for uses other than the ones for which they have been approved. (This is known as "off-label" use). It does mean that any woman who considers HRT to prevent heart disease must bear this fact in mind.

So when a new reason to use the drug surfaces, the tendency to prescribe it becomes even greater. This has led to a powerful bias in favor of HRT among medical practitioners. All too often, physicians (and women as well) easily accept that it is the best or even the only choice. In most cases, this outlook springs from a mindset which is simply to medicate rather than investigate underlying causes or work toward helping the woman prevent those problems using lifestyle strategies such as diet or exercise.

We need many more studies to answer a whole range of questions: How long should women take ERT/HRT? What impact does a woman's age have upon the therapy's effectiveness and risk? What are the advantages of using natural forms of estrogen and progesterone instead of synthetics? The truth is that none of these therapies have been used or studied long enough to know for sure.

In many instances, the doctor (or the patient) is unfamiliar with many of the more natural alternatives to prescription hormones which can yield equivalent benefits without the risks. In others, the benefits of drug treatment have been heavily marketed as a sort of chemical fountain of youth by the pharmaceutical companies that manufacture them. Even the news media often base their reporting on accounts generated by publicity-hungry medical journals, which often send out press releases in advance of peer-reviewed research.

Much of what women hear and read about hormone replacement therapy is shaped by these and other biases, and the tragedy is that by believing HRT is the "right" answer for everyone, some women suffer needlessly from its side effects. As with many prescription drugs, sometimes the side effects are worse than the original symptoms. Five to 10 percent of the women who take estrogen report bloating, headache, breast tenderness, and diarrhea; and weight gain, irritability, and depression with synthetic progesterone.

It all comes down to this: *quality of life issues are the most important factors in making the HRT decision.* Remember, every woman— and this includes *you*—has a unique health profile and needs to choose an approach which fits her risk level and symptoms. And as you evaluate and balance out all of your options, be aware that your choices are not limited to taking HRT or doing nothing.

I advocate *what works* for each individual. Because of the possible protective effects of conventional HRT, *I believe that it is appropriate as a heart-disease preventive for certain high-risk women and can be a helpful adjunct treatment for women who already have coronary artery disease,* particularly those with major risk factors such as increased Lp(a)—a deadly form of cholesterol—or high fibrinogen. Nor would I rule it out for some women who have menopausal symptoms that create an unsatisfactory quality of life.

But for many other women, including those who already take conventional HRT, I have often found that natural (bioidentical) estrogen and/or progesterone preparations are a better choice. If they start with or switch to the milder natural products, sometimes they will find that these preparations relieve their menopause symptoms while still providing some of the possible cardioprotective benefits of prescription hormones. In other women, simply adding nutritional supplements and foods with phytoestrogens provides all the estrogenic activity they need while balancing menopausal symptoms with protection against heart disease and osteoporosis.

The route you take will depend upon your risk profile for heart disease, osteoporosis, and cancer and, most important for some, the wild card—your menopausal symptoms. The aim is to match your level of heart disease risk with preventive benefits and to balance the risks of the hormone therapy (such as increased risk of breast cancer) against your risk of heart disease. The higher your cardiac risk, the greater the risk you may be willing to assume from hormone therapy. If your symptoms are extreme and truly diminish your quality of life, you may opt for relief from conventional or natural HRT, whether or not it matches your risk for heart disease.

Every woman must ultimately "choose her risks" in deciding whether or not to take hormones and, if so, in what form to take them. Any form of HRT will raise a woman's breast cancer risk, however slightly. However, based on available evidence to date, I believe that short-term use (one to two years) for relief of menopausal symptoms should *not* be influenced by fear of cancer.

A woman who has had a hysterectomy, however, should avoid combined use of estrogen and synthetic progestins. I also do not recommend estrogen replacement for women at high risk for breast cancer.

As you can see, the hormone decision is one that every woman must make carefully, with unbiased information, and *it is not a decision that should be made in a fifteen-minute office visit.* Doctors frequently make choices about treatment based on standardized decision pathways (algorithms) modeled upon research and decades of clinical data in which the physician follows a series of questions and answers about a patient's symptoms and condition, which leads to a consistent answer: prescribe this drug or that treatment. The great dilemma with hormone replacement therapy in general, and for prevention of heart disease in particular, is that there is no reliable clinical model for making this decision. Every woman must be evaluated as an individual and anyone, physician or otherwise, who attempts to force a standardized decision upon a woman is doing her a great disservice—and perhaps even putting her in harm's way.

Your Hormones: The Light Side, the Dark Side

Your hormones are prime examples of the mysterious elegance of the human body—how so many intricate processes work as well as they do staggers the imagination. At the most basic physical level, hormones are what differentiate women from men, and this distinction is especially true when it comes to heart disease risk.

Women have "built-in protection" against heart disease through the cyclic release of natural estrogens and progesterone during a woman's menstrual cycle. Problems may arise if these protective hormones diminish due to natural or surgically-induced (hysterectomy) menopause. A double whammy for heart disease risk happens when a woman with decreased protective hormones also has several risk factors for heart disease. The time may come when you will have to decide whether to opt for hormone replacement therapy—not only to quell heart disease, but other diseases as well. Hormone replacement therapy, or HRT, does not come without its own risks. But knowledge is power—and I will arm you with as much information as possible about hormones and your heart so you will be able to make informed choices about your own health.

The Brighter Side of Estrogen

The history of estrogen use in medical therapy has been a roller-coaster ride of tremendous promise followed by deep dives of disappointment as new risks and side effects come to light. Some of estrogen's most significant actions in reducing the risk of heart disease stem from its direct effects on the heart and its blood vessels as well as the brain. We know that the action of estrogen is critical to healthy functioning in these organs by the presence of estrogen receptors in the aorta, heart, and brain tissues.

Researchers have learned over the years that estrogen keeps a woman's overall cholesterol level lower than a man's, reduces her LDL "bad" cholesterol, and raises levels of protective HDL cholesterol. In postmenopausal women, estrogen replacement therapy lowers LDL and raises HDL by 10 to 15 percent, for a reduction of 40 to 50 percent in the overall risk of heart disease. Estrogen also prevents oxidation of LDL cholesterol—an important distinction, because, as previously mentioned, the real danger isn't just how high your LDL level is, but whether or not that LDL is *oxidized*; it is only when LDL has gone through this decomposition process that it begins to form the substrate for arterial plaque.

Estrogen also lowers a dangerous type of cholesterol called lipoprotein(a) or Lp(a). As we discussed in Chapter 3, elevated Lp(a) is associated with an increased risk of premature coronary artery disease (CAD) in men and women. Like overall cholesterol and harmful LDL cholesterol, Lp(a) increases after your estrogen production falls at menopause.

Estrogen also appears to improve your body's ability to dissolve blood clots by breaking down strands of fibrin which hold them together. In the process, this may help to avoid the formation of artery-clogging cholesterol plaques and prevent strokes.

More of Estrogen's Positive Effects
on Your Cardiovascular System

ESTROGEN HELPS TO KEEP YOUR BLOOD VESSELS ELASTIC AND FLEXIBLE.
Your arteries have muscular walls capable of widening and narrowing the central channel, or lumen, through which blood flows. Arteries are constantly dilating (widening) or constricting (narrowing) their lumen diameter in order to regulate blood pressure, volume of blood flow, and other critical factors.

While your arteries need to both dilate and constrict in order to function properly, heart disease, particularly coronary artery disease (CAD), usually involves arterial *constriction* which is too frequent; too great; lasts too long; occurs too strongly in the form of a spasm; or occurs inappropriately, when the artery should actually be dilating to allow increased blood flow. Research indicates that most of estrogen's actions on the cardiovascular system help the arteries to dilate, and that overall, estrogen tends to increase blood flow. This may be related to estrogen's powerful action on the endothelium, the innermost lining of the arteries that forms the smooth, slippery surface against which blood flows.

The endothelium is one cell layer thick, a veneer so thin that it can be seen only under a microscope, but its cells exert a powerful influence on the arteries. These cells release substances called *factors* which cause the smooth muscle walls of the artery to relax, so the vessel can dilate and blood flow increase. The most important of these is called *endothelial cell releasing factor,* or EDRF. Estrogen stimulates endothelial cells to release EDRF.

Without adequate EDRF activity, arterial walls fail to dilate, and blood flow to the heart is compromised. Arteries that are clogged with plaques do not dilate normally, most likely due to some disturbance in the release of EDRF. Studies have shown that estrogen enhances EDRF dilation in the coronary arteries of post-menopausal women with atherosclerosis.

As a result of this key role in protecting and enhancing the endothelial cells that line your arteries, I call estrogen "endothe-lial-cell friendly." L-arginine, an amino acid I frequently recom-mend for chest pain, coronary artery spasm, and cholesterol low-ering, works in a similar way. Antioxidants such as vitamin E and N-acetylcysteine also positively affect EDRF as well as the miner-als magnesium and selenium.

ESTROGEN PROTECTS THE DELICATE, THIN ENDOTHELIAL LAYER FROM INJURY. This is a critical function, because the plaques which block arteries often begin with injuries to the endothelium. Such dam-age can be initiated by high LDL cholesterol, elevated blood sugar and insulin, high blood pressure, and toxic chemicals which enter the bloodstream from smoking.

ESTROGEN DECREASES THE LEVEL OF BLOOD SUGAR, which reduces the damage that elevated blood sugar can do to the endothelium. It appears to do this without increasing the level of insulin in the blood, possibly because it prevents the breakdown of insulin. This is important because along with diabetes, one of the causes of CAD is the prediabetic condition called insulin resistance (see Chapter 2). Estrogen's ability to reduce blood sugar without increasing the blood level of insulin helps to prevent this cycle of damage.

ESTROGEN INCREASES BLOOD FLOW IN VARIOUS ORGANS AND REGIONS OF THE BODY, including the thyroid, breast tissue, hands, and forearms. Studies suggest that, either directly or indirectly, estrogen increases the flow of blood through the muscular tissue of the heart and causes the coronary arteries to dilate, which in turn augments blood flow and oxygen delivery to the heart muscle. Estrogen also acts as a natural calcium channel blocker, further helping to keep the arteries dilated.

IN WOMEN WITH CORONARY ARTERY DISEASE, ESTROGEN TREATMENT HAS BEEN ASSOCIATED WITH A SLOWING OF THE ONSET OF ISCHEMIA—diminished blood flow to the heart muscle caused by blocked coronary arteries, which can lead to symptoms of angina.

ESTROGEN IS AN ANTIOXIDANT, protecting your cells from the byproducts of the breakdown of oxygen molecules. Just as rust damages and "ages" iron, over time cellular oxidation "rusts out" or damages tissues at the cellular level and is one of the causes of age-related health problems, including atherosclerosis and even aging itself. New research also shows that topical estrogen may delay aging of the skin.

Even endothelial cells themselves, along with many other cell types in the arteries and bloodstream, produce free radicals which may damage cells and create the initial injury that eventually becomes an arterial plaque. These free radicals also inactivate EDRF before it is able to dilate the artery. Estrogen counteracts these effects: it protects the endothelial cells from oxidative damage and preserves the functioning of EDRF.

But What Is "Natural" Estrogen?

"Natural" estrogen refers to the sex hormones that have the same molecular structure as those derived from or made by the human body. There are only three forms of estrogen which are "natural" or native to a woman's body: estrone (E1), estradiol (E2), and estriol (E3). In terms of potency, estradiol (E2) is the strongest and estriol (E3) the weakest. When estrogen replacement is delivered in any of these forms, it is considered *natural* estrogen replacement therapy.

Some postmenopausal women in effect make their own hormone "therapy." A woman's body continues to produce estrone in her adrenal glands and fat cells. Estrone is then converted into estradiol, which can supply estrogen-dependent tissues, such as the brain, to help maintain mental clarity and emotional stability. But it also stimulates cell growth in the breast and uterus and may be a contributing factor to the higher incidence of breast cancer in *some* overweight women.

Other women produce more estradiol than can be balanced by their progesterone levels. They become what is called *estrogen dominant*, a condition characterized by headache, fatigue, irritability, bloating, and breast tenderness. Such women may also wish to find a way to rebalance their progesterone-to-estradiol ratios and eliminate these quality-of-life issues.

In contrast, women who are naturally slender or who have kept their weight down and maintained their lean body mass through exercise may be producing very little estrone in their fat cells. This leads to low levels of estradiol circulating in the body. In such cases, a woman's tissues may be estrogen-starved. Since estrogen performs approximately four hundred known functions in a woman's body, the effects of its precipitous decline in some women can prove highly disruptive to their quality of life, upsetting their physical and emotional balance. This situation requires a different sort of approach.

Estrogen can be taken by such women in a form which exactly matches their own natural estrogens—from botanical sources such as soy and Mexican wild yam (*Dioscorea composita*). A more accurate term for these botanical estrogens is *bioidentical*, indicating an exact match with your own native hormones. However, the raw botanical material is natural but the plants' biochemicals do *not* naturally match human forms of estrogen. Instead, the plant precursors must be carefully treated in a laboratory to create an exact match for the human body's own hormones and a perfect fit for the body's estrogen receptors.

These bioidentical estrogens are available in delivery systems which can provide just one hormone (estradiol), two hormones ("biest" preparations including estrone and estradiol), or three hormones ("triest" preparations including estradiol, estrone, and estriol).

Estradiol is available by prescription as tablets, (i.e., Estrace), patches (i.e., Climara or Estraderm), or a cream. Biest and triest preparations must be made to order by a compounding pharmacy and can only be obtained by prescription. A common starter preparation is estriol 80 percent, estrone 10 percent, and estradiol 10 percent ("triest"). One of the advantages of topical estrogen is that this form bypasses the liver and does not stimulate an increase in triglycerides sometimes seen with oral estrogens. Oral estrogens also increase the risk of gallstones and occasionally may increase blood pressure. Oral estrogens also suppress production of the immune factor IgF-1 in the liver, a protein that carries out many of the important functions of growth hormone. Topical estrogens are not associated with such side effects and have more of an antioxidant effect as well.

How Does "Natural" Compare with "Synthetic"?
XENOESTROGENS: A MIXED BAG

Xenoestrogens are hormones not naturally found in the human body, some of which may be synthetic. This category includes conjugated equine estrogens (CEE)—Premarin, which is derived from the urine of pregnant mares. It also includes Cenestin, which is derived from a plant source and contains a mixture of nine estrogens. This term also encompasses the newer group of *selective estrogen receptor modulators*, or SERMs.

Conjugated estrogens refer to a mixture of different forms of estrogen that are present in a single preparation. Conjugated estrogens—such as Premarin, the best known form; and Cenestin, used for short-term treatment of menopause symptoms such as hot flashes—are *derived* from natural sources but are not *considered* "natural" estrogens because they contain numerous other forms of estrogen which have no natural place in the human body and whose fate within the body is still uncertain. No one is entirely sure what happens to the other estrogens that don't find a match with the body's receptors. Neither the plant precursors for Cenestin nor the salts formed in pregnant mare's urine for Premarin are fit for human supplementation without laboratory purification and conversion.

Because conjugated estrogens contain numerous forms of estrogens, they can be very potent. Each form of estrogen requires its own metabolic pathway, taking weeks to be eliminated from the body. Over a period of many years, this adds up to increased potential for DNA damage, which in turn may cause mutation leading to abnormal cell growth. Also, some women—whether from increasing age, illness, or genetic predisposition—may have difficulty eliminating the byproducts of estrogen metabolism resulting in a buildup of toxic amounts in the body. (This can even happen with the body's own estradiol.) The use of natural estrogen involves far fewer metabolic pathways and, therefore, less oxidative stress and free radical damage to DNA. Natural forms of estrogen usually are administered through the skin, which also metabolizes estradiol to a much more limited extent.

SELECTIVE ESTROGEN RECEPTOR MODULATORS (SERMS)

The newest category of HRT includes selective estrogen receptor modulators, or SERMs. These laboratory-created, completely synthetic "designer" preparations target specific estrogen receptors to stimulate certain processes and block others, meaning it could have positive or negative effects at different places within the body. The best known SERM, *tamoxifen* (Nolvadex), is prescribed to women with estrogen-dependent breast cancer to reduce their risk of recurrence of the disease.

Tamoxifen has well-documented breast protective effects, blocking estrogen's damage to breast tissue. It can bind to estrogen receptors in breast tissue like a key fits into a lock. But, unlike the estrogens found in replacement therapy, this key can't *turn* the lock—it doesn't "open the door" to cause stimulation of the breast receptor, and it even keeps the body's own estrogens from reaching the receptors it occupies. However, tamoxifen doesn't block estrogen's damage elsewhere in the body. Thus, while reducing a woman's risk of breast cancer, it can double or even triple her risk of uterine cancer. Unfortunately, present preparations also increase the risk of blood clots in the lungs and legs.

Tamoxifen's breast protective effects also tend to lessen over time. Recent findings indicate that after approximately five years of use, the estrogen receptors on breast tissue occupied by tamoxifen start to change their shape, diminishing its benefits.

A second SERM in use today is *raloxifene*, approved by the FDA for prevention of osteoporosis under the brand name Evista. It has selective estrogenic activity for bones but not on uterine tissues. Some recent data on Evista suggests that it can decrease risk of breast cancer by up to 50 percent in postmenopausal women and up to 75 percent in women over age seventy. It can, indeed, increase bone density although the maximum benefit in a two-year study was 2 percent, considerably less than the protection provided by estrogen replacement therapy. An unfortunate side effect of raloxifene is hot flashes.

Overall, raloxifene and tamoxifen lower total cholesterol by about 5 percent and LDL "bad" cholesterol by about 10 percent. But they fall short when it comes to triglyceride lowering and HDL "good" cholesterol boosting compared with standard HRT. If further research on SERMs, especially in their ability to prevent osteoporosis while reducing breast cancer risk, continues to be positive, they hold great promise for the future due to their ability to target specific tissues. Until then, however, I recommend starting with bioidentical estrogen preparations such as those discussed earlier in this chapter, and/or dietary sources of phytoestrogens.

Phytoestrogens: The Power of Plant Therapy

The term "phytoestrogen" refers to a category of biologically active chemicals occurring naturally in plants which can act like estrogens in the body. These substances have much weaker activity than either the body's native estrogens (E1, E2, E3) or those compounded by pharmaceutical companies. Nevertheless, phytoestrogens bind to estrogen receptors in the body and prevent more potent forms of estrogen from gaining access, thus blocking their activity. They are nature's version of SERMs. These compounds promote bone formation in some women. They also appear to have cardioprotective qualities.

For a number of women, phytoestrogens may be sufficient to relieve menopausal symptoms such as hot flashes, night sweats, vaginal dryness, and urinary incontinence. At the same time, they are probably not potent enough to increase a woman's cancer risk, unless she already has an estrogen-dependent cancer. They are readily available from dietary sources such as soy milk, tofu, and soybeans. Phytoestrogens can be found in components of red clover, chaste berry, soy, wild yam, and whole ground flaxseed.

Phytoestrogens are substances found in plants and have a chemical structure similar to estradiol, the dominant form of estrogen before menopause. Because they are chemically similar to estrogen, they fit into the estrogen receptors on the cells of various tissues. This allows them to have an estrogen-like effect on the body, which, according to research, can be one one-hundredth

(1/100), one one-thousandth (1/1,000) or one one-hundred-thousandth (1/100,000) of the effect of estrogen, depending on which phytoestrogens are consumed.

Because they have these attributes, like SERMS, phytoestrogens fool the cells into thinking there are estrogen molecules in their estrogen receptors. Think of the receptor as a lock, and the estrogen or phytoestrogen molecule as a key that fits only that lock. In the case of estrogen, the key actually turns the lock—that is, has a chemical effect on the cell. Phytoestrogens work like a dummy key: they fit the lock but the lock doesn't turn—the chemical effect of estrogen does not take place, or takes place at a minuscule level.

Your goal is to balance out fluctuating levels of estrogen in the body. When estrogen levels are high, phytoestrogens will fill some receptor sites and block the effect of the estrogen in the system. If a woman's estrogen levels are low or falling, phytoestrogens will fill the receptor sites and trick the cells into thinking there really is estrogen present. There is also some evidence that phytoestrogens help to boost the blood estrogen levels of postmenopausal women. If a woman is suffering from menopausal symptoms, this may improve her quality of life.

The highest concentrations of phytoestrogens are contained in lignan, which are found in flaxseeds. There are also high levels in the isoflavones genistein and daidzein, all of which come from soy, and which are easy to get in tofu, tempeh, soy milk, roasted

---

Hormones at a Glance

HORMONES CAN BE *native*—produced by the human body; *natural*—derived from plants or animals but not necessarily a match for your body's receptors; *bioidentical*—a perfect match for your body's receptors, be they synthetic or natural; or *synthetic*, compounded in a laboratory and not an identical match for your body.

soybeans, and other soy products. Other phytoestrogens are found in plants and herbs such as ginseng, a widely used tonic herb, and dong quai, long used in Asia to treat menopausal symptoms and PMS. Black cohosh root such as Remifemin is a phytoestrogen used by herbalists for menopausal symptoms. A phytoestrogen diet rich in nuts, carrots, seeds, soy, lignans, legumes, and whole grains is a good dietary adjunct for any menopausal woman.

Not much research has been carried out into the specific cardioprotective effects of dietary and supplemental forms of phytoestrogens; however, it is likely that their estrogenic effect delivers some cardioprotective benefits, and women with diets high in phytoestrogen foods have fewer menopausal symptoms. For example, difficult menopause is virtually unknown in Japan, and there is no word for "hot flash" in Japanese. Several comparative studies have shown that 55 percent of American women complain of menopause symptoms while only 9 percent of Asian women do. Menopause problems are rare across East Asia, probably because the people eat a

What About Wild Yam?

MANY OVER-THE-COUNTER PRODUCTS CONTAIN "ESTROGEN" made from the wild yam. However, before you buy any wild yam product, it is important to know the type of yam that was used in its manufacture. The one to look for is *Dioscorea composita,* a.k.a. Barbasco—the true Mexican wild yam. The active ingredient it yields is *diosgenin*. Next, look for the percentage of diosgenin the product, usually cream, contains. A concentration of at least 0.1 percent is currently recommended.

BUT EVEN IF THE CONCENTRATION IS clearly stated on the label, you still may not get what you pay for. These preparations are not held to the same standards as prescription medications and preparations. Some independent analyses of their contents have yielded levels far below those promised. Know that even if the formula is up to snuff, for some women its estrogen-like activity will not be strong enough to preserve bone mass, relieve menopausal symptoms, or maintain brain function.

diet that is extremely high in phytoestrogen-rich foods: they consume 40 to 100 grams of soy foods per day, in contrast to Western women who eat less than five grams of soy per day.

Research has indicated that among premenopausal women, consuming high levels of soy protein lowers blood cholesterol, significantly lowers serum estradiol levels (the level of estrogen circulating in the bloodstream), and prolongs the menstrual cycle. These last two effects may help prevent breast cancer. How? Current thinking is that one cause of breast cancer among American women is their exposure to decades of repeated, elevated monthly estrogen levels due to early age at start of menstruation, giving birth to few children (pregnancy and breast-feeding stop the cycle of menstruation), and giving birth at later ages. Soy's effect of lowering estrogen levels might counteract this. Soy proteins also reduce the formation of tumors in animals, again, probably due to their anti-proliferating effect on blood vessels. There is some evidence for this among humans, too: Japanese women have a much lower incidence of breast cancer than American women, and those who do develop it tend to have better prognoses than American women.

Please note, however, recent research indicates that soy is *not* indicated for certain women diagnosed with breast cancer. As we will discuss further in Chapter 15 women with a positively expressed p53 gene should *not* take soy. In these women, soy can feed an estrogen-dependent tumor and cause it to grow faster.

Progesterone in Hormone Replacement Therapy: Double-Edged Sword?

Progesterone is the second piece of the HRT puzzle. Progesterone, alone or in combination with estrogen, is frequently used for hormone replacement therapy in women with an intact uterus. As with estrogen, there is considerable controversy over the relative value, risks, and side effects of "natural" compared with "synthetic" preparations.

"Natural" (native) progesterone refers to progesterone made by the human body. But preparations which are bioidentical to those produced in the human body are also considered natural progesterone replacement therapy. The source of such products may be either plant- or animal-derived, then modified in a laboratory. Most "natural" forms of progesterone replacement therapy are made from extracts of the Mexican wild yam. This yam (*dioscorea composita*) does not itself contain progesterone, estrogen, or any other hormone. Yam extracts called saponins and sapogenins (diosgenin) form the basis for the manufacture of progesterone and other hormones.

Neither the yam in its unprocessed state nor the raw extract diosgenin can be converted to progesterone within the human body; women lack the necessary enzymes to bring about such a conversion. Instead, it takes five chemical conversion steps carried out in a laboratory to yield progesterone that is bioidentical to the human body's. Technically, neither Mexican wild yam nor diosgenin are "natural" or bioidentical to humans. If you want to raise your levels of progesterone (or its cousins DHEA or pregnenolone) you must use a pure, pharmaceutical-grade compound that has gone through this conversion process.

Interestingly, synthetic progesterones (progestins/progestagens) are derived from the same botanical source as natural progesterone. This conversion process, however, yields a molecular structure which is *not* bioidentical to the body's own progesterone.

Until recently, the only form of progesterone replacement therapy available to women has been *medroxyprogesterone acetate* (MPA), a synthetic progestin marketed under the brand name Provera or combined with Premarin in a product called Prempro. Because it prevented the overgrowth of cells of the uterine lining, Provera quickly became a standard part of HRT for women who had not undergone hysterectomy.

However, evidence is building against this hormone. Recent research has linked long-term use of synthetic progestins with an increased risk of breast cancer. In an analysis of 52,705 women with breast cancer and 108,411 without it, the risk of breast cancer was 53 percent higher for combination therapy and 34 percent higher for estrogen alone, compared with no hormone use.

A study published in the January 26, 2000, issue of the *Journal of the American Medical Association* suggested that the risk of developing breast cancer increases by about 80 percent after ten years of combined hormone replacement therapy; after twenty years, 160 percent. In the study of 48,355 women who participated in the Breast Cancer Detection Demonstration Project, 2,082 women developed breast cancer. Among those women, researchers found that combined estrogen/progestin regimens were associated with greater increases in breast cancer risk than estrogen alone. The risk above and beyond "normal" breast cancer risk was estimated to be 8 percent per year for combination therapy and 1 percent per year for women taking estrogen alone.

Although our understanding of this complex relationship continues to evolve, it is still not fully understood exactly *how* hormones raise the risk of breast cancer. We do know, however, that estrogen stimulates the growth of breast cells and that certain types of cancer are sensitive to estrogen. It has also been suggested that cyclical use of progestin increases rather than decreases abnormal cellular activity in the breast.

It appears that rather than directly transforming normal cells into cancerous cells, estrogen promotes the rapid growth of cells which have already become cancerous. But this is probably not the only metabolic process involved. There is a growing body of evidence supporting the "metabolite theory" of cancer. Estradiol and estrone break down into metabolites called *semiquinones*. As the body ages, it becomes less efficient at ridding itself of these breakdown products, which also are free radicals capable of damaging cellular DNA. In addition, semiquinones promote tumor growth and blood vessel development, or angiogenesis.

I have found that synthetic progestins can lead to serious cardiac side effects in my patients, including shortness of breath, fatigue, chest pain, and high blood pressure. One of my patients, Jen, began to experience increasing spells of shortness of breath for which we could find no reason. Despite various tests for heart trouble, my colleagues and I were beside ourselves trying to figure out the cause of Jen's problem and alleviate her suffering.

She was preparing to seek a second opinion in Boston when she casually mentioned that she had been taking Prempro, a combination of Premarin and Provera, to prevent osteoporosis. We immediately called a halt to the Prempro, as Provera is known to cause coronary artery spasm. Within a few days, Jen's shortness of breath resolved almost completely. I suspect that this drug caused spasm or constriction of her blood vessels, thus increasing the resistance and pressure in her heart, and make breathing difficult. In my patients, I always recommend a natural progesterone over a synthetic progestin. The effects are considerably less harsh. In fact, I no longer use any synthetic progestins in my patients at all.

My concerns were validated in the March 8, 1997, issue of *Science News* (among other publications), in which researchers stated that Provera poses a huge risk compared to natural progesterone. The synthetic progestin (Provera) appears to nullify the beneficial effects of estrogen (estradiol) on blood flow to the heart. Natural progesterone does not have this negative effect on blood flow.

A much safer (although not entirely risk-free) progesterone is now available under the brand name Prometrium. Because it is *micronized*—broken into tiny coated particles that resist enzymatic action—it is protected from destruction in the digestive tract.

While this is good news, we're not home-free yet.... Natural micronized progesterone may have side effects similar to synthetic progestins and progestagens—such as acne, oily skin, bloating, depression—but they are generally milder.

But then There's Natural Progesterone

John Lee, MD, author of *What Your Doctor May Not Tell You About Menopause* and *What Your Doctor May Not Tell You About Premenopause*, has researched and written extensively about the benefits of "natural" progesterone replacement therapy. His work has found that using natural progesterone skin cream lowers cholesterol and triglyceride levels in postmenopausal women. Lee cites other actions of natural progesterone, including its anti-inflammatory effects, the fact that it promotes the burning of fats for energy, and its action in protecting the integrity and functioning of cell membranes. All of these work to protect the endothelium and prevent plaque and atherosclerosis—indications that using natural progesterone, in the form of a cream or micronized, may protect against heart disease.

Increasing numbers of women, especially those who are estrogen dominant, have been using natural progesterone instead of conventional HRT and ERT to alleviate symptoms of perimenopause and menopause—with excellent results. Among its benefits are enhanced libido, increased energy and stamina, and stimulation of the body's own production of estrogen, progesterone, and testosterone. Again, it is important to monitor your hormone balance, preferably with saliva testing, to avoid any potential overdose. Some progesterone creams are extremely potent. I agree with Dr. Lee that the role of natural progesterone is misunderstood by mainstream medicine and poorly understood relative to heart disease. Much more research is needed in this area and also in the area of cardioprotective effects of natural progesterone. I also agree with his concerns that foreign hormones—

The HERS Study

RESULTS FROM THE FIRST LARGE-SCALE, RANDOMIZED STUDY of estrogen plus progestin for secondary prevention of coronary artery disease in postmenopausal women were published on August 19, 1998, in the *Journal of the American Medical Association*. The study cast a shadow on the widely held belief that hormone replacement therapy could assuage the cardiovascular effects of dwindling estrogen at menopause.

THE HEART AND ESTROGEN/PROGESTIN REPLACEMENT STUDY (HERS) of 2,763 women with coronary artery disease and with no hysterectomy were given hormone replacement therapy (synthetic estrogen and progesterone) and monitored for four years.

THE STUDY CONCLUDED THAT THIS FORM OF COMBINATION HRT improved lipid profiles but did *not* reduce the overall rate of coronary heart disease events during the treatment period. This was surprising because previous observational studies had indicated that estrogen replacement therapy gives a cardioprotective benefit to women who already have coronary artery disease—up to a 50 percent reduction in cardiovascular events. Of additional concern, the women showed an increase in blood clots and gall bladder disease.

THE HERS STUDY IS A GOOD FIRST STEP TOWARD understanding the value of HRT for secondary prevention of coronary artery disease events in postmenopausal women, but I do have concerns about some of the background characteristics of the study's participants, and I don't think its results invalidate the body of research that supports estrogen's role in heart health. Like most good research, it raises as many or more questions than it answers. There have yet to be well-controlled clinical trials on the use of estrogen with *natural* progesterone used as secondary prevention. This would be important to know.

MEANWHILE, WE EAGERLY AWAIT THE RESULTS of the Women's Health Initiative which includes HRT treatment of 28,000 women and will provide more broadly applicable results. The results should become available in 2005. For now, we must exercise caution whenever we use HRT in women with documented coronary heart disease.

from pesticides, solvents, plastics, and hormone- and antibiotic-laced meats and dairy—can further upset your delicate hormonal balance, and that we all need to avoid these environmental pollutants as much as possible. To get natural progesterone in a topical form, you will need your doctor to write a prescription.

Like synthetic and micronized progesterone, natural progesterone is taken ten to fourteen days per month. Natural progesterone is also available as a skin cream or gel and is usually applied once or twice daily in one-quarter to one-half teaspoon amounts. Start with a 2 percent progesterone cream yielding one-half teaspoon of progesterone twice per day for the first two months, then reduce to one-eighth teaspoon twice per day. Working with your physician, you may need to regulate this dose up or down depending upon how you feel.

Have You Heard of DHEA?

Dihydroepiandrosterone (DHEA) is a hormone produced by the adrenal and sex glands of the human body. It is a building block or precursor for the sex hormones. DHEA levels decline as we age; low levels of this vital hormone are associated with numerous diseases, including cancer, heart disease, and disorders of the immune system. Supplementation with DHEA has been reported to improve memory, increase stress resistance, decrease joint pain, decrease body fat, increase lean muscle mass, and improve sleep. Dosing for women should be conservative—10 to 25 mg every other day if indicated by low saliva or blood hormone levels. It may be taken orally, under the tongue or as a skin gel. Side effects of overdose may include acne, increased facial hair, sleep disturbances, fatigue, irritability, and deepening voice. Use DHEA with caution. It may promote estrogen-like activity and contribute to the development of hormone-dependent cancers. If you have a family history of breast or ovarian cancer, consult your physician before trying DHEA as it may not be your safest option.

Pregnenolone for Mentality and Mood

Pregnenolone is a hormone produced in the adrenal cortex and brain from cholesterol. It is a precursor of both DHEA and progesterone. Like many other hormones, levels of pregnenolone decline with age. Low levels seem to be associated with depression, memory loss, and diminished mental clarity. It also appears to enhance the interaction between nerve cells. This is linked with an antianxiety effect. Pregnenolone is used primarily for its benefits in mental function and mood regulation and is not usually the first choice for relief of menopausal symptoms such as hot flashes and vaginal dryness, although it can be used for this purpose. Side effects are the same experienced with progesterone and DHEA. Supplementation at doses of 20 to 25 mg per day may enhance concentration and reduce mental fatigue.

If You Decide to Try HRT....

Your mental, emotional, and physical well-being during the perimenopausal period—before, during, and after menopause—largely depends on maintaining a balance between fluctuating (and ultimately, declining) levels of estrogen, primarily estradiol, and progesterone. Many women breeze through this "change of life" without giving it a second thought. Others find they can manage quite nicely with dietary changes, most notably phytoestrogens such as soy and flax. Still others, especially those with serious, poor quality-of-life issues surrounding menopause, consider prescription medications, some derived from plant, some from animals, some from molecules synthesized in the laboratory. Another way of balancing the progesterone/estrogen ratio includes hormonal building blocks such as DHEA or pregnenolone.

This balancing act must be tailored to each woman, working in conjunction with her physician. If your physician is unwilling to work with you on making these critical choices, *find one who will.* Don't try to go it alone! Effective therapy requires regularly monitoring hormone levels. Before beginning any HRT regimen (even a totally "natural" one), it is also important to have a thorough physical exam including a pelvic exam, professional breast exam, and PAP smear. A Blood Chemistry Profile, which includes blood count, liver function, thyroid function, and lipid profile, should also be done. Saliva hormone levels could be extremely helpful in gauging the type and dosage of therapy to be taken. A mammogram is another test that needs consideration, and a baseline bone density scan is also in order to judge the effectiveness of the therapy in preventing osteoporosis. These important tests can help you to create a comprehensive program to keep your hormonal ratios in optimal physiological balance.

If you decide to try HRT, don't expect a "perfect fit" on the first try. The right dosage often requires fine tuning and adjustments over time. A regimen designed in your 40s when your risk of breast cancer is relatively low and your risk of developing osteoporosis over your next three to four decades of life is relatively high may not be the optimal regimen in your 80s, when your risk of breast cancer is higher and the risk to your bones from living without estrogen for fewer years is lower.

Finally, be honest with your physician about your family history, your own medical history, your fears and expectations as well as your family's fears and expectations. Promptly report any side effects that occur during your therapy, and let the doctor know when something just isn't working for you. Be precise in describing both your physical and emotional symptoms. Even the most dedicated and insightful physician will have difficulty getting to the root of a problem described as "I just don't feel like myself."

Clear, detailed communication is important: "I can't concentrate for more than ten minutes." "I feel bouts of depression without warning several times every week." "I have gained five pounds and feel bloated." "My skin broke out in acne." If your needs aren't clearly presented to your physician, it is unlikely that you will get

---

HRT at a Glance

- Hormone replacement therapy (HRT) is appropriate as a heart-disease preventive for certain high-risk women and can be a helpful adjunct treatment for women who already have coronary artery disease;
- The HRT decision often comes down to a quality-of-life issue—if you find you are turning on the air conditioner in the middle of winter to deal with hot flashes, for example, you are probably having "quality-of-life issues;"
- For most women, a year or two of HRT is perfectly safe, to usher them through the transition of perimenopause to a better quality of life until their body's fluctuating hormones have rebalanced;
- No woman should take *any* form of synthetic progesterone if she has had a hysterectomy;
- Natural micronized progesterone (Prometrium) is far safer than synthetic Provera;
- If you have had a heart attack and are postmenopausal, your risk of recurrent heart disease is probably much higher than your risk of breast cancer: While *one in three* women will die of a heart attack or stroke, one in eleven will get breast cancer during their lifetime;
- If you are at high risk for breast cancer with a poor qualify of life due to menopausal symptoms, go with natural phytoestrogens over prescription HRT;
- Bioidentical estrogens, such as triest gels, and natural progesterone, such as progesterone creams can often reduce menopausal signs without resorting to "heavy artillery" such as Premarin, Provera, and Prempro;
- Prescription ERT and HRT often have unpleasant side effects including weight gain, breast tenderness, cramps, and blood clots;
- Duration of estrogen use is the key: If you cannot tolerate being without HRT due to poor quality-of-life issues, you must know that the longer you take it, the greater your risk of breast cancer. *Any* type of HRT will eventually increase your risk of breast cancer.

what you need. Likewise, if your physician's responses aren't helpful or clearly understandable, make it known and ask for clarification, even if it takes extra effort. It's *your* life and your health at stake!

Whatever form of estrogen replacement you select—including none at all—I advise you to have your hormone levels regularly monitored, especially when you are beginning therapy or wish to change your form of therapy, (i.e., discontinuing Premarin to start a yam-derived preparation). The object of monitoring hormonal levels is not to obtain any particular numerical target; the absolute value is less important than the *ratio* of key hormones to one another. The aim is to obtain an optimal balance between your estradiol (E2) and progesterone levels. In my opinion, the best method of doing this today is through saliva testing. It is noninvasive, usually less expensive than other methods, and accurately reflects tissue levels as well as the hormone's biologically active amounts. (See Appendix B for more on saliva testing.)

It is generally agreed by most researchers and clinicians that estrogens can assuage menopausal symptoms, reduce bone fractures, and probably reduce the incidence of coronary artery disease. The evidence is strong that estrogen confers these reductions in risk by restoring the beneficial effects of naturally produced estrogen.

Despite this impressive resume, the value of hormone replacement therapy for secondary prevention—that is, in women who already have established coronary artery disease—remains less clear. As a result, I count myself among a group of clinicians and researchers who are becoming increasingly conservative when it comes to recommending HRT in women. While I wouldn't hesitate to recommend estrogen to a woman at high risk for a recurrent heart attack, who has a clear-cut risk factor such as high Lp(a) or high fibrinogen or who has unacceptable quality-of-life issues surrounding menopause, I do advise caution when it comes to this important midlife choice.

For most women, I now recommend natural estrogen first,

along with lab tests to see what effects the estrogen is having on HDL "good" cholesterol, homocysteine, and Lp(a), then reassess her progress within the next three to six months. Balance is the key: Start with the least invasive approach, such as a natural or bioidentical estrogen/progesterone, and work up until you find the right balance.

Assessing Your Individual Risk Profile

As you probably have gathered by now, I believe the best way to prevent and treat heart disease is through a balanced approach, one that uses both conventional and alternative methods where each is appropriate. I always recommend using natural, noninvasive, non-pharmaceutical methods first, whenever possible. I extend this philosophy to hormone replacement therapy and favor the use of bioidentical estrogens and progesterone derived from plants over the use of potent formulas like Premarin and Provera. I will even choose dietary management, nutritional supplementation, and herbal remedies over naturally derived hormones, when such an approach seems safe and appropriate.

Just as every woman must assess her unique set of needs, risks, and symptoms to come to her own decision about using hormone replacement therapy, it may also be necessary for a woman to try more than one method of hormone replacement before she finds the one which works best for her. This is not always easy in our "all or nothing" healthcare world: Many physicians routinely prescribe potent hormones such as Premarin and Provera, and if a woman has side effects, simply take her off the medication and offer no other alternatives. Even after a woman finds the right type of hormone replacement therapy, she may have to work with the dosage for weeks or even months until she finds her ideal balance.

Therefore, knowing all the risk factors of HRT and how it relates to heart disease will allow you to be well prepared to make the right decision.

CHAPTER TWELVE

Women's Choice: A Decision Tree

**Cynthia: How One Woman Took Control of
Her Own Health Care**

Cynthia grew up in Poland in a family of highly trained professionals who placed great emphasis on education. She met her husband-to-be while in nurse's training, and they emigrated to the United States.

At thirty-three, Cynthia had a total hysterectomy and was started on 2.5 mg Premarin daily—a dose two times higher than the highest dosage currently used for estrogen replacement. Even a young resident questioned the treatment plan because she was so young. Cynthia still spoke only limited English at the time, but she believed that her gynecologist knew best because he was a doctor, and so she followed his instructions to the letter.

From the beginning of Premarin therapy, she could not sleep. She developed heart palpitations and swelling in her ankles. The doctor's only response to her discomfort was to restrict her fluid intake because she was "just retaining fluid." Cynthia suffered with her symptoms for fifteen years, rarely sleeping more than an hour at a time. Eventually she developed migraine headaches lasting as long as three days. The headaches started clustering in different locations and increasing in frequency.

She started to experience buzzing and pounding in her ears. Her libido was gone, and her marriage was suffering. Cynthia even considered the possibility that she might have a brain tumor. When she sought an evaluation, the physician for her new HMO would not give her a thorough examination to find the cause of her pain.

The only one to question the Premarin was Cynthia's mother. But Cynthia believed that she was protecting herself from heart disease and osteoporosis. Her doctors were so committed to the Premarin therapy that they never even considered it a possible culprit for her symptoms.

I can only speculate that they had bought into the theory that high-dose Premarin is appropriate for all women after total hysterectomy and that all women would assuredly feel better on estrogen replacement. I can only believe that her doctors sincerely believed that all Cynthia's symptoms had to be attributed to other factors, the most obvious of which was her stress level.

But in looking at her cardiac risk profile, there was *no family history* of cardiac disease or cancer. Her father and mother were still alive at ages eighty-seven and seventy-six. Since Cynthia was so young, age could be scratched off as a risk factor. Her blood pressure was on the low side, and she was a nonsmoker. But, after years on Premarin, her blood pressure was rising. Despite a history of diphtheria at three years of age, I considered Cynthia to be at low risk for heart disease at the time her ERT was started.

It took an educational program to shift Cynthia's awareness and cause her to start questioning ERT. She was watching a television show about headaches, menopause, and natural remedies. Although she knew nothing of such treatment, Cynthia was at the end of her rope. She realized that something natural could be her last resort and, possibly, her best hope. She got a book on the subject and looked up the side effects of Premarin. She was shocked. She had every one! For the first time, she considered that even her exhaustion might be connected to ERT.

She started to make things happen for herself. Her doctor agreed to let her cut the dose back to 1.25 mg. Immediately, her headaches disappeared. But her doctor refused to let her discontinue Premarin altogether. By now Cynthia knew she was on the right track, so she changed her insurance company and found herself a gynecologist who would work with her. Together, they mapped out a new plan of hormone therapy that included natural phytoestrogens.

After fifteen years of misery, she now has about one headache a month and no longer retains water. Her energy level has returned to what it was when she was twenty, and her libido is back.

With age, however, Cynthia developed other problems. At age fifty-six, she had developed high cholesterol and a rise in blood pressure as well as osteoporosis; and she was overweight, occasionally short of breath, and continued to have occasional palpitations. To further screen these concerns, she took a Nuclear Cardiolite Stress Test (see Appendix A for more information on this and other diagnostic heart tests). Her results were within normal parameters. Her preventive plan now includes a Mediterranean diet and natural cholesterol-lowering nutrients such as garlic and the Ayurvedic herb *guggulipid*. Nutritional supports like coenzyme Q10 (CoQ10) have also helped decrease her palpitations and lower her blood pressure. I encouraged her to develop an exercise program to maintain optimal body weight, which will also help to lower her blood pressure and moderate stress and tension.

It is Cynthia's hope that her story may send a message for other women who also have symptoms that they have not thought to attribute to hormone therapy. Cynthia brings a message that there is often no therapeutic panacea in any medical situation. We need to participate in our treatment plans and challenge the treatment when our gut tells us that something is wrong. It is never too late to change the game plan. And, of course, the final lesson is that no matter how old you are, there are times when you should listen to your mother.

At the same time, there are cases in which the option for HRT is perhaps too easily dismissed. There is also a bias *against* hormone replacement therapy. Many women's health advocates, including physicians, point their patients toward natural approaches which will bring relief of menopausal symptoms and offer protection against osteoporosis, but they often carry their contention to extremes. If one were to subscribe to the negative bias about hormone replacement therapy, women like Janet would needlessly suffer.

Janet: How Hormones Saved the Day

At fifty-one, Janet was in love and anticipating her upcoming marriage. Her nuptials would involve leaving her long-time home in Texas to move to sunny California with her new husband John, and she was sure that she was up to the challenge. Everything was falling into place beautifully—a new marriage, a new private psychotherapy practice, and a new location.

But just before her wedding, Janet's usually regular menstrual cycle stopped abruptly. Her periods had never been erratic unless she was adjusting to jet lag, and Janet had never been one to experience any symptoms she would have called PMS. She kept her weight at an optimal level and enjoyed good health. So Janet was perplexed at her weepiness and bouts of depression, with no apparent reason. She sought help from her internist, questioning him about whether her depressed state could be related to her sudden menopause. She was advised of the improbability of her theory but encouraged to see a gynecologist.

Following up with her gynecologist, Janet explained that she had no emotional source for her depressive symptoms. She strongly felt that the culprit was physical, and a recent onset of menopause seemed like the most likely cause. Her gynecologist agreed, and started her on a combination therapy of Premarin with progesterone. At this point, Janet was at low risk for heart disease and cancer. As a result, HRT was an appropriate choice to improve her quality of life.

Within one week, Janet felt better. For her, hormone therapy seemed to be the answer. But, things were not as simple as she would have hoped. Gradually, her blood pressure, usually low at 90/70, also changed with menopause, creeping up higher and higher. Now, with one risk factor for heart disease, Janet faced a moderate risk for coronary artery disease. Just in case her Premarin was contributing to her new hypertension, Janet's gynecologist tried changing her from the pill form of estrogen to a patch application when it first became available in 1987. Janet had some skin irritation and she found that her depression returned. As soon as she switched back to the oral estrogen prescription, she felt fine again.

By 1990 Janet's internist told her about a French gel product, not yet FDA approved, that showed promise. A compounding pharmacy made up a hormonal preparation for her. She found that she preferred this method to her previous one.

She experienced no side effects until 1995 when she had some blood spotting and was referred to her gynecologist for a uterine biopsy, which was negative. But the physician was concerned about the gel product and recommended that she go back to the Climara patch. The adhesive still irritated her skin a little, but she accepted this minor annoyance. Although she has yet to find the perfect solution, for Janet HRT was the best solution for the abrupt onset of depression she experienced with menopause. But it was a decision she will need to revisit regularly.

Keeping these different scenarios in mind, it is important to address the risk levels for heart disease in a format that enables you to get a sense of where your own risks and quality of life issues might fit into the big picture. This is where the "Decision Tree" comes in. Here are a series of case studies—(I) very high risk, (II) high risk, (III) mod-

Computing Your Risk for Heart Disease

YOUR HEART DISEASE RISK IS VERY HIGH IF YOU HAVE ANY ONE OF THE FOLLOWING:
1. known coronary artery disease (CAD)
2. angina
3. a history of a previous heart attack
4. a history of angioplasty
5. a history of coronary artery bypass graft surgery (CABG or CABS)

YOUR HEART DISEASE RISK IS HIGH IF YOU HAVE TWO OR MORE OF THESE TRADITIONAL RISK FACTORS:
1. family history of heart disease
2. natural menopause before age 40 or menopause before age 45 induced by surgery, illness, or medical treatment
3. history of smoking
4. high blood pressure (above 140/90)
5. diabetes
6. obesity
7. elevated blood cholesterol (above 240 mg/dl is high, above 200 mg/dl is borderline high)
8. low HDL cholesterol (below 35)
9. a poor diet
10. a sedentary lifestyle
11. elevated Lp(a)
12. elevated ferritin
13. history of a TIA (transient ischemic attack or temporary lack of circulation to the brain)

erate risk, and (IV) low risk—that will illustrate some of the choices and challenges inherent in developing an individualized program.

I—If Your Heart Disease Risk Is Very High

If you have angina or coronary artery disease, or have had a previous heart attack, angioplasty, or coronary artery bypass surgery, you are in the highest risk group for additional cardiac events.

Estrogen's protective effects are important for women at this level, especially for those who have already developed significant

---

14. elevated homocysteine
15. elevated fibrinogen

YOUR HEART DISEASE RISK IS MODERATE IF YOU HAVE AT LEAST ONE OF THE FOLLOWING TRADITIONAL RISK FACTORS:
   1. family history of heart disease
   2. early menopause
   3. smoking
   4. high blood pressure
   5. diabetes
   6. obesity
   7. elevated blood cholesterol
   8. low HDL cholesterol
   9. elevated Lp(a)
   10. elevated ferritin
   11. elevated homocysteine
   12. elevated fibrinogen

YOUR HEART DISEASE RISK IS LOW IF:
   1. you have no family history
   2. you have no known risk factors

atherosclerosis. Estrogen's cholesterol-moderating effects, endothelial protection, and other benefits may reduce the likelihood, or slow the process, of further clogging of the coronary arteries. Women with coronary artery disease who have other high-risk conditions, such as diabetes or high blood pressure, need this kind of protection far more than women at moderate or low risk. For such women, taking HRT or ERT may literally be a lifesaving step. I also suggest HRT for a high risk woman if she has high fibrinogen, high Lp(a), or low HDL.

On balance, the gains from using synthetic hormone replacement for a woman in this category will in most cases outweigh the risks. If you have not had a hysterectomy, your risk of endometrial cancer can be almost virtually eliminated by also taking progesterone; if you have had one, you have no risk of endometrial cancer and can take unopposed estrogen. Following is a satisfactory treatment plan for one woman in this category.

Deborah: Story of a Very High Risk Woman

What are the options for a very high risk woman when estrogen therapy is clearly indicated, there is no family of breast, uterine, or ovarian cancers, but the side effects of ERT are intolerable?

Deborah did have a history of colon cancer many years ago, but because this was not a hormone-dependent cancer, such as cancer of the uterus, ovaries, fallopian tubes, or breast, this did not present a risk for Deborah in terms of considering HRT.

Deborah is sixty-three years of age, postmenopausal, and has a history of heart disease, high blood pressure, and high cholesterol. She has no cardiac symptoms such as chest discomfort, shortness of breath, or lightheadedness. I was greatly relieved to find that her homocysteine was normal, but I did discover that she had a high Lp(a). For the first time, I understood why her vessels were progressively clogging.

Together we agreed that estrogen therapy was appropriate to try to knock down her Lp(a) and halt her advancing heart disease. I prescribed an estrogen (Climara) patch of 0.05 mg per week along with 100 mg oral micronized progesterone daily during the last two weeks of the month. Prior to bedtime, Deborah also takes traditional cardiac medication for her high blood pressure and high cholesterol. For supplements, she takes CoQ10 (30 mg, three times daily) and an antioxidant vitamin/mineral formulated to ensure that she gets enough folic acid, plus B6, B12, and other important nutritionals.

Two months later, Deborah sent me a fax to let me know how she was feeling. In two words, it was "not good." She stated that the hormonal therapy was not working well for her. After following our game plan for one month, she developed heavy cramps, then very heavy bleeding that lasted almost two weeks. She felt weak and tired and her breasts had become tender and painful within a few days on the estrogen. Finally, Deborah decided "enough was enough."

She let me know that she was taking a month off, during which time she would recommit herself to an exercise program and be judicious about her diet. She did not want to consider daily natural estrogen and progesterone cream in which menstruation would not occur. Deborah also told me that she wasn't getting much support at home and that with all her medication and trying to maintain her house, she felt overwhelmed.

Deborah had known heart disease, and needed to treat her Lp(a), but simply couldn't live with the side effects. So we had to go to "option B"—strengthening her alternative medical program. I recommended several other approaches to help lower her Lp(a). First, Deborah agreed to take phytoestrogens daily in a shake of ground flaxseed and soy milk.

She also agreed to take niacin, starting with 100 mg twice daily and working up to 500 mg, adjusting it slowly for the flushing or "hot flash" sensations that niacin generates. I also included DHA (docosahexaenoic acid), a fish oil preparation that helps lower Lp(a) for women and men alike. Like niacin, the best way to take DHA is to start with low doses daily and increase weekly to 1,000 mg per day. Since Deborah likes to eat fresh fish, she also agreed to consume more fish meals in her diet. And, because elevated Lp(a) creates an inflammatory reaction in the blood vessels, it was important to have Deborah include in her plan supplements with anti-inflammatory properties, such as garlic and ginger. She can use fresh garlic or take a supplemental form if fresh garlic taste and odor are a problem. A cup of ginger tea every day will provide her with adequate ginger support. In light of research showing a 22 percent lowering of Lp(a) with CoQ10, we increased her CoQ10 dosage to 240 mg daily and added 500 mg vitamin C.

This combination gave Deborah the best possible game plan for her, and one that she could live with. Periodic retesting of her Lp(a) showed gradual improvement. If her blood level did not come down satisfactorily, I would add 250 to 500 mg bromelain three times daily to her program. (Bromelain comes from the pineapple plant and also has anti-inflammatory properties that can help neutralize some of the deleterious effects of Lp(a).)

Despite her struggles with her health and personal life, Deborah is able to collaborate equally with her physician, express her emotions, and follow her own good sense about what is "right" or "not right" for her as an individual. It is easier for me to treat women like Deborah because she is an active participant in her own health and is not afraid to give me feedback on my recommendation, even if it's not working for her. She accepts responsibility to decide when to change the game plan, and lets me know what she's changing so that I can give her my professional take on her decision. And, of course, ultimately it's up to Deborah to choose her best option once we have both shared our perspectives. This, for me, is the cornerstone of a healthy relationship between physician and patient.

Balancing the Concerns of the Very High Risk Woman

The ERT/HRT decision becomes even more complex for a woman in a high heart-risk group who is also at risk for breast cancer. A woman's age and the length of time she takes ERT/HRT affect her breast cancer risk, and should be taken into consideration. Other breast cancer risk factors include:

❖ a first degree relative (mother or sister) with breast cancer;
❖ alcoholic intake greater than 2 drinks per day;
❖ repeated exposure to insecticides and pesticides;
❖ early onset of menstruation (before age 13);
❖ late menopause (after age 50);
❖ not having children, or having a first child after age 35;
❖ not having breast-fed;
❖ obesity;
❖ a breast biopsy suggestive of increased risk.

However, even with increased risk, a woman's lifetime probability of developing breast cancer would rise only moderately with ERT/HRT, while her chances of prolonged health and survival due to protection from heart disease would increase significantly (therefore, her life expectancy would still increase).

According to the most recent research, women who take HRT for three years or less show no significant increase in risk for breast cancer; beyond five years, the longer a woman takes hormone replacement therapy and the older she is, the greater her risk of developing breast cancer.

If a woman has a higher-than-normal risk for breast cancer, many physicians will recommend against ERT/HRT, no matter what the cardiovascular benefits. If a woman chooses that route, she may still decide to derive some of the protective benefits of estrogen by using a dietary strategy and nutritional supplements that provide high levels of phytoestrogens. And, if a woman already has a history of breast cancer, I do not recommend that she take ERT/HRT or topical estrogen at all, but choose a dietary phytoestrogen approach (as long as her tumor is not estrogen dependent, see Chapter 15).

The other downside of ERT/HRT is its potential side effects, which affect 5 to 10 percent of women who take it. These include bloating, headache, breast tenderness, and diarrhea from estrogen; plus weight gain, irritability, and depression from progesterone in the combined therapy. Again, there is no easy answer for this: the side effects of progesterone may be reduced by adjusting the dose, but if these side effects are unbearable, a woman may have to choose another course. This was certainly the situation in Deborah's case.

Of course, a woman at very high risk for heart disease should also be taking steps to minimize her controllable lifestyle risk factors such as not smoking, eating a Mediterranean-type diet, keeping weight down, exercising, and following a dietary and supplement regimen.

II—If Your Heart Disease Risk Is High

You are at high risk for cardiovascular disease if you have two or more of the traditional risk factors discussed in Chapter 2, such as family history of premature heart disease; natural menopause before age forty or menopause before age forty-five induced by surgery, illness or medical treatment; history of smoking; high blood pressure (above 140/90); diabetes; obesity; elevated blood cholesterol (above 240 mg/dl is high, above 200 mg/dl is border-line high); low HDL cholesterol (below 35); poor diet; or sedentary lifestyle. Other important risk factors (as discussed in Chapter 3) are elevated levels of blood Lp(a), C-reactive protein, high oxidized LDL, fibrinogen, homocysteine, serum ferritin, as well as a history of TIA (transient ischemic attack).

In some views, women in this group should also consider conventional hormone replacement therapy or bioidentical topical therapy, depending on quality-of-life issues. While it's true that ERT/HRT will lower the elevated risk for these women, especially those with high Lp(a) or fibrinogen, it pays to observe that of the risk factors above, most can be diminished or even eliminated by changing diet and lifestyle, or by taking simple preventive steps. While nothing can be done about family history or early menopause, any woman who is seriously concerned about her risk for heart disease can quit smoking, lose weight, begin to exercise, and adopt a low-cholesterol, heart-healthy diet. If necessary, she could also begin taking cholesterol lowering or anti-hypertensive medications, although I would recommend lifestyle changes and some nutritional and herbal approaches first. If you have diabetes, taking these steps will reduce its severity or may even eliminate it altogether.

Women with an elevated Lp(a) should also follow my modified Mediterranean diet, including fresh coldwater fish two to three times per week, fresh fruits and legumes (chickpeas, lentils, etc.) daily, and monounsaturated fats like olive oil and oils with omega-3 essential fatty acids such as flaxseed oil or fish oil. You should also take targeted supplements similar to those that I recommended for Deborah in the very high risk category.

A postmenopausal woman with high serum ferritin (iron) can lower her stored iron by beginning to donate blood—every other month at first, if necessary—while continuing to have her ferritin levels tested. As the bone marrow manufactures new red cells to replace those that are removed, it draws from the body's supply of stored iron, gradually diminishing it. Once your ferritin level returns to normal, donating blood three to four times per year will help keep ferritin levels within the safe range. Obviously, I recommend that this be done under a physician's guidance and monitoring.

Overall, I would work with a high-risk woman to eliminate the risks before recommending hormone therapy. However, if alternative methods are tried but unsuccessful, then a woman may want to begin hormone therapy. Following is an example of how one high risk woman came to me for treatment and how we worked out her strategic plan.

Ellen: Story of a High Risk Woman

Ellen is a sixty-six-year-old woman who has dual residences in New Jersey and Florida. She is well informed and diligent about finding health care solutions that work for her individual needs. Ellen's active lifestyle and conscientious exercise program includes swimming three-fourths of a mile several times per week and lifting light weights. She consulted me about her hormone dilemma after hearing me lecture at a Florida health show. Ellen had good reason to be concerned.

When she hit menopause, Ellen had opted for HRT; she was at low risk for cancer but had a family history for premature heart disease. She had lost one brother to coronary artery disease; "it was like losing my best friend." Her other brother, a health professional, had struggled with congestive heart failure. Her own cholesterol was high, but she had been advised "not to worry about it." Ellen followed a Mediterranean diet and rarely "cheated." But she decided to dig a little further. She also had her coronary calcium score checked (for more on high-frequency calcium CT scanning, see Appendix A) to see if there were any early changes in her coronary arteries. A perfect score is zero, suggesting no calcium deposits in the arteries; Ellen scored 319. The mean score for healthy women in her age group is 97, while a typical woman with coronary artery disease has an average score of 469.

Ellen knew that she needed to become more aggressive with cardiovascular prevention. Her physician recommended HRT. But after only seven days on Premarin, she experienced shortness of breath, especially at bedtime when she felt as though she needed to "suck air" in to get enough. Her back ached, her memory was blunted, and she felt depressed. She found her quality of life to be so compromised that she took herself off the medication and requested a saliva test to see where she stood. It documented that her hormones were within normal range. While her spirits lifted, she still was not completely satisfied.

Ellen decided to consult an orthomolecular (nutritional) psychiatrist. He gave her B12 shots for her fatigue, which she learned to administer herself. She asked him about hormone therapy and followed his recommendation to try 100 mg natural micronized progesterone for ten days a month. She took the product for a few cycles but was so afraid of "having a heart attack" that she stopped in light of tremendous anxiety about her heart. She simply did not have trust in the system.

When Ellen sought my advice on HRT alternatives, I agreed that she might be wise to consider some form of HRT because of her coronary calcium score and her strong family history—she was at high risk. She was satisfied with my opinion. I also recommended that she have a "new millennium" blood test to screen for other risk factors such as Lp(a) and homocysteine elevations that may be familial, as well as to check her levels of CoQ10 and other antioxidants.

The results of Ellen's bloodwork were excellent. Her blood showed that she had good antioxidant protection. She is now taking 100 mg micronized progesterone daily two weeks per month and low-dose natural estrogen in the form of a topical patch once a week. She is also pleased with her quality of life and reports no side effects on this combination. When I last spoke to Ellen, I also encouraged her to take a calcium/magnesium formula to protect her from osteoporosis. Her natural hormone therapy—when added to her healthy lifestyle and diet, exercise, and targeted nutritional supplements—puts her on a program that offers promise for preventing coronary artery disease *and* osteoporosis.

Balancing Breast Cancer Risk for the High and Moderate Heart Disease Risk Woman

Women in high and moderate risk categories who do *not* have heart disease need to think a little differently about breast cancer when balancing risk with benefit. Under normal conditions, a woman has about an 11 percent chance of developing breast cancer during her lifetime. Even if ERT/HRT raises that risk by 40 percent, it still means that her risk of developing breast cancer would not be more than 15.4 percent.

At the same time, hormone therapy may reduce her far higher risk of heart disease and other cardiovascular diseases. Since the risk of breast cancer is considerably lower than the risk of coronary artery disease, this might tip the balance in favor of ERT or HRT for many high- and moderate-risk women.

When the High Risk Woman Should Consider Natural Hormone Replacement Therapy

If a high risk woman manages to reduce or eliminate some of her risk factors or if she experiences intolerable side effects from Premarin like Ellen did, there is still another option: the natural, plant-derived hormone preparations. These are available in the form of a topical patch, which is applied to the skin above the buttocks or below the navel. The two patches I prescribe to my patients are Estraderm and Climara. Both are made from soybeans and may offer cardioprotective benefits similar to those from a woman's naturally produced estrogen. They are less potent than Premarin, and because they are natural, they have fewer side effects. Some women do develop skin rashes in the area where the patch is applied, which is often an allergic reaction to the adhesive.

The natural estrogen patch contains estradiol, one of the three forms that estrogen takes and the form which has the predominant effect in premenopausal women. The patches are effective for about one week, after which they must be changed: this makes them more convenient to use than daily medication. Like oral estrogen, topical estrogen also alters blood lipids but only after continuous treatment for at least four to six months. Because it is absorbed directly into the bloodstream and does not pass through the digestive system and the liver, topical estrogen does not stimulate the liver to raise blood triglyceride levels as oral estrogens do, and some studies have found that it actually lowers triglyceride levels. This makes the patch especially good for women who have high triglycerides, although it does not increase beneficial HDL as oral estrogen does.

Other studies have indicated that like oral estrogen, the estrogen patch increases the production of prostacyclin, which helps dilate arteries and also improves the efficiency of the heart by enhancing the functioning of the myocardium and the walls of the aorta. Topical patches also have an added bonus for women: an antioxidant effect.

However, like oral estrogen, the estrogen patch carries an increased risk of endometrial cancer. If a woman has her uterus, she must also take progesterone to protect her from endometrial cancer. The appropriate choice is micronized progesterone, a product which is also extracted from soy, and whose action approximates natural progesterone. Micronized progesterone is usually prescribed in oral form, 100 mg once to twice per day for continual daily dosing, and 100 mg one to three times per day for ten to fourteen days per month if taken cyclically. Natural micronized progesterone may cause some of the same side effects as synthetic progesterone, including bloating, acne, and depression.

Like all forms of estrogen, the natural estrogen patch carries some increased risk for breast cancer. A cardiac high-risk woman with a family history of breast cancer may still want to consider the patch because her risk of heart disease is still significantly higher than the risk of breast cancer. Any woman who has had breast cancer should not consider an estrogen patch.

Another alternative which I find women accepting more and more is a combination of topical estrogen gels (biest) which contain 80 percent estriol and 20 percent estradiol along with 10 to 25 mg progesterone cream used on the 16th to 25th day of the cycle.

III—If Your Risk of Heart Disease Is Moderate

A woman is at moderate risk for heart disease if she has at least one of the following traditional risk factors: family history of heart disease, early menopause, smoking, high blood pressure, diabetes, obesity, elevated blood cholesterol, low HDL cholesterol, elevated Lp(a), elevated homocysteine, a sedentary lifestyle, or other "new millennium" risk factors discussed in Chapter 3.

As with high risk women, before considering any kind of hormone therapy to prevent heart disease, I first strongly recommend that a moderate risk woman take steps to eliminate her risk factors: reduce cholesterol, exercise, quit smoking, lose weight, and take targeted nutritional support in vitamins, minerals, and phytonutrients.

If poor quality-of-life issues such as palpitations, night sweats, hot flashes, and insomnia are present, I recommend starting with the estrogen patch or topical triest or biest gels. These less potent forms of estrogen act on a woman's body in much the same way as the native estrogen she produces herself before menopause and will cause fewer risks and side effects than full-blown HRT.

I see many moderate risk women in my practice. Usually, they have sought a cardiology consultation because they are aware of one or more cardiac risk factors and are looking for preventive guidelines.

Maggie's is a story of a moderate-risk woman treated successfully with synthetic ERT. Her cardiac risk factor: hypertension. Incidentally, her blood pressure readings at home reflect well-controlled high blood pressure (around 120/60), but when she comes to the office to be checked, we get sky-high readings like 168/98, indicating that she has documented White-Coat Syndrome.

But Maggie was really struggling a few years ago when she was confronted with symptoms of menopause. She complained of hot flashes as well as chest tightness and heart pounding under stress. She would wake up in the middle of the night soaking wet, feeling an irregular heartbeat. Menopause, with its accompanying random fluctuations in estrogen production and release, is a primary cause of these disconcerting changes that Maggie experienced. Her sensation of chest tightness most likely was associated with periods of higher heart rates. I told Maggie that her hormones were most likely the cause of her symptoms, not her heart.

For the last few years she has remained symptom-free on a combination of Premarin 0.625 mg and progestins (Medroprogest 1.5 mg) to ease the fluctuating estrogen levels that were kicking off her vasomotor system. In addition to a calcium channel blocker (Isoptin), Maggie also takes 1,000 mg calcium with vitamin D every day.

For optimum health, she also takes a multivitamin, B complex, and vitamins C and E. HRT worked for Maggie in this instance, but not every woman may need—or tolerate—HRT. Jobeth's is a case where a targeted nutritional program was the answer.

Jobeth's husband had consulted me for advice about a good recovery strategy after his bypass operation. When he was hit with heart disease at only fifty-seven years of age, his wife decided that the whole family should be evaluated for cardiac risk. She knew that she herself had a high cholesterol level. And, at fifty-two, she was starting to experience some "skipped heartbeats" while she was lying down. Her seventy-eight-year-old father was being treated for palpitations, but there was otherwise no obvious family history for coronary artery disease. But she wanted to be sure, so Jobeth followed her intuition.

When she consulted with me, Jobeth was already seeing a naturopathic physician, so she was already on a sound preventive program. Her practitioner had felt that zinc and copper should be balanced in the body. She was surprised to hear me tell her that you could get too much of the heavy metal copper, which is oftentimes found in some multivitamins. She quickly exchanged the multivitamin she was taking for another formula containing minimal copper.

I did a complete cardiac evaluation for Jobeth, who had started perimenopause five years earlier at forty-seven. She had been somewhat symptomatic with hot flashes and sweating, but she experienced these changes as tolerable. Although she had a history of a low thyroid (her present thyroid function was normal), I felt that her elevated cholesterol and palpitations were most probably due to the hormonal swings of menopause.

We found that a simple program was helpful for Jobeth. The plan included a multivitamin-and-mineral combination, 60 mg CoQ10 three times a day, a magnesium (400 mg)/calcium (1,000 mg) formulation, and a "phytoestrogen shake" of soy milk and ground up flaxseeds. This combination should help to stabilize her heartbeat irregularity directly as well as provide her with the phytoestrogens from the flax and soy to help balance her hormone levels and indirectly reduce her symptoms. Jobeth reports feeling much relief of her symptoms on this simple dietary and supplemental combination. Many patients will achieve a favorable response with just magnesium and CoQ10. For annoying palpitations or if symptoms persist, I frequently add 1 to 2 grams of L-carnitine. A sound multivitamin/antioxidant formulation, along with CoQ10, is also great cardiovascular prevention for the future.

Balancing the Risk for the Moderate Risk Woman

Multiple considerations often play into the decision for a moderate risk woman. Although Maggie showed dramatic improvement on Premarin, another moderate risk woman with a different profile—for example, only one risk factor, no known risk for osteoporosis or breast cancer, and no menopause symptoms—might even consider bypassing the topical estrogens and use dietary sources for estrogen replacement. Again, every woman is different, and each must choose the solution that works best for her.

IV—If Your Heart Disease Risk Is Low

A woman with no family history and no known cardiac risk factors is considered at low risk for heart disease. However, low risk does not mean no risk: she will still experience the loss of cardiovascular protection that comes with the declining estrogen production of aging and should take steps to protect herself. Fortunately, she can do this easily by integrating phytoestrogens into her diet, via foods, nutritional supplements, and herbs. (See Chapter 11 for more on phytoestrogens.)

Joan: Story of a Low Risk Woman

Joan came to see me for a consultation after hearing me speak on nutritional alternatives in Boston. At forty-eight, Joan had a history of mitral valve prolapse (for more on MVP, see Chapter 8) since she was eighteen. Eight months prior to her office visit, she had been diagnosed with hyperthyroidism and told she was in menopause.

Tuning in to her own good sense and using a lot of her own intuition, she set out on her own path until she found the answers that she needed.

Joan had been told she had asthma at age thirty. When she was thirty-eight, she had a subtotal hysterectomy. Hormone therapy was never even a consideration at that time. But all in all, she felt that things were going smoothly. She was told that doctors heard the classic "click" of MVP, but she was unaware of any symptoms except some occasional fatigue.

Then, at age forty-seven, Joan started having heart palpitations and often awoke in the middle of the night with a racing heartbeat. She struggled with bouts of intense anxiety, hot flashes, and swollen feet. Her blood pressure was up. Joan's tests indicated that her thyroid was working overtime. The thyroid medication her doctor started did relieve the rapid heartbeat episodes and the hypertension, but she still continued to experience anxiety and middle-of-the-night anxiety attacks.

Another specialist took her off her long standing asthma medication, which may have been another culprit behind Joan's racing heartbeat. When she sought answers from a well known medical center, her physician felt her symptoms were "just menopause" and wanted to medicate her with estrogen for the fast heartbeat and lump-in-the-throat sensation that plagued her. Another physician told her that she had an ulcer in her throat and sent her to a throat specialist.

Joan felt frustrated. She had grown tired of the medication merry-go-round. She was gaining weight on the thyroid medication, and it was aggravating her asthma as well. She felt that everyone was trying to medicate her. Joan started to search for new alternatives. She read the data on breast cancer for women on estrogen: ERT was a treatment plan she felt she wanted to avoid if she could.

Joan next went to see an Ayurvedic physician. He told her that her iron was very low. She started on a three-month program that included Ayurvedic herbs, supplements, and a bowel cleansing program to detoxify her body and build up her blood. As Joan's energy improved, her other symptoms began to subside. Because her spouse had experienced relief of his circulatory problems on my recommended plan of ginkgo biloba, Joan consulted me to see if there was anything more she could do for her residual palpitations. Her family history for heart disease was negative, and her cholesterol, triglycerides, and blood sugar were all normal.

Joan's recent exercise stress test had been within the normal range, and her echocardiogram showed only a mild MVP. One of the tricks in Joan's evaluations has been isolating which symptoms were attributable to her overactive thyroid and MVP, and which ones may have been related to the hormonal changes of menopause.

For Joan, I added 30 mg CoQ10, three times daily, to treat her arrhythmia. Research has confirmed my own clinical experience with irregular heartbeats that respond well to simple CoQ10 supplementation. Studies have shown CoQ10, acting as what we call a "membrane stabilizer" on the heart's electrical conduction system, can make it harder for arrhythmias to get triggered in the first place. In one study of twenty-seven patients with a type of arrhythmia called PVCs (premature ventricular contractions), the PVC activity was significantly reduced after only four to five weeks of CoQ10 and was effective for up to 25 percent of the research participants. In my cardiology practice, I have found that 25 to 50 percent of the patients that I place on CoQ10 for arrhythmia control have had very positive results.

Also, Joan agreed to incorporate an antioxidant vitamin/mineral formula containing magnesium, a phytoestrogen shake, garlic, and ginkgo into her Ayurvedic plan. After three weeks on this nutritional program, Joan reported that her palpitations had subsided. She doesn't care much for the taste of the flax shake, so instead takes flaxseed oil and adds soy milk to her cereal each morning. For Joan, adding her own individualized, alternative approach to assuage her symptoms has made all the difference in her quality of life. And the good news is that Joan was very satisfied. A low-risk profile for heart disease coupled with absence of serious menopausal symptoms did not require any HRT.

What If You Have Pronounced Menopausal Symptoms?

For some women, the main issue is not whether or not to use hormone replacement for possible protection from heart disease but the desire to alleviate menopause symptoms so intense that quality of life is ruined. Susan, a nurse at my New England Heart and Longevity Center, has had this experience. Susan's early onset of menopause during her mid-thirties hit her very hard. She had all of the classic symptoms at amplified levels, including hot flashes several times an hour, day and night. These were accompanied by drenching sweats, racing heart rates, and "air hunger." She experienced not just "fuzzy thinking" but a profound loss in her ability to concentrate and think clearly. Susan is very gifted, and at the time her menopausal symptoms hit she was thinking about completing her studies for a PhD in neurophysiology. The early onslaught of symptoms made it impossible for her to continue.

Susan brought all her capabilities to bear on her problem: she is a licensed massage therapist and an expert in natural healing methods. She did not want to begin taking Premarin, so she tried to boost her estrogen levels using every natural remedy mentioned earlier. Nothing worked. She couldn't function: she was miserable physically and psychologically. Out of desperation, Susan began taking Premarin, and it worked a miracle for her. Within two days, she was sleeping through the night. After four days, the hot flashes stopped and so did the palpitations and air hunger. After three weeks, her brain came back on line. Her life completely changed, her symptoms disappeared, and she was able to function at her normal level. Then she started progestin (Provera) to lower her risk of endometrial cancer.

Within two days she was exhausted, achy, bloated, depressed, and her mental faculties and memory again began to fail—classic side effects of synthetic progesterone replacement. Her gynecologist cut her dose in half. Later, he reduced it by half again. He reduced the number of days she had to take it from fourteen to ten days per month. He also tried her on several other progestins—all with the same disastrous results. Additionally, her dose of Premarin was increased twice to counter the effects of the progestins.

On the advice of a reproductive endocrinologist, Susan tried oral micronized progesterone. She still had the same side effects, but to a lesser degree.

That was nearly ten years ago. Susan currently continues on Premarin 1.25 mg daily combined with 100 mg micronized progesterone twice daily for ten days each month. She still dislikes taking progesterone and is considering a further reduction in the dose. And, as she has learned more about botanically derived, bioidentical estrogen replacement, she is considering a change from Premarin. Until then, Premarin continues to be her biochemical lifeline. Without it, neither her body nor mind can maintain normal functioning. For her, the breast cancer risk was overridden because the

---

Anatomy of a Hot Flash

1. Sudden feeling of heat
2. Increased heart rate, palpitations
3. Flushing of skin
4. Sweating
5. Insomnia

Premarin, as with Janet earlier in this chapter, gave her back her quality of life. And, with Susan's small body frame and delicate bone structure, she is also a high-risk candidate for osteoporosis. Luckily for her, the hormone therapy that agrees with her so well will also offer her some protection from developing osteoporosis.

Because of its abrupt onset, Susan recognized her symptoms as being related to menopause, but not every woman will put the picture together so easily. *Many women mistake severe menopausal symptoms for heart disease.* I see this often in my practice: a woman

---

HORMONES: Quick Wrap-up

- **HRT IN ANY FORM, BE IT NATURAL OR SYNTHETIC,** for two to three years, may be your ticket to relieving menopausal symptoms and a bridge for you to achieve a better quality of life. Be reassured that unless you are already at high risk, your increased level of risk for breast cancer will be minimal. SERMs may be the answer for many women in the future, as they become more refined and natural.

- **FOR WOMEN WHO HAVE HAD A HYSTERECTOMY,** estrogen alone or estrogen with natural progesterone may be considered. Synthetic progestins should be absolutely avoided.

- **CONSISTENT RESEARCH DEMONSTRATES** that the longer the duration of HRT use, the greater the risk of breast cancer. (For example, a recent article in the January 26, 2000, *Journal of the American Medical Association* cites that in a new study of 48,000 women, 2,082 more cases of breast cancer were found in women on a estrogen/progestin regimens than on estrogen alone. The statistical analysis found that the "excess risk increased by 8 percent for each year of combined hormone use and by 1 percent for each year of estrogen-only use." The aggregate effect is an increase in breast cancer risk of 80 percent after ten years and 160 percent after twenty years.) For many women who have been on HRT for a decade or longer, the signal is clear: it's time to stop.

- **THE BOTTOM LINE FOR WOMEN** who may still be on the fence about hormonal use: A healthy diet, avoidance of smoking, regular exercise, nutritional supplements, and emotional healing may hold the answers for you.

comes to me complaining of heart palpitations, skipped heartbeats, rapid heartbeat—sometimes with sweating and insomnia. She's frightened and thinks she's having heart problems. We examine her and find no indication of heart disease, but we do find fluctuating estrogen levels. Her age is forty-five or a little older, and it turns out she is having classical menopausal symptoms.

I call this the "sheep in wolf's clothing" syndrome: a woman thinks her menopause symptoms are heart disease. Luckily, these women can get relief with most types of hormone replacement therapy. In such cases, I usually suggest starting with the gentler natural phytoestrogens or topical estrogen gels before progressing to the stronger topical patch. Finally, if that does not work, conventional HRT may be considered.

There's no getting around the fact that as we age, our risks for all kinds of problems increase, whether it's for breast cancer or heart disease or osteoporosis or any other chronic, age-related disease. Your best bet is to never lose sight of the big picture. Ask yourself: What is my greater risk? What do I want my quality of life to be? What risks can I live with in order to come out ahead for the most number of years? One thing is for certain: the controversy over HRT will go on. But we look forward to research now under way that will refine our knowledge and help women and their physicians make more informed choices. We expect women to become increasingly savvy about their choices, and insist on a true partnership with their health care providers. Do your homework, know your risks, invest in your own health, and you'll reap the rewards of a long, healthy life.

SECTION V

Heart Health for a Lifetime

CHAPTER THIRTEEN

Depression and Your Heart:
How to Break Through

Did you know that anyone who suffers from depression is *four times more likely* to get heart disease? Although the precise correlation isn't clear, some clinicians and researchers have speculated that depressed people are more likely to engage in self-destructive, addictive behaviors such as cigarette smoking, alcohol abuse, and overeating. Depressed people, who typically also have low self-esteem, are also less likely to engage in health-promoting activities such as exercise or to follow a healthy diet.

Researchers have also theorized that some of the chemical alterations involved in depression may also be implicated in the development of cardiovascular disease. We know, for example, that the physiology involved in depression stimulates the central nervous system, causing an increase in heart rate and blood pressure that over time can lead to excess wear and tear on the cardiovascular system.

Women appear to be more vulnerable to depression than men. For example, in the Nurses' Health Study, women who turned their anger inward instead of expressing it outwardly were more likely to develop depression. Some women may not consider venting their anger "feminine," but if it's not released, this emotion can become toxic and lead to clinical depression.

Although depressive disorders have a high prevalence in the general population, physicians have historically done a poor job recognizing subclinical signs of depression (where the individual is apparently able to function normally), perhaps because they have been unaware of its profound impact on health. Depression can be difficult to evaluate in a brief office visit, especially if the patient is compensating for it, acting "perky" when seeing the doctor in hopes of getting a cleaner bill of health. And another large component is that the individual may not even realize that she *is* experiencing depression. Denial is a major defense mechanism.

On any given day, it is estimated that 80 percent of patients seen in any physician's office are complaining of somatic symptoms—chest pain, arrhythmia, stomach upset, migraine headaches, various pain states, bowel irregularities, etc. I find this statistic to be a staggering reflection of how underdiagnosed depression is. Oftentimes, these complaints are physical manifestations resulting from an underlying depression.

As a consumer of the medical system, you must be aware of the signs and symptoms of depression so that you can be proactive in getting treatment for yourself or a loved one. I believe this awareness is critical to the health of every woman's heart and health.

Are You at Risk for Depression?

How can you recognize depression in yourself, a friend, or family member? And who is most at risk? First, *anyone recovering from a heart attack or bypass surgery is a serious candidate for depression.* Research has demonstrated that not only do depressed individuals suffer more heart attacks, they also have a higher incidence of sudden death as well. And for those recovering from heart attack or bypass surgery who are struggling with untreated depression, the risk of re-infarction or sudden death increases by 50 percent.

Many people are complacent, believing that "feeling low" is normal after a cardiac event. While fatigue after a heart attack or surgery is to be expected for the first month, *persistent feelings of sadness, loss of hope*, and other emotional states are not. Identifying and treating depression in cardiac patients is a key feature of primary prevention and a critical component in long-term recovery and quality of life.

I have learned that looking for the causes of depression is equally important in a *preventive* approach to cardiovascular disease. Women seem to be more vulnerable than men when it comes to depression. Research has also shown that these statistics may be skewed because, overall, more women report depressive symptoms. For example, the psychological impact of a *surgical scar* alone has a different effect on the emotional health of women recovering from heart surgery. Women generally tend to feel they have been violated; they often fear their partners will no longer find them attractive (see "Healing the Wound That Saved You" on page 266).

After a heart attack or cardiovascular surgery, *recovering women living alone* and/or those who perceive themselves as *lacking social support* are at greater risk for depression as well. In fact, lack of social support is correlated with higher complication rates for both men and women. And, for both sexes, a *previous history of depression* appears to be the strongest predictor of depression following a heart attack or any other cardiac event.

Many of the *drugs prescribed* for a variety of medical problems have also been reported to cause or be associated with mood symptoms as side effects. These medications include antihypertensives, antiarrhythmics and cardiovascular drugs, hormones (including steroids and birth control pills), histamine-2 receptor blockers (such as Cimetidine/Tagamet), anticonvulsants, Levodopa, antibiotics, and chemotherapeutics. Possible medication side effects need to be evaluated by your health care provider. Your pharmacist is another good resource for information about medications and interactions.

Because the affected individual may not recognize symptoms, it is also extremely important for family members and friends to be on the watch for these telltale signs of depression which are often part of a cluster of symptoms:

❖ excessive fatigue;
❖ lack of motivation;
❖ sleep disorders (over/under-sleeping, disrupted sleep due to premature awakening);
❖ loss of appetite (or overeating);
❖ weight loss (or gain);
❖ lack of pleasure in life;
❖ disinterest in hobbies, activities, and relationships.

If you, or a loved one, exhibit one or several of these symptoms, I urge you to talk to them about it. Perhaps she has been afraid to discuss the possibility of depression and will be relieved to have someone else take the initiative. You and/or your loved one will need to consult a physician and share your concern. Sometimes the doctor who knows you best, such as an internist you have had for years, is the best person to help.

Support, Nutrition, and Light:
Three Steps to Lifting Depression

I'm sure that many of you are familiar with the popular drugs Prozac and Paxil, or *selective serotonin reuptake inhibitors* (SSRIs). Prozac and other SSRIs are widely prescribed because of their effect on serotonin levels. Serotonin is a brain neurotransmitter that carries signals from one brain cell to the next via specialized receptors. It does many things: in addition to regulating your moods, appetite, and sleep patterns, it enhances your optimism, mental focus, and sense of control. Stress, along with poor diet, lack of exercise, and excess caffeine and alcohol consumption, can further deplete your serotonin stores. Another important neurotransmitter is *beta endorphin*, whose main job it is to ease physical and emotional pain. This natural opiate can also control anxiety, reduce anger, and even relieve certain types of depression. Without adequate levels of these two key neurotransmitters, chemical deficiencies in the brain can result in anxiety, depression, carbohydrate cravings, food bingeing, mood swings, and sleep disorders.

Drugs like Prozac and Paxil work by blocking the absorption of serotonin at the nerve synapse, thus prolonging its effects in the brain. Now, while there are many people who need these drugs because of chemical imbalances in the brain, they can have a host of side effects, including rebound anxiety, tingling in the extremities, and dependence, and are intended to be used only as a short-term bridge to better health. I believe there are better ways of overcoming serotonin deficiency using family support, nutrition, and light.

Family Support Can Save Your Life

Family support and strong social ties are extremely important elements for supporting depressed family members. If the depression is more severe, antidepressant medication may be needed. One or more family members or even a close friend may need to spend time with the depressed person so that she feels less isolated. This is usually a short-term arrangement until the depression begins to lift. Psychotherapy or counseling may be recommended to explore the possible unconscious roots of the depression and reshape cognitive behavior. In some cases, short-term hospitalization may be necessary.

Combat Depression with Nutrition

My nutritional plan for depression is quite simple. I recommend that you follow a low-sugar, adequate-protein diet to provide essential amino acids necessary to support the formation of critical nervous system chemical transmitters. This translates into about four to five ounces of protein with every meal in order to stimulate steady production of tryptophan, which is the building block of serotonin, or the "happy" chemical in the brain. In addition, there is increasing evidence that many depressed women are "sugar sensitive"—when they consume sugary foods, the result is heightened release of beta endorphin, the opiate-like, pain-blocking brain chemical. Unfortunately, for such people, eating sugar can be like drinking alcohol. It provides a short-lived "high," followed by a crash, rebound cravings, and relapse—not unlike an addiction.

WARNING:

IF YOU ARE PRESENTLY TAKING AN SSRI MEDICATION, MAO inhibitor, or any other antidepressant drug to increase your mood, then do *not* take St. John's Wort or any other herb unless you consult with your personal physician. Many people need medication for treatment of their symptoms, and your doctor is the one who knows you best. But if you already take a prescribed antidepressant for a depressive disorder and want to consider the possibility of taking any herb, *do not stop your medication abruptly* and switch to this or any other herb. It is necessary to time a transition period carefully for proper absorption and symptom management.

IF YOU TAKE ST. JOHN'S WORT IN COMBINATION
with any of these drugs, you may produce serotonin excess which may result in symptoms such as confusion, sweating, diarrhea, and/or muscle discomfort. If you are taking MAO inhibitors such as Parnate, Marplan, and Nardil or SSRIs like Prozac or Paxil, you must stop these drugs for at least five weeks before changing over. And remember that caffeine is also a drug that could counteract the effects of any herb you are taking.

If you suffer from mild depression from time to time or are recovering from heart surgery, incorporate a Mediterranean diet (see Chapter 4) into your lifestyle with these enhancements:

❖ **EAT MORE EGGS.** Eggs contain all the basic amino acids necessary to produce essential neurotransmitters such as dopamine and serotonin. They are also rich in sulfur and magnesium, both good for your heart. Eat up to six per week—and don't worry about the notion that eggs contribute to LDL "bad" cholesterol. That's an unfounded myth.

❖ **INCLUDE PROTEIN WITH EVERY MEAL.** In addition to salmon, I encourage you to eat a bit more meat and fowl because they are excellent sources of amino acids which support neurotransmitter function. Organic, range-fed meats are best. Turkey, chicken, and tofu as well as salmon, milk, soy milk, and scrambled eggs are all high in neurotransmitter-boosting tryptophan.

❖ **DON'T SKIMP ON ESSENTIAL FATTY ACIDS (EFAS).** These healthy fats are especially important for proper brain function. Prime sources are fish and flax. Eating two to three cold-water fish meals per week or using flaxseed oil (one teaspoonful daily) either drizzled on salads or mixed in a phytoestrogen shake (see recipe on page 365) are good ways to get your EFAs.

❖ **EAT A POTATO.** Researcher Kathleen DesMaisons, PhD, author of *Potatoes Not Prozac*, found that eating half a baked potato (with skin) before bed puts the biochemistry in motion to increase serotonin levels naturally. Potatoes, which have a moderately high glycemic index create a precisely timed, intentional "hit" of insulin to escort serotonin- and sleep-inducing tryptophan into the brain, yet due to their high satiety index are not likely to trigger carbohydrate cravings.

Healing The Wound That Saved You

"THE DOCTORS TOLD ME THAT SURGERY was absolutely necessary... the pain was my "message"... nothing else would help... my life was on the line... now, I have a second chance... so why can't I learn to love this scar?... I feel so different about me."

IF YOU ARE A WOMAN EXPERIENCING THESE FEELINGS of an altered body image, please take some comfort in knowing that you are not alone. Coming to terms with a chest scar can be very difficult for a woman. Many of my female patients have told me their scars make them feel very self conscious, especially those who derive a good deal of their self-esteem from the appearance of their chest, neckline, and legs. Some will no longer wear low necklines or short skirts because of it. Research has shown, in fact, that a surgical scar can lead to a prolonged adjustment for women, thereby affecting their ability to heal quickly. I'm sure it also can be an underlying reason for depression after cardiac surgery. After all, this sense of personal assault that women often experience isn't something they could have anticipated before surgery.

INTERESTINGLY, SOME MEN REPORT THAT, AFTER HEART SURGERY, they have found themselves crying for the first time at what seems to them to be at unusual times, such as watching a sad movie or reuniting with a loved one. They have felt dismayed, disarmed, and embarrassed by their new vulnerability. But they soften when I remind them, as I would you, that someone has literally and metaphorically "touched your heart," and your emotional life may never be the same. You've had your heart "opened" for you, though it may even have been the unplanned outcome of an emergency situation... and now you can really *feel*.

SO, IF YOU ARE A WOMAN TRYING TO COME TO TERMS with your scar, you may be using up a lot of psychic energy that you could be investing in feeling better. But now it's time to reframe your experience. I offer you the following imagery process. It has helped many women to accept their body as beautiful, just the way it is. Using a relaxation technique, allow yourself to tune out your external environment and tune in to your own inner voice.

FIRST, ASK YOURSELF THESE QUESTIONS AS YOU PONDER YOUR SCAR: "Why has this been placed in my path? What do I need to learn about myself? And what new path shall I choose now?"

CLOSE YOUR EYES AND THINK ABOUT THESE QUESTIONS, and, as you talk to your scar, see if a thought or an image arises as you go through this process. If you are fortunate enough to have something come to you, you may want to think about exploring its message. With time, the emotional attachment to your scar will recede, and the wound will soften. But the new "you" may chose to live in the world in a different way. The truth is that the scar is your blessing in disguise. Learn to honor it and cherish it, for it's given you a gift... and with this process of reframing... maybe it's not so bad after all.

Baked potatoes (or even a small slice of whole-grain toast or noninstant oatmeal) can be used as tools to control weight and depression, and induce sleep. Research has shown that severe carbohydrate cravings can be a result of serotonin deficiency, often exacerbated by trendy low-carb diets. One study showed that appetite was reduced in people taking Prozac, Paxil, or other SSRI drugs; in fact, some doctors were prescribing these drugs for weight control, regardless of the person's mood. Dr. DesMaisons has found that potatoes have a similarly positive impact on eating and mood behavior without the side effects.

❖ **EXERCISE AWAY THE BLUES.** Exercise is another intervention that I prescribe, particularly for mildly depressed people. I recommend a low-level exercise program, with simple walking twice a day. You can start with as little as five- to ten-minute periods and increase gradually to thirty minutes as it feels comfortable for you. Just try it and see your mood gradually elevate to higher levels. Take a partner and share the walk when you can! And remember, walking outdoors is a great double play to combat depression because you're also getting exposure to natural light (which I'll mention again later).

You may even consider a group endeavor, such as a cardiac rehabilitation program or a health club, to add the element of camaraderie and social support to some of your workouts.

There, trained professionals can assist you to develop an exercise prescription, gradually increasing your exercise tolerance over time. I highly recommend that if you do try a health club, find one with an exercise physiologist on staff to supervise your program. They have advanced training in the special considerations for exercising cardiac patients.

Natural Supplements for Depression

The development of supplemental and herbal treatments for depression has been an exciting advance in nutritional healing in the 1990s. Over the last few years, I have grown quite comfortable recommending herbs such as St. John's Wort and *ginkgo biloba* as nutritional support systems to relieve underlying depression as well as to improve sleep quality.

The Medicinal Properties of St. John's Wort

Medical research both in Western Europe and America have demonstrated in controlled double-blind studies that St. John's Wort *(Hypericum perforatum)* is an effective treatment for mild depression with minimal side effects. In other studies, sleep quality was improved with St. John's Wort. The mechanism of action for St. John's Wort appears to be similar to the pharmacological drug Prozac. In fact, many alternative health professionals call St. John's Wort an "herbal Prozac." In my practice, I recommend St. John's Wort as a natural therapeutic approach and herbal alternative to drugs such as Prozac, Zoloft, and Paxil for mild to moderate depression and in the treatment of seasonal affective disorder (SAD). Several flavonoids give St. John's Wort its medicinal properties.

St. John's Wort is native to many parts of the world, including North America and Europe. It grows especially well in the climate of northern California and Oregon. The herb comes from a perennial plant, two to six inches high, with yellow petals and is harvested for its medicinal purposes in July and August. It can be purchased year-round from most health food stores in either a tincture or capsule form. The usual recommended dose is 300 mg (3 percent Hypericin), up to three times daily. Look for a product that includes *standardized* Hypericin to be sure you are getting the full benefits.

Because cases of photosensitivity have been reported, it is recommended that you avoid long periods of sun exposure if you are taking St. John's Wort. In a study of 1,592 patients, mild gastric irritation was reported in a scant 0.55 percent.

In addition, this herb should *not* be used with SSRIs such as Prozac or MAO-inhibitors such as Nardil and Eldepryl, the "smart drug" that enhances dopamine in the brain. In fact, you should never use St. John's Wort and Eldepryl—or *any* MAO-inhibitor and SSRI—together. That's because you run the risk of "serotonin syndrome"—excess secretion of serotonin which can trigger agitation, confusion, severe shivering, sleepiness, rapid muscle contraction, over-reactive reflexes, sweating, and even coma and death.

Ginkgo Biloba

Another nutritional supplement I've had success with in treating mood disorders is *ginkgo biloba*. Ginkgo is frequently used as a medicinal in Europe; in fact, more than five million prescriptions were written for this herb in Germany alone in 1988. Within my philosophy of treating the "whole" person, I have been recommending ginkgo to my patients for almost a decade for a wide range of conditions, including age-related memory loss, dementia, cardiovascular disease, arterial disease in the lower limbs, dizziness, ringing in the ears (tinnitus), impotence, and depression. This powerful herbal medicine has made a difference in the quality of life in many of my patients without the side effects of potent toxic drugs.

One of the most fascinating findings about ginkgo biloba is its tendency to concentrate in the brain tissues. Although I recommend ginkgo principally for cardiovascular health, it amazes me how many of my patients comment on clearer thinking, improved mood, alertness, and better memory. Many of my elderly patients also report a marked reduction in anxiety.

The ginkgo tree is one of the oldest living plant species, tracing back more than two hundred million years. Its medicinal aspects come from ginkgo biloba extract (GBE), containing active ingredients ginkgo flavone glycosides (bioflavonoids) and terpene lactones (ginkgolides and bilobalide). The actions of these bioflavonoids are responsible for the antioxidant action of ginkgo as well as its ability to help prevent platelet stickiness leading to blood clotting.

Research suggests that the primary actions of GBE include a blood-thinning effect by inhibiting platelet stickiness, dilatation of blood vessels, and better utilization of glucose and oxygen uptake, even under situations of vascular insufficiency. All of these actions improve blood circulation and sugar metabolism in various tissues, including the brain.

More than forty scientific trials have confirmed that GBE derived from the leaves of the ginkgo tree is an effective treatment for a host of medical conditions. In many of these trials, daily doses of 120 to 240 mg resulted in improvement of symptoms in six to twelve weeks. Ginkgo biloba has been effective in geriatric patients with resistant depression, and there is excellent research to show that GBE therapy may be effective in delaying the onset of Alzheimer's disease and even improving cognitive skills.

A study published in the *Journal of the American Medical Association* looked at the effect of ginkgo in 309 Alzheimer's patients with dementia. Most of the patients who took 120 mg ginkgo extract a day experienced no deterioration in cognitive skills over a six-month period, and more than 20 percent improved. However, most of the patients who took the placebo did deteriorate over time. The researchers concluded that the medicinal and antioxidant properties of ginkgo biloba extract protect brain cells from free radical oxidative stress. I typically recommend doses between 120 and 240 mg daily.

This herb is essentially free of serious side effects. According to recent research, less than 1 percent of people studied experienced a mild gastrointestinal upset and a few had an occasional, mild headache when taking ginkgo. However, I do not administer ginkgo to patients using Coumadin (a blood thinner) because of the compounded blood thinning effects. I would also not advise ginkgo for diabetics with severe retinopathy, or inflammation of the retina, because of the remote possibility of bleeding. I would also not recommend ginkgo in those patients taking chronic aspirin therapy because of some isolated case reports of bleeding. In most people, however, the health benefits of ginkgo far outweigh the risks.

"Lighten" Your Spirits

In addition to family support, psychotherapy, exercise, diet, and supplemental support, there is also another major approach to depression, and that includes light. Environmental lighting systems have been used to combat depression in psychiatric settings. Now they are available for use in your home or office.

Environmental lighting can also help with a milder form of depression that is chronic and occurs at particular times of the year: seasonal affective disorder (SAD). It is helpful to be aware of this condition so that you can take steps to intervene if you think it may be happening to you. Look for products that offer "full spectrum" lighting (see Resources, page 407).

Seasonal Affective Disorder:
A Source of Depression

I STILL REMEMBER RECEIVING THAT LATE NIGHT PHONE CALL from my younger sister, Maria, when she was living in the upper peninsula of Michigan. It was in the middle of a long, dark, cold northern winter. She called seeking the comfort of a close family member, sharing with me her feelings of sadness and despondency. I stayed up joking and reminiscing with her to ease what we then thought was a simple case of the midwinter "blues." She would later admit that this was to happen on two to three more occasions until she left this heavily wooded area with only limited sunlight and moved south. Once in sunny Florida, Maria no longer struggled with bouts of depressive-type symptoms.

MY SISTER WAS A TYPICAL CASE OF what is called *seasonal affective disorder* or SAD. This mood disorder is usually cyclic or seasonal and is often associated with a type of depression. Lack of natural light appears to be a precipitating factor. Long, dark winters, punctuated by late sunrises and early sundowns, are a major cause of the SADs that affect the majority of northern populations worldwide. Seasonal affective disorder rates are extremely high in Sweden, Denmark, Alaska, Maine, Wisconsin, Michigan, and Minnesota. It appears that climate and geography play major roles in this type of depression regardless of your genetic disposition for depression.

IN FLORIDA AND TEXAS THE REPORTED PREVALENCE is very low—about seven cases per 100,000. However, in the northern latitudes of Massachusetts, Minnesota, and Maine, up to one in ten people may be affected by SAD, especially during the holidays and in the depth of winter.

IT IS TRUE THAT THE END OF DAYLIGHT SAVINGS TIME can trigger the seasonal blues. Those who work indoors, driving to and from work in the dark, fail to "see the light of day." This lack of natural light exposure causes many to feel depressed. And, because the mind and the body are so connected, when you are depressed emotionally, your immune system also becomes depressed, increasing your overall risk of illness. What's really needed is *more light*. When "turning on" to light in its natural form is limited, we can find a helpful substitute in the form of light therapy.

FOR MY SISTER, A SIMPLE MOVE TO FLORIDA, with its longer, sunny days, cured her depression. But for others of us living in the higher latitudes, including myself, an environmental source of natural light is definitely the way to go. I believe that the right kind of light can make a difference in your physical and emotional health and well-being.

NATURAL LIGHTING IS LIKE INDOOR SUNLIGHT. Sunlight or natural light possesses the "full spectrum" of different light wavelengths, resulting in photochemical reactions that enhance emotional and physical well-being. If you, too, want to nurture your body and your mind, and help prevent the negative impact that darkness has on your life, consider installing natural lighting in your home or office as a way of improving your mood, and ultimately your cardiovascular health.

LIVING IN THE NORTHEAST, MY WIFE JAN AND I make sure to have natural light in both our office and home. In fact, we've noticed that even our plants at home with the winter "droops" perked up and greened up when we accidentally placed them in the path of our environmental desk lamps.

CHAPTER FOURTEEN

Cultivate the Mind-Body Connection

"But Doctor! I did everything right! I changed my diet, added supplements, started an exercise program, lost weight, stopped smoking, and cut my stress level at work. Why isn't my heart getting better?"

I hear this kind of frustration in my office all too often. Some of my patients have invested heavily in their physical recovery, only to require more medication, yet another angioplasty, or bypass surgery. What's missing? I believe strongly that there are powerful "conversations" going on between the heart and the head... something I refer to as the "heart-brain hotline."

"See a Therapist? What for? I'm Not Crazy!"

Looking at the emotional component of disease, as we did in Chapter 13, is something I believe in with my whole heart, but addressing this often-overlooked aspect of healing may require more than simply lowering your "stress level"—especially if you already have a heart condition. Many times your sensitivity to external stressors is just the tip of the iceberg. What often lies just beneath the surface are more deeply ingrained behavior patterns that usually go all the way back to early childhood.

These old knee-jerk responses may show up as maladaptive behavior patterns—like overworking, overeating, or excessive drinking. Oftentimes, simply *identifying* your habitual patterns just isn't enough to dig you out from under them. Insight is one thing, but action is another, and as I've said before, turning your health risk around requires that you take a very proactive stance. We *all* have blind spots, living out familiar stories based on unconscious decisions made years, even decades ago. There are countless dialogues that we have with ourselves every day, and some of them can be the roots of our myths about life. What you *think* can affect how you act and what you feel. How many of these self-talk phrases do you hear going on in your head?

"If folks knew who I really am, they might not like me."
"If I really work hard, then they'll value and appreciate me."
"Deep down inside, I know I'm not really good enough."
"If an uncomfortable feeling comes up, I don't have to feel it if I don't want to. I can just keep busy, or take another drink."
"Having something to eat always makes me feel better."
"Ugh! I screwed up again! I can't do anything right."
"I know my schedule is too busy, but if I'm alone with myself, I feel depressed."
"Nice girls (women) don't ever lose their temper or get angry.... at least not in public."
"Assertive women are too aggressive; you might get labeled a bitch."
"If I don't risk being vulnerable, at least I won't get hurt again."

Like shorthand for a way of life, such secret narratives do more than limit your future possibilities—over time, they can take a toll on your health as well. When their health is at stake, I often recommend that my patients try psychotherapy. I have found that what is most difficult for my patients to realize is that their physical disease may be an emotional symptom that is traveling incognito. It may be a disguised issue with psychological roots that are just as significant as any medical illness. In my experience, it helps to explore these life issues with a trained professional, be it a competent counselor, a professional therapist, or coach.

Perhaps you're thinking: "Who me? See a therapist? What for? I'm not crazy!" You may have been misinformed about what psychotherapy is all about. Maybe you think you have to be deeply depressed, desperately anxious, or so stressed out that you are having trouble functioning before therapy is warranted. You may think that it will take years to get anywhere in therapy, and that medication is inevitably a part of the picture. Nothing could be further from the truth. It is important to explore the hidden subconscious issues we all have in order to truly heal, mind, body, and spirit.

How Badly Do *You* Want to Get Well?

Arlene was a forty-six-year old executive who was still depressed one year after her myocardial infarction and bypass surgery. Like many women and men, she found out abruptly that she had heart disease: her heart attack had come on "out of the blue." Although now back to work full time, she was napping on her lunch hour, and again before dinner. Arlene continued to have occasional bouts of crying and her love life was still "on hold."

Now that she had returned home to her domestic roles as wife of a workaholic husband, mother of a teenager seeking his own identity, daughter to an ailing mother, and school educator to classes overfull with students, she encountered a sense of despair and sadness that she didn't really understand.

Arlene also struggled with regular bouts of anxiety, leaving her exhausted much of the time.

In short, Arlene was stuck in a combination of stressors, many of which had predated, and possibly had even contributed to, her heart attack. But she was also unaware that some of this sadness was really grief—and it was blocking her recovery. Not only was she still grieving the loss of her previous health status, she was filled with losses and heartbreaks that went back to an infidelity in her early marriage, and even beyond to her childhood. The problem with grief is that, as each one of us grieves a recent loss, it also brings up all the old losses we have ever had over our lifetime, many of which may never have been grieved fully. Many people suppress their grief or push through it rapidly, either because it is too uncomfortable or because they feel driven to get on with their lives, perhaps for the sake of others. Living in denial is a time-tested way to avoid feeling grief or heartbreak. The problem is that old, unresolved hurts and losses accumulate and can influence how we handle a current loss.

For Arlene, as for many others, going through a heart attack and bypass surgery had provoked some old areas of psychic pain. But her operation also had the potential to start her on an even deeper journey of emotional healing. I suggested to Arlene that she consider working with a psychotherapist for a while. She readily agreed.

Only a few months later, she shared what she had learned about her response to heart disease. Her heart attack had come on the anniversary of her father's death. Arlene's father had been forty-six when he had his first myocardial infarction. In therapy she recalled her father's long recovery. Arlene's sixteen-year-old son was now the same age that she had been when she was first dealing with her father's heart disease, and the illness had seemed catastrophic to her.

Patients were hospitalized for much longer periods when Arlene had been a girl, and oftentimes they had overly strict guidelines on physical exertion. The limitations her father's "bad heart" placed on him and the family had impressed her deeply. In many ways, her father had never been the same after his heart attack; it was as if his spirit had been broken. Arlene realized that she had started to lose her dad right after that very first myocardial infarction when he had become emotionally distant and preoccupied with his own concerns.

It was through therapy that Arlene finally understood that her father had suffered from clinical depression after his heart attack. In the process, she realized that she still carried a lot of old beliefs—"baggage"—about the meaning of the diagnosis of heart disease. Her unconscious expectation was that life would "never be the same" for her or her family. She began to understand the power of an "anniversary" reaction: her heart had reenacted the hurt she had experienced with her father's death so many years before. Our bodies have a way of "remembering" and recreating scenarios that go beyond anything we can explain with science.

Arlene's first response to her diagnosis had been colored by an experience that had happened long ago at an impressionable age. (If Arlene's dad had had a speedy recovery and a more positive outcome, she probably would have had a more positive expectation for herself.) Becoming aware of her expectations and beliefs through therapy began to turn her recovery around. She used her discoveries to reach out to her own son so that he could have a different experience than she had lived through. She vowed to break the cycle of depression that she realized was coloring her own world view before it tainted her son's emotional growth.

Arlene was dismayed at first to acknowledge the depth of her spouse's underlying depression and negativity, but started to identify ways to address her home environment. She was able to reframe her own beliefs and expectations by having conversations with positive-minded people—especially women—who were using heart disease to turn their lives around and redefine their priorities. She sought out upbeat people to spend time with, modeling their attitudes and beliefs until her new way of life started to feel more natural than her habitual way of "seeing the glass as half empty."

Learning that depression could put her at risk for future cardiac problems (people with untreated depression are twice as likely to have another cardiac event) was an added motivation for Arlene. Finally, she was ready and willing to "take charge" of her own healing. She started unearthing the myths she had about life and love, heart disease and recovery, and confronted and dismantled them one by one.

Understanding the Value of Doing Inner Work: A Paradigm Shift

Increasingly, health care practitioners see "disease" as a process that emerges from a chaotic imbalance in the *whole* person. Ultimately, I view the heart as a pulsating jewel, a metaphorical and physiological core of the energies and conversations linking body, mind, and spirit. Take a moment to picture your own heart in this way— it could change how you think about your heart.

Recall a time when you were "falling in love." Was there not an unexplainable "melting" in your chest when you saw your beloved? Or, if you think about someone you have loved deeply in your life—parent, child, friend—do you not feel a warm sensation in your chest? And what about negative emotions such as anger, anxiety, and fear? Most of us know what we are most afraid of, but how do you determine, for instance, that you "feel afraid?" Is it just from the mind's recognition of a bodily sensation? What about all the times your fear is activated by your thoughts, your anticipation of that which you dread? There is a growing body of evidence to support the concept that *what you think does affect what you feel.* And whatever one feels affects the heart at its most fundamental level: how fast it beats, how well it pumps.

Fear and Love: the Most Visceral of All Emotions

Fear often causes the heart to beat rapidly and forcefully. Fear may even cause palpitations, a sensation of pounding and irregularity of the heartbeat, which is often interpreted as distressful by the individual. I have seen this cardiac response occur when fearful patients were attached to cardiac monitors. Those who have experienced panic attacks will tell you that their greatest anxieties originate from rapid heartbeats and sensations in their heart that they identify as overwhelming.

Emotions such as fear and panic set up a type of negative feedback loop in the heart. Fear can trigger an adrenaline release which, in turn, overstimulates your heart, increasing your heart rate and causing it to fire off extra beats. As you feel your heart speeding up or beating irregularly, you become even more anxious, prompting your system to pump out even more stress hormones—and the vicious cycle continues.

Love may also cause an increase in heart rate and pumping action, but in this instance its effects are perceived as nurturing rather than threatening. Ask anyone who has ever been in love, and he or she will tell you that their heart beat faster when they saw, embraced, or even thought about the one they loved. Correlated with such positive emotion, the awareness of the heartbeat is overshadowed by the pleasurable sensations of deep excitement and passion. And so, the same symptoms of "heart flutters" are attributed to a positive source, and we feel "lighthearted," carefree, exuberant, and joyful.

As you can see, perception has a lot to do with how we interpret what may be going on in our hearts. And whether one perceives a particular experience—such as speaking to a large group—as threatening or satisfying is actually a very personal experience. Whether we are filled with excitement or dread in the moments before we stand up to speak is also a reflection of our early life experiences, belief systems, and expectations. The "heart-brain hotline" involves both conscious and unconscious dimensions—and it can be explained in terms of physiology.

When Your Sympathetic Nervous System Is Not Always so Sympathetic

You've probably heard of people who performed superhuman feats, such as lifting a car off a child's foot. What's happened in this instance is that the sympathetic nervous system (SNS) has kicked in, releasing hormones like adrenaline and norepinephrine. This release of physical power, negation of pain, and mobilization of energy—expressed as strength, speed, or struggle—are all part of the classic "fight-or-flight" response to stress. In such an emergency, the SNS can actually save your life.

This physiology worked extremely well for our ancestors—like the cavemen who needed to get out of the path of a charging woolly mammoth in a big hurry. Blood is shunted to the heart, to pump faster; to the brain, to think faster; to the eyes, to see more keenly; and to the skeletal muscles to fight or flee. Capillary beds clamp down to prevent bleeding. When a caveman's SNS was activated, energy was quickly mobilized and discharged in the service of self-preservation. But today, more modern anxieties have replaced the woolly mammoth: traffic jams, fear of downsizing at the office, overwork—the list goes on.

Chronic activation of your SNS from these daily stressors has tremendous potential to harm you, for two reasons. The first is wear and tear on your heart and circulation. The second happens when body systems "shut down" to fuel states of hyperarousal—

digestion, immune-system activity, sexual drive, and repair of tissues are all inhibited. In fact, research has shown that staying in SNS "overdrive" increases your risk of developing one form of diabetes, and there is evidence that stress-induced high blood pressure can encourage the formation of atherosclerotic plaques.

But wait! The parasympathetic nervous system (PNS) is standing by to balance the SNS by initiating actions that bring SNS functions back down to earth. The PNS lowers blood pressure, reduces heart rate, returns blood to the extremities, and restores calm. Such softening, expanding, and letting down are components of what Dr. Wilhelm Reich called his model of expansion and contraction.

According to Reich, a contemporary and colleague of both Sigmund Freud and Albert Einstein, the parasympathetic nervous system operates in the direction of expansion, "out of self toward the world," including emotions of pleasure and joy. Reich viewed the sympathetic nervous system as operating in the direction of contraction, pulling the individual "away from the world, into the self," and contributing to emotions such as sadness and suffering. At a cellular level, Reich viewed what he called our "life force" as being in a continuous health-promoting rhythm, alternating between expansion and contraction.

Reich introduced his concept of "body armor"—patterns of chronic muscular tension that form an elaborate defense mechanism and protection from both the outside world and one's own interior pain—in the 1940s. In his book, *Character Analysis* (1938), Reich proposed that there are "energetic blocks" in the body, reflecting unconscious defense mechanisms where the body has armored, or defended itself, against psychological (emotional) assaults. It is these areas of contraction or stagnated energy, he suggests, that lead to psycho-physiological imbalance and eventually disharmony or illness. According to

Reich, the fragmented parts of the self must be reintegrated to reestablish health and balance. His studies and research led to a type of psychotherapy grounded in working directly with the body that would later be known as bioenergetic therapy.

Bioenergetic Therapy—Best-Kept Secret for Healing the Heart

In a nutshell, bioenergetic therapy uses the language of the body to heal the problems of the mind. "The life of an individual is the life of his body," concluded Alexander Lowen, MD, a student of Reich's who expanded his mentor's research into a broader understanding of the connection between emotional conflict and physical expression. Lowen described all therapy as an adventure in self-discovery. As the founder of bioenergetic therapy, he offered a body-mind approach that has a liberating and positive effect on emotional, physical, and psychic distress. Here's how it works:

The bioenergetic therapist first "reads" the client's body, using information about the physical to understand the personality behind the character structure. The goal of therapy is to reveal the client's core issue(s) so that, with awareness, insight, and body work, he or she may experience more feeling—more life.

The next step is to assist the client in discovering how his or her body works energetically, by pointing out chronic areas of tension that create muscular "blocks," the result of long-suppressed emotions. These tensions can then be addressed through direct body work, such as bioenergetic exercises or emotional release.

Bioenergetic therapists often work with those grappling with physical illness, such as asthma, high blood pressure, heart disease or chronic back pain, and assist them to understand the messages the body may be trying to send about their emotional health. For example, both men and women with heart disease often have a high, inflated chest that rarely moves freely, even with conversation. The bioenergetic therapist may interpret this type of body structure as indicating an old hurt or heartbreak, so longstanding that the body has literally "armored" itself to avoid being hurt again. The client's core issue may involve being unable to take love in—or be loved—so frequently the therapist needs to help the patient release deep heartbreak with crying and sobbing so that it will not contribute to heart disease.

An individual with high blood pressure might be evaluated as having excessive tension in the arms, shoulders, and upper back. This posture signifies unresolved anger that needs to be acknowledged, addressed, and released to restore physical and emotional health. A firmly held, jutting-out jaw suggests over-control and an excessive will to dominate. These and other habitual body postures can lead to an excessive stimulation of the sympathetic nervous system and a subsequent energy drain on the heart, causing cardiac vulnerability.

Bioenergetic therapy is *experiential*—it goes beyond "talk" therapy in that the therapist will often use specific body positions designed to first encourage deep, free breathing and later release emotional expression. The physical posture used in any session is selected to be appropriate to that particular client at that particular moment.

Emotional release in bioenergetic therapy is designed to bring a new sense of freedom and confidence to those looking to heal anxiety, depression, workaholic tendencies, stress, medical problems, sexual issues, and cardiac illness. This therapy can truly be the gateway to emotional, physical, and spiritual healing.

However, other types of therapy, such as gestalt, which strives for an understanding of conscious "here and now" behavior; and cognitive behavioral therapy (CBT), which looks at your beliefs and expectations, are also excellent interventions for the cardiac patient. Many times, a patient will first explore these forms of therapy before going to a higher level with bioenergetics.

There is a deeper, more spiritual place waiting to be discovered in each of us, a place of knowing that some refer to as an inner healer or advisor. One of the therapies that delves further into this realm is Reiki, which taps into spiritual energy. Reiki is often used to help people take the "leap of faith" to enter therapy. As we discussed in Chapter 7, it may take praying or quieting yourself through meditation to get in touch with this part of yourself, but cultivating the spiritual dimension is essential to true healing.

Seek out sound advice, first and second opinions, and plan the strategy that works best for you. When you truly believe in the plan of action you are directing for yourself, you will see that investing in exercise programs, vitamin supplements, and therapy are of equal importance as spending your money on dining out, new clothes, a new hairdo, or decorating your home. Your health care choices are an investment in your future. When you take charge of your own healing process, your new sense of purpose will enhance your quality of life.

Changing your stance from one of reaction to one of action will pay off in long-term benefits for yourself and others around you. Sometimes it involves learning to trust yourself to know what you need, and sometimes it means trusting another who has the courage to speak up and confront you with "the truth" you don't want to see.

"But How Do I Know Who to See? Who to Trust?"
Maybe you have already made the decision to explore psychotherapy but have no idea who to tell or where to begin. Choosing a therapist may seem like a challenging task. But here are some guidelines that can make the process easier for you. Most importantly, remember—you're in charge.

1. AVOID WAITING UNTIL YOU ARE IN CRISIS TO SELECT A THERAPIST. While crisis does not preclude seeking assistance (there are crisis counselors trained to work with those in this type of traumatic situation), it is easier if you can go through this selection process thoughtfully.

2. ASK FOR REFERRALS. Start with your physician, who may already have a satisfactory relationship with one or more therapists. By satisfactory,

---

Ten Tips for Psychological Well-Being

1. Surround yourself with people who believe in you and what you are doing.

2. Avoid those who are sharply critical or negative toward your plan to collaborate with your care providers.

3. Choose health care providers who are caring, take the time to inform you of treatment options, and support your participation in planning your own care.

4. Decline some treatment options if, after extensive information gathering, it doesn't feel like the right path for you to take.

5. Take a serious look at health care providers who have a negative bias toward adjunctive therapies such as nutritional supplements, psychotherapy, prayer, etc.

6. Create in your home a healing atmosphere. Don't avoid confrontations, but do openly share and discuss your feelings, even if anger comes up. Enjoy quiet music, make one room a "safe" place to rest, or read. Or just be still.

7. Take a risk. Do the thing that may seem the hardest to do. Go off the beaten path when you need to. Try acupuncture, massage, Reiki, energy work.

8. When selecting strategies for yourself, stick with the ones that feel right or helpful. Discontinue any route you explore if it doesn't feel right for you as an individual even though it may have worked for others.

9. Learn to love yourself. And nurture loving relationships in your life. Take in the love of others... it's life affirming and healing.

10. Above all, learn to listen to and trust your own intuition. Believe that no one knows *you* better that *you* do. You are the best person to plan your own care.

I mean that their patients are seen in a timely fashion and have given the physician positive feedback about their experience. Your physician may recommend a social worker (MSW), a marriage/family therapist (MFT), a psychologist (PhD), a nurse-psychotherapist (MSN/CNS/ APRN), psychiatrist (MD), or a clergy/counselor depending on his/her assessment of your individual need. You may have a personal preference as well. I recommend psychotherapists trained in bioenergetics because they work directly with your body and its energy blocks. Be confident that you can collaborate in this process with your doctor to be sure that you are comfortable and find the type of therapist with whom you would work best. Also, check your insurance coverage to see what training level may be necessary to receive reimbursement. Check to see if there is a co-pay amount, or a list of providers from which to choose. However, don't be afraid to invest your money in a therapist who's not "on your plan" if you feel that person may be the best match for your needs.

Ask friends for referrals. Oftentimes psychotherapists in your area may have reputations for being helpful. Therapists may often have special areas, so don't be afraid to inquire.

Check the Yellow Pages under counselors, therapists, or psychotherapists. They are listed under specialties and may have brief descriptive ads.

3. BRIEFLY INTERVIEW YOUR POTENTIAL THERAPIST ON THE PHONE. Most therapists will define their specialty or scope of practice during a brief phone call. This is a good time to discuss issues of fees and potential insurance reimbursement. You will both get a rough idea of whether or not you could work together. You should feel free to ask about the therapist's type of licensure, where they trained, and their experience level.

4. SCHEDULE A ONE- TO TWO-HOUR INITIAL ASSESSMENT SESSION. This is an opportunity for therapist and client to meet personally and explore their comfort level for working together. The therapist can describe his or her usual style as well as help you to assess your particular goals from the therapeutic process. In this session you can both see if you feel like a "good fit." During this initial session, ask yourself the following:

❖ What is my overall goal for seeking assistance?

❖ Does this individual feel like someone with whom I could build a trusting relationship?

❖ Do I feel intimidated by this person? Or, do I feel "seen" as an individual and understood as a person?

❖ Does this person seem relatively confident that he or she has the skills to work with my particular problems, needs, and goals?

❖ Does this office feel like a safe, supportive environment?

Choose a therapist as you would a friend and work partner. Rest assured that a psychotherapeutic relationship is a highly confidential one. You are in control of who you see, how often, and for how long. The hardest part is always just taking those first few steps... but if you can break through that initial resistance, the rewards can be life-changing and the growth enormous.

CHAPTER FIFTEEN

Secrets of Aging Gracefully: Staying Fit and Healthy for a Better Life

With the passage of time, changes inexorably occur in the human body. From the minute we are born, we begin to age. The signs range from the obvious—weight gain, loss of height, muscular weakness; to the hidden—loss of elasticity in blood vessels, slowsut, and, most significantly, cellular damage from free radical activity.

I've seen a wide variety of physiological responses to the aging process. Some eighty-year-olds physically appear fifty to sixty. Conversely, I see middle-aged men and women who look like they are ready for retirement. Why do some people "age" faster than others? Remarkably, it turns out that aging is only about 30 percent genetic and 70 percent lifestyle! This is very good news indeed, for it means that *you* have a lot to say about how you age.

I like to attack aging both from the inside and the outside. While creams and lotions can help, to truly delay aging you need to address what's going on at the cellular level—the biochemical basis of aging.

Much research is now focusing on this biochemical/molecular aspect of aging. Investigators in California and Italy, for instance, have discovered that when mitochondria, the energy-producing part of cells, are impaired by free radicals banging around, they can't do their job effectively. This is especially important because mitochondrial DNA has no defense mechanism to repair itself like nuclear (cellular) DNA does. And mitochondria don't have many genes to spare, leaving them at high risk for early cell death, known as *apoptosis*. Researchers now believe that the areas of the body that are rich in mitochondria, such as the heart, pancreas, eyes, and muscles, are those most prone to the ravages of age-related diseases.

The newest anti-aging strategies seek to rein in free radicals in order to delay mitochondrial impairment. Provocative research points to the merits of "fertilizing" mitochondria with L-carnitine, coenzyme Q10 (CoQ10), alpha lipoic acid, vitamin E, and vitamin C. These targeted nutrients are able to get inside the mitochondrial membrane and support their function, thus preserving the life of these organelles. If you can delay premature loss of mitochondria, you can delay aging of the entire organism.

Even before the latest research came out, I was convinced that these five nutrients are major keys to unlocking the mystery of anti-aging medicine. I take them as supplements every day and suggest that you do, too. These five nutrients are a must for anyone interested in preventive and anti-aging medicine.

Some of the more serious consequences of premature aging—and the most insidious and damaging diseases of aging in women—are osteoporosis, breast cancer, and macular degeneration of the eye. Here are my specific strategies for preventing these diseases and minimizing your risk.

You *Can* Prevent Osteoporosis

Osteoporosis is one of the most damaging of all threats to post-menopausal women. Not long ago, Helen, a patient of mine, was scheduled to undergo surgery for a fractured hip due to osteoporosis. She didn't trip over a phone cord or fall down the stairs. Nor was she involved in an automobile accident. She was simply straining while lifting a window.

Stay Away From Diet Sodas

ALTHOUGH THERE HAVE BEEN VOLUMES OF BOOKS suggesting various diets for women of all ages, keep in mind that any particular style of eating may seriously affect your health. And one concern I have is that you may choose some products thinking that you are doing the right thing for your health, when just the opposite may be true. For example, consider the impact of one food product commonly consumed by women—young and old alike—to keep their calorie intake down and maintain their weight: diet sodas.

MOST SODAS, ESPECIALLY DIET DRINKS, CONTAIN PHOSPHORIC ACID, which can leach out calcium from your bones. This is not only crucial for all women, but all of us, including our young children. When I was a football coach for the team my younger son played on, I was shocked to see so many fractures occurring in young teens. It was almost like watching them take a not-so-nasty tumble and end up with a major bone break. At first I was baffled—but then I realized the probable source of many of these fractures. These twelve- to fifteen-year-olds had weakened bones, and I would bet that many of these kids were big-time soda drinkers, ingesting more phosphorus and phosphoric acid than their young bodies could manage.

ALTHOUGH MANY WOMEN ARE EXTREMELY KNOWLEDGEABLE about maintaining an adequate calcium intake to support good bone health, many do not know that phosphorus/phosphoric acid overload can be one of the major factors in facilitating osteoporosis. So if you are watching your calcium but slugging down those diet drinks, it's like pouring precious fuel into a tank that has a huge hole at the bottom.

This woman was one of many I have seen over the years who fractured a hip doing routine activities such as carrying groceries or climbing stairs. My own mother fractured her tibial bone as she abruptly shifted her weight when she was startled by a ringing telephone.

Although fractures may appear suddenly, osteoporosis, like heart disease, often develops silently and insidiously. Just as a heart attack may be the first symptom of heart disease, a spontaneous fracture may be your first sign of osteoporosis. Approximately twenty million Americans have fragile bones that are susceptible to fractures. Osteoporosis is the direct cause of more than 1.3 million fractures per year, including 250,000 hip fractures. Consider:

❖ Women are much more vulnerable than men to develop this degenerative process
❖ Osteoporosis is not an inevitable consequence of aging
❖ Contrary to previous teaching, osteoporosis is treatable
❖ Diet, exercise, and targeted nutritional support are vital steps to slow down bone loss.

What Are the Risk Factors for Weakened Bones and Fractures?

High risk is prevalent among thin, fine-boned women with a family history of osteoporosis. Other risk factors include excessive caffeine or alcohol use, cigarette smoking, adult-onset diabetes, inactivity, hormone deficiency, long-term use of thyroid medication or corticosteroids, overuse of phosphoric acid (common in diet soft drinks), and excessive protein in the diet. Dietary deficiencies, particularly of calcium, vitamin C, and vitamin D, also play an important role.

How Do You Know if Your Bones Are Developing Osteoporosis?

If you have one or more of the previously mentioned risk factors, it's best to have your bone density evaluated for early changes.

Knowing your baseline bone density measurement can give you valuable information about your vulnerability to bone loss and osteoporosis. One such bone test is called the SEXA (single electron X-ray absorptometer), which reads the bone density at the heel of your foot. Although this is a highly worthwhile screening mechanism that is becoming very popular, it is not as accurate as a full scale DEXA.

The most reliable test of bone density is the DEXA (dual energy X-ray absorptometer). This technique provides fast, precise measurements with minimal radiation-exposure risk to the patient. DEXA can

---

How Free Radicals Accelerate Aging

THE SEARCH FOR A UNIFIED VIEW OF AGING HAS BEEN THE FOCUS of considerable research. In my own research and study, I found the most compelling theory to be one proposing free radical oxidative stress as the primary agent responsible for accelerating the aging process. Here's what happens...

IT IS NOW WELL-DOCUMENTED THAT UNSTABLE MOLECULES known as free radicals can do considerable damage to cell membranes. Normally, these molecular marauders are neutralized by sufficient levels of antioxidants within the cells. But many factors—such as a poor diet of over-processed, nutrient-depleted foods, excessive stress or exercise, exposure to toxic chemicals in your everyday environment, or excessive radiation—can give free radicals a free rein to roam and damage like tiny terrorists.

NEITHER YOUR VASCULAR SYSTEM NOR YOUR HEART CAN completely escape this insidious process. The result is that the incidence of heart disease and other degenerative conditions increases with age—unless you fight back! Remember, rapid aging isn't inevitable. To minimize free radical damage and slow the rate of aging, use weight-bearing exercise, healthy foods found in a modified Mediterranean diet, and targeted nutritional support involving vitamins, minerals, and herbs.

be used to measure any part of the skeleton, including the forearm, hip, and spine, the most common fracture sites in those with osteoporosis. DEXA is valuable for menopausal women, and particularly for any woman who has sustained a fracture after relatively minor trauma.

The DEXA test should be performed only by experienced personnel. According to Robert Lang, MD, of Hamden, Connecticut, a nationally recognized authority on osteoporosis, errors in interpretation are not unusual, so it's important to have a well-qualified expert interpreting the DEXA. Follow-up measurements are usually recommended to ensure that bone density has been maintained or is increasing.

What Do You Do if the Test Results Show You Are at Risk for Osteoporosis?

Here are some easy steps to follow to help minimize your chance of developing the disease:

❖ **MAINTAIN A DIET ADEQUATE IN CALCIUM.** The National Institutes of Health (NIH) recommends the following approximate daily calcium levels:

Adolescents—1,200 mg
Adults—1,000 mg
Postmenopausal women—1,500 mg if *not* on estrogen replacement therapy (ERT); 1,000 mg if on ERT.

Although the average American diet supplies between 500 and 800 mg calcium daily, adding one to two glasses of skim milk or, better yet, one to two glasses of calcium-fortified soy milk daily should provide you with all the calcium you need.

Green leafy vegetables, asparagus, broccoli, and sea vegetables are all excellent sources of calcium. Tofu and other soy products are outstanding sources of calcium, and many contain other phytonutrients that support bone mass. If you cannot fulfill your calcium requirement from dietary sources alone, supplementation may be a suitable alternative.

But do not be overzealous—excess calcium, paradoxically, can also promote bone loss due to its interference with the absorption of another important mineral, manganese. Research has demonstrated that *calcium intake of more than 2,000 mg per day may be detrimental to your health* because of its negative impact on the absorption of magnesium. To avoid constipation from calcium supplementation and improve bone mineralization, be sure to take adequate magnesium, preferably in a 2.5:1 ratio of calcium to magnesium. A 1,000 mg calcium formula with 400 mg magnesium would be an ideal combination. I also recommend 1 mg boron to further enhance bone support.

❖ **TAKE IN VITAMIN D.** Inadequate vitamin D can be a problem for those who are confined indoors or have limited or no exposure to sunlight. This presents a dilemma for many women who reside in nursing homes or are just too fragile to go outside. Inadequate sunlight may also be a problem for many people who live in the northern latitudes. Just fifteen minutes of sunlight a day on exposed areas of the body—particularly the hands and legs—along with a healthy diet, should be enough to get your basic require-

---

What Causes Bones to Become Brittle?

THE CONSERVATION OF BONE DEPENDS UPON A DELICATE BALANCE between two types of cells. In healthy bone tissue, *osteoblasts*, the cells that support the protein matrix of new bone, are in a state of equilibrium with *osteoclasts*, the cells that clear away old bone. This dynamic relationship of bone formation versus bone resorption can be disrupted by many factors. When bone resorption outpaces new bone formation, osteoporosis occurs.

ment of vitamin D. Most high-quality multivitamin/mineral supplements also contain 200 to 400 I.U. vitamin D. The RDA for
vitamin D is 400 I.U. per day. Older people may safely take up to
800 I.U. per day.

❖ **MOVE!** Weight-bearing exercise is paramount in the prevention
of osteoporosis. There's no doubt about it—people who are sedentary are much more prone to osteoporosis. Walking at least twenty
minutes every day will help prevent bone loss in your hips. I also
recommend weight-bearing aerobic exercise to strengthen the heel
of the foot.

Walking to a supermarket with a backpack and filling it up
with some groceries is a great way to help bone density in your
hips, ankles, and heels. Swimming should not be your predominant
form of exercise as it is *not* weight-bearing; however, aquatic aerobics are fine. Warm up with twenty minutes of stretching for the
hamstrings and lower back. Remember, regular exercise not only
helps conserve bone but also maintains flexibility, erect posture,
and muscle strength.

❖ **CONSIDER HORMONAL REPLACEMENT THERAPY (HRT).** Some studies
support estrogen's role in preventing bone loss in women. Estrogen
slows down the rate of bone cell death. Although estrogen therapy
only helps restore bone integrity for about one to two years, it can
help to support bone density relatively quickly. And, although the
increase is only modest, some studies suggest the risk of hip fracture can be reduced during that time by as much as 50 to 80 percent. But remember, ERT is not for everyone. You must consider
all the variables previously discussed (see Section IV), including
natural progesterone, in building bones.

Natural topical progesterone cream in doses of 20 to 25 mg
daily may stimulate osteoblastic activity, causing new bone formation.
Remember, estrogen slows down bone breakdown, but progesterone

actually builds new bone and should be considered by all peri- and postmenopausal women. I recommend progesterone cream that can be formulated by most compounding pharmacies; usually one quarter teaspoon, the equivalent of approximately 25 mg, will suffice.

For perimenopausal and menopausal women, using progesterone cream for the last two weeks of your usual cycle is very easy to do. You can rub it into your hands, chest, arms, face, or breasts, where it is readily and quickly absorbed. This unbound type of progesterone enters the bloodstream quickly, and since it is not taken orally, it is not readily broken down by the liver.

Are There Other Alternatives to Hormonal Therapies?

If estrogen replacement therapy is not an option for you, and you are at risk for osteoporosis, consider *salmon calcitonin,* a synthetic version of a natural hormone. Salmon calcitonin, available only by injection for over fifteen years, is now formulated as a nasal spray. Although associated with a 1 to 3 percent incidence of nausea, this is more tolerable than the 10 to 15 percent rate of nausea experienced in patients treated with the injectable form. And this side effect usually decreases over time.

The nasal formulation is recommended for patients with low bone mass who are more than five years postmenopausal and who can't—or won't—take estrogen. Although the bone-enhancing benefits of salmon calcitonin are less dramatic in some women, the drug has an additional analgesic effect that may be quite beneficial for those with chronic pain from fractures.

Medical and traditional therapy could also be appropriate. Newer medication approved by the FDA for osteoporosis treatment includes *alendronate* (Fosamax). Alendronate has been shown to increase bone density for at least three years after the treatment period. In a study of nine hundred women, alendronate administered daily over three years significantly increased bone density of the spine, hip, and total body. This study also demonstrated a 50 percent decrease in the number of women with new vertebral and hip fractures, suggesting an effect comparable to estrogen.

However, alendronate must be taken according to strict directions to minimize side effects (nausea, diarrhea) reported in up to 30 percent of users. This drug may offer another option for those who will not consider HRT and have low bone mass and a history of fractures attributable to osteoporosis. Remember, you must be under a doctor's care if you want to consider alendronate, which should be used only in advanced cases of osteoporosis.

Also, prevent falls. Check your home and workplace for hazards—loose rugs, exposed electrical cords, and other clutter underfoot—that may increase your chances of a spill. Wear low-heeled, soft-soled shoes to reduce your risk of tripping, and watch those stairs.

Like all diseases of aging, osteoporosis isn't inevitable. Give your bones a boost by doing weight-bearing exercise, eating the healthy foods found in a Mediterranean diet, and taking nutritional supplements.

Keeping Your Eyes Healthy and a Whole Lot More

Your eyesight is precious and irreplaceable. Two of the greatest threats to vision as we age are macular degeneration (MD) and cataracts.

I watched my own mother gradually have her vision stolen away by macular degeneration, a thief of eyesight. Many of my patients also suffer from this heartbreaking disorder. About 30 percent of people over the age of sixty-five seek medical attention for various degrees of acute macular degeneration (AMD), which is characterized by light sensitive cells in the macula—a part of the retina—deteriorating and causing a loss of central vision and, eventually, complete blindness.

Acute macular degeneration occurs when the macular tissue begins to deteriorate or when new blood vessels develop adjacent to the retina. If these newly formed blood vessels leak, vision declines progressively and may lead to total loss of vision over a short period of time.

But the good news is that *lutein*, an antioxidant and carotenoid, has been found to have specific medical applications for the eye. Several studies have demonstrated that a higher level of lutein in the blood is significantly correlated with a reduced risk of macular degeneration. A study performed at Harvard University showed that subjects who consumed 6 mg lutein per day had a 43 percent lower risk for macular degeneration compared to those individuals whose consumption was beneath this level. Because lutein is a powerful antioxidant, it may protect the retina by preventing the oxidation of the many polyunsaturated fatty acids which people knowingly and unknowingly ingest in their diets.

In addition, lutein filters out visible blue light which causes free radical damage in the retina. Besides preventing macular degeneration, lutein and another carotenoid, *zeaxanthin*, also reduced cataract formation. In one study, presented in the *British Medical Journal* in 1992, researchers examined cataract formation among 50,000 women over an eight-year period. The results showed that women who consumed more spinach, an ideal source of both lutein and zeaxanthin, had much lower cataract formation than those whose consumption of vegetables consisted predominantly of only beta carotene. And, in the Nurses' Health Study of 77,000 nurses over a twelve-year period, a 22 percent lower risk of developing cataracts was realized in women with a high dietary intake of lutein and zeaxanthin.

What Can You Do to Prevent AMD?

Since the only carotenoids that have been observed to be absorbed directly by the eye are lutein and zeaxanthin, and there is no cure or treatment for age-related macular degeneration, it is imperative to include these two specific carotenoids in your diet or take them in the form of supplements. First, get enough lutein in your diet by eating foods such as green-leafy vegetables, kale, broccoli, and spinach. Corn and peas are high in zeanxanthin. If AMD runs in your family, then along with your vegetables, take at least 6 mg lutein daily as a nutritional supplement to ensure you are getting enough.

Lutein Prevents Cancer

While most of the research in lutein looks at the benefits for the eye, researchers have also studied its relationship to cancer. At the University of Michigan, scientists found that lutein was the single most predominant carotenoid in the cervix of healthy women. Lutein is rapidly metabolized or recycled in the woman's cervix. A woman's cervix undergoes considerable oxidative stress which changes not only cells, but DNA itself. The researchers at the University of Michigan concluded that women who consumed diets high in fruits and vegetables that were also high in lutein had a lower prevalence of cervical cancer.

Lutein's cousin, *beta-cryptoxanthin*, was also shown to prevent cervical cancer in a fifteen-year study that involved approximately 15,000 women. Women who ate fresh yellow fruits and vegetables had a lower incidence of cervical cancer, presumably due to beta-cryptoxanthin and lutein, preventing free radical damage in the tissue.

It also seems that women with active breast cancer have an improved prognosis when their intake of lutein is high. Once again, researchers believe a high consumption of yellow and green vegetables rich in lutein had a positive impact on estrogen receptors in the breast and had a direct effect on improved prognosis.

Lutein's protection against cancer doesn't stop with cervical and breast cancer. There is impressive data documenting that lung cancer rates are also lower among those who consume more lutein. For example, people in the Fiji Islands, who eat an average of 18 to 23 mg of lutein per day, have considerable fewer cases of lung cancer than those on other South Pacific Islands, where inhabitants consume much less lutein and the rate of smoking is the same.

Tips to Slow the Aging Process

OF COURSE, THERE ARE MANY MORE CHRONIC degenerative diseases, from arthritis to diabetes to Alzheimer's to allergies. However, following are tips and techniques to further slow the aging process and strengthen your resistance to free radical stress:

- Follow a modified Mediterranean diet, with special attention to consuming more fresh organic fruits and vegetables, especially red, yellow, and dark-green varieties—the more colors, the greater the nutrients.
- Avoid tap water and drink only filtered or spring water.
- Exercise every day, even if it's just a fifteen-minute walk around your neighborhood.
- Limit your alcohol consumption to no more than two 6-ounce glasses of wine every other day.
- Reduce excessive exposure to high UV-light (from 10 AM to 3 PM—at least fifteen minutes of sunlight a day for vitamin D metabolism is recommended), toxic chemicals including pesticides, and heavy metals. Consider use of an air filtering system in your home or workspace.
- Avoid eating any beef or foods that have begun browning, which means it is already oxidizing.
- Curb your intake of trans-fats, such as are contained in margarine, most crackers, and "snack" foods.
- Get plenty of sleep. Whether it's six or eight hours, don't short-change yourself.
- Relieve stress and relax every day; engage in self-reflection about where you are going in life; maintain a positive attitude towards health and aging; remain active in body, mind, and spirit.

Strengthen Your Immune System to Defeat Breast Cancer

My sister, Pam, was terrified the day she called to tell me about a large lump she had found in her breast. With a positive history of breast cancer—my mother had a mastectomy—my sisters have always been watchful. Now, Pam knew to move quickly, asking our younger sister Maria, a registered nurse, to check her findings. Maria confirmed Pam's lump, noting its size, shape, and texture, and suggested a prompt biopsy. Thankfully, Pam's biopsy was negative for cancer, and we all breathed a deep sigh of relief.

But the biopsies of approximately 180,000 women in this country will be positive this year. And of these women, 46,000 will eventually lose their lives to this dreadful disease. Although many more women still die of heart disease, breast cancer is projected to become the leading cause of death sometime during this next century.

What can you do to prevent breast cancer? First, lay the foundation for a lifetime of health by eating a modified Mediterranean diet (discussed in Chapter 4). Second, take targeted nutritional supplements (discussed in Chapter 5). Third, sharpen your awareness of environmental toxins, which I believe are a *major* contributor to breast cancer. Fourth, exercise—it can reduce your risk of cancer by 25 percent (see Chapter 6). Fifth, be committed to staying healthy from this day forward. All of these factors work together to maintain and/or rebuild your immune system, the single most important factor in maintaining breast health.

Prevent Cancer *or* Help Heal Yourself

I learned so much from Joan, a fifty-three-year-old nurse who elected to go on chemotherapy when she learned she had breast cancer; but she didn't stop there. Joan sought my advice on how to complement her program with targeted nutritionals. Here are some of the options that I discussed with her, which I recommend for optimal prevention of breast cancer:

BREAST-CANCER-FIGHTING FOOD STRATEGIES THAT HEAL:

❖ Maintain a *hormone-residue-free diet* with organic range meats and dairy whenever possible.

❖ Juice with *raw fruits and vegetables* at least twice per week.

Lifestyle Tips

- **AVOID USING CHEMICAL ANTIPERSPIRANTS.** They prevent you from eliminating toxins, which may be deposited via the lymph nodes in the armpits. Most breast tumors develop in the upper outside quadrant of the breast, where the lymph nodes are located. Use a natural antiperspirant instead or consider a mineral-salt "stone" deodorant found in health food stores.

- **BEWARE OF XENOBIOTICS.** These ubiquitous compounds are found in hair spray, perfumes, soaps, plastic wraps and food containers, household cleaners, dry cleaning, gasoline vapors, insecticides, and pesticides. Like xenoestrogens, they mimic estrogen and lock onto receptor sites in the breast, causing abnormal cell division. While it's impossible to avoid all of these products, the more you're aware of their potential impact on your health, the more ways you can figure out how to skirt the problem. For example, try to buy as many foods as possible from small markets that use old-fashioned butcher paper to wrap meats and seafood. If that's not possible, remove the plastic wrap from your foods as soon as you get home and place in glass containers. Do not microwave food with plastic. If you're over forty, you should also consume squalene, which is found in extra-virgin olive oil, rice bran oil, wheat germ oil, and shark-liver oil, available at health food stores. These oils neutralize many petrochemicals and are one of the hallmarks of my modified Mediterranean diet. Consume at least one tablespoon of extra-vigin olive oil per day in salads or on veggies.

- **INVEST IN A WATER FILTER.** Remember, massive amounts of industrial detergents and other chemicals can make their way into the ground water. I use filters that remove chlorine in my house. Chlorine may contribute to breast cancer and lung disease.

❖ Add *garlic* and *ginger* to foods for great flavor as well as antioxidant activity.

❖ Eat *phytonutrient-rich foods* such as broccoli, cabbage, cauliflower, brussels sprouts, and kale. Also, cruciferous veggies like cabbage and brussels sprouts contain indole-3-carbinol, which are proven breast-cancer fighting agents.

❖ Drink *green tea,* which can suppress the formation of new cancer cells, daily.

❖ Increase your intake of *healthy fats* through omega-3-oil-rich fish like salmon, cod, and haddock, as well as monounsaturated extra-virgin olive oil. Olive oil contains squalene, which neutralizes the effects of chemical *xenoestrogens,* substances which could stimulate estrogen receptors in the cells and change genetic messages, stimulating abnormal growth of cells and tissues and setting the stage for breast cancer.

❖ Eat *soy and flax* daily, *unless* you have estrogen-dependent cancer. Research shows that flax can reduce the growth of breast tumors by more than 50 percent in animal models; as little as 1.6 to 3 grams of soy daily is correlated with a reduction in the risk of breast cancer in Asian women.

❖ Avoid eating well-done, burned, or charred meats.

❖ Limit your intake of alcohol.

CONSIDER THESE SUPPLEMENTS:

❖ *Alpha lipoic acid* is a powerful and versatile antioxidant that is both fat- and water-soluble. It has the ability to neutralize the toxic effects of radiation and chemotherapy as well as recycle other antioxidants such as vitamins C and E. I recommend 100 mg daily for all women.

❖ *Antioxidant vitamins A, C, D, and E* offer protection against cancer. You can get all four in a quality multivitamin mineral complex. Research also shows that women who live in climates with lots of natural sunlight—and therefore high levels of vitamin D—may be less vulnerable to breast cancer than women who live in Northern climates.

❖ *N-acetylcysteine (NAC)*, is an amino acid that, when broken down to glutathione, can inhibit the growth of breast cancer cells. In fact, there's an interesting relationship between cancer cells, whey protein concentrate, and glutathione, the universal antioxidant that protects you from both toxic chemicals and the oxidation of LDL "bad" cholesterol.

The Mitochrondria-Free Radical-Aging Connection

MITOCHONDRIA CREATE MORE THAN 90 PERCENT OF THE ENERGY needed to support metabolism and growth, and sustain life, in the form of ATP, or adenosine triphosphate. ATP is a form of stored energy necessary to fuel all cellular functions—the energetic force necessary for life. Think of it as "high octane fuel" for all the energetic transactions in your body. You may think that you eat only to satisfy hunger or your taste buds or to socialize, but the truth is you consume food to get the energy sources required to generate ATP, the body's major form of stored energy. Inside the mitochondria, fatty acids (fats) are oxidized by oxygen, which releases electrons to travel down the respiratory chain and make ATP. The ATP is eventually transported to various parts of the cell to supply energy on demand.

DURING THIS PROCESS, NOT ALL OF THE OXYGEN IS METABOLIZED to water and carbon dioxide. As a result, some oxygen molecules, as many as 2 to 5 percent, leave a trail of unstable, highly-reactive molecular fragments known as free radicals. Although free radicals play a role in supporting a number of life processes, they are better known as the "bad boys" of molecular biochemistry. Among other misdeeds, these tiny vandals have been incriminated as a cause of extensive damage to lipid membranes, mitochondria, and even DNA itself. Their mayhem has generated enormous interest among health care professionals, especially those on the front lines of preventive and anti-aging medicine. Recent investigations suggest that free radicals may be involved not only in the origination and development of degenerative diseases but also in the very process of aging itself.

Researchers report the concentration of glutathione in tumor cells to be higher than that of normal cells surrounding them. This difference is believed to be an important factor, making antioxidant-rich cancer cells "resistant" to the oxidative stresses of chemotherapy. As a result, a higher concentration of glutathione in cancer cells is *not* good during chemotherapy.

Here's the catch: it's difficult to remove glutathione from tumor cells without jeopardizing healthy tissue. (This is basically the same dilemma faced in traditional cancer treatment: killing cancer cells without damaging healthy ones.) What's been needed is a compound that can selectively strip cancer cells of their glutathione while maintaining health-promoting levels of glutathione in normal cells. And remarkably, whey protein can do that.

❖ *Whey protein* has the ability to selectively deplete cancer cells of glutathione while increasing this antioxidant's level in normal, healthy tissue. Clinical studies have demonstrated tumor regression in patients fed 30 grams of whey protein concentrate daily. Although researchers have yet to understand *how* whey protein works, they report that its supplementation may represent an effective strategy to starve cancer cells of a nutrient that promotes their growth and expansion. Consider 30 grams of whey protein daily for both prevention and treatment of breast cancer.

❖ *Melatonin* is one of the most promising supplements for both prevention and treatment of breast cancer. In Europe, high dosages of this hormone, which declines with age, have been used extensively for breast cancer treatment. Dosages as small as 3 mg and as high as 50 mg taken at bedtime have been reported to have a positive impact on survival.

Melatonin blocks estrogen receptors, much like the drug tamoxifen but without the toxic effects; it also boosts overall immune response that can help neutralize metastasized cancer cells. Studies have shown that women with low melatonin levels are at higher risk of breast cancer, prompting some scientists to hypothesize that melatonin *deficiency* may play a role in the development of cancer.

As a result, some physicians recommend that all women over the age of forty, especially those with family histories of breast cancer, take at least 3 mg melatonin prior to bedtime. In addition, melatonin has been shown to defend against malignant melanoma—and as a bonus, it will help you sleep better. Melatonin should not be taken by anyone suffering from leukemia, Hodgkin's disease, or multiple myeloma. Since melatonin is one of the best free-radical scavengers known, and particularly since it helps to neutralize the hydroxyl radical—the most damaging radical for cancer—its use as a cancer preventive is most promising.

I recommend a dose of 1 to 3 mg melatonin prior to bedtime for women concerned about breast cancer. You can work your way up in 3 mg increments to about 12 mg, keeping in mind the potential for side effects such as vivid dreams, headaches, and depression.

❖ *Immunomodulators* include a class of nutritional supports that literally "turn on" the immune system defense by stimulating white blood cells to attack foreign bodies, including cancer cells. Transfer factor has been known to increase immunoglobin and killer cell activity, which can help squelch breast cancer cells. *Beta-1,3/1,6-Glucans* have been known to increase killer cell activity, supporting overall immune response and stifling breast cancer. And some patients with advanced breast cancer with clinical metastasis have had complete remission on doses of 400 mg or more of CoQ10. Since CoQ10 has absolutely no down side, it should be considered a vital agent for both prevention and treatment of breast cancer. I recommend 180 mg per day for maintenance and 400 mg per day for breast cancer patients (120 mg if you are taking a hydrosoluable form).

❖ *Essiac Tea* was developed by Canadian nurse Renee Caisse, who successfully treated thousands of breast cancer patients from the 1920s until her death in 1978. In fact, Essiac (Caisse spelled backwards) came within just three votes of being legalized by the Canadian Parliament in 1938. Although Essiac is not approved as a cancer aid in the United States or Canada, its appeal and use remain strong. Many health food stores and distributors claim to offer the "original" Essiac formula. The formula containing herbs including burdock root, sheep's sorrel, slippery elm bark, and others is regarded as a potent tonic and detoxifier, theorized to reduce tumor growth as well as support the body's natural defenses. Although Essiac is not likely to prove a "magic bullet" against cancer, its long history of use in thousands of patients has given testimony as a powerful adjunct in the treatment of breast cancer. You can find it in most health food stores.

❖ *Poly-MVA* combines alpha lipoic acid and other vitamins with the trace element palladium to create a unique, nontoxic form of "nutritional chemotherapy." This combo gets inside the cancer cell without damaging surrounding healthy cells. Once there, research indicates that palladium and alpha lipoic acid interfere with the energy metabolism of cancer cells by changing the tumor's cell proteins, and thereby destroying the cells. Since "normal" cells are not impacted by Poly-MVA, no harm occurs outside the tumor.

Conventional chemotherapy and radiation therapy kill cancer cells, but they also take out normal cells. One goal of medical research is to find treatments that selectively kill only cancer cells. We have heard of many case studies in which patients with advanced cancers have survived following the use of Poly-MVA. It is currently being used in Canada, Mexico, Australia, South America, India, and throughout Europe. Clinical trials are now being conducted in the United States. Since Poly-MVA has no known downside, its use as a cancer preventive or even as a non-toxic anti-cancer nutritional should be considered in the battle against breast cancer. It has also been employed to help assuage the toxic side effects of radiation and chemotherapy. (For further information visit the website at www.polymva.com.)

Soy and Breast Cancer—Unraveling a Complex Relationship

You may recall from earlier chapters that naturally occurring flavonoids, such as *genistein* and other soy products, are phytoestrogens. They are great for "tricking" estrogen receptor sites if you want to relieve symptoms of menopause or reduce your breast cancer risk, but the latest research reveals they are helpful in inhibiting only specific types of breast cancers.

Turns out that soy is appropriate only if you have a breast cancer that is *not* hormone dependent—that is, one that doesn't "feed" on estrogen. Estrogen can combine with genistein to cause some breast cancer cells to grow faster. Although soy isoflavones and their cousins, the flax lignans, have been known to prevent cancers, the research is mixed as to whether supplemental soy isoflavones are safe *if you already have breast cancer.* Therefore, I advise that *women with any type of breast cancer test their blood estrogen levels to see if they have high levels of estrogen before making their supplement decisions.*

Another way to see if you would be starving or feeding your breast cancer with soy products is to have a blood test commonly used to evaluate breast cancer patients called p53. If the test is positive, then you have mutant p53 and are more likely to benefit from soy extracts. If the test is negative, it indicates that you have functional p53 and you're less likely to benefit from soy extracts. The bottom line is: anyone with breast cancer *must* do her homework before adding soy in the form of genistein to her program. (To test your p53 level, have your physician contact Impath Laboratories at 800/447-5816.)

In addition, *soy supplements should not be taken one week before, during, or after radiation therapy.* That's because soy blocks protein kinase-C activity in cancer cells, and radiation therapy depends upon this enzyme to help generate the free radicals that kill cancer cells. The theory is that you need localized pro-oxidant activity to kill cancer cells. This raises the argument that many of you may have read about—that antioxidants may interfere with cancer treatment. The research continues, but for now I'd like to focus on the evidence that large amounts of genistein in breast cancer cells could paradoxically protect them against radiation-induced, free-radical–mediated destruction. The bottom line is: *soy products are contraindicated during active radiation treatment for breast cancer.*

Despite these concerns, don't be scared away from soy. Genistein has a great deal of anti-cancer activity and remains a powerhouse of cancer prevention. Genistein also helps cut off the blood supply to the tumor. As a result, it's extremely beneficial *if* you have a non-estrogen–dependent cancer.

Fight Back Against Breast Cancer: Roundup

What can a woman do if she receives the life-changing news that she has breast cancer?

Most often, the first line of treatment is a lumpectomy, or even radical mastectomy if the cancer is particularly invasive. But then what? How does one handle the possibility that cancer cells can spread (metastasize) to the lung, liver, bone, brain, and other vital organs? What if there are already signs that cancer cells are seeding themselves elsewhere? How does a woman choose among chemotherapy, radiation, more surgery, or alternative therapies like melatonin? I asked my wife Jan what she would do if she was ever confronted with the news of a malignancy in her breast and was surprised to learn that she had often wondered about the same thing. Of course, few people know with certainty what they would do until they're faced with the situation, but just pondering these questions made us realize how difficult it can be to gather the information needed to make wise decisions.

While surgical intervention may initially be the clear path to choose, the decision-making process becomes much more difficult when it comes to radiation and/or chemotherapy. For example, some chemotherapeutics are known to be very stressful on the heart. If you choose this course of therapy, you will need to be mindful of supporting your heart as well. Every woman needs to sit down with her physician and her family before making her choice. Ultimately it will be her decision, but enlisting support and feedback from others can make it easier. As I have seen in my own practice, some women elect conventional medicine, while others embrace alternative therapies. And another group may integrate the two with an emphasis on diet, supplements, and lifestyle modifications.

To reiterate some of the guidelines in this chapter, begin by sharpening your awareness of all the toxic components in your environment—pesticide residues in foods (eat organic); sprays in your yard and neighborhood (avoid using them); air and water quality (invest in an air and water purifier—and a juicer).

Secondly, eat a diet that helps to inhibit breast cancer. Review the Mediterranean diet, and include soy isoflavones and flax lignans. (However, if you do develop breast cancer, soy isoflavones, as discussed, may not be indicated.) Use as many of the targeted nutritional supports discussed above and in Chapter 5.

Most importantly, *remain steadfast in your battle.* Remember, if you are going to survive breast cancer, you must fight back. This includes using your anger as a motivating and healing force in your body. I agree with one of my colleagues, Bernie Siegal, MD, who has often said that people who "fight back" are the ones who often win the battle against cancer. Remember, even long-simmering emotions of rage and resentment may contribute to cancer. A powerful mind/body approach may include emotional release work, mental imagery, self-discipline, and a deep awakening of your spirituality.

Since one out of nine women will someday develop breast cancer, it's important that every woman become informed about this complex condition. If you or someone you love is ever given a diagnosis of breast cancer, be assured that there are many complementary options to explore in addition to conventional therapies.

The breast cancer epidemic can be stopped, but first women need to be aware of all the ramifications of prevention and the many treatment options.

CHAPTER SIXTEEN

The Female Advantage: Stories of Healing and Hope

Even though, throughout this book, we have focused on the obstacles women must overcome when it comes to diagnosing heart disease—and women must be aware of these special dilemmas—there is a positive side to the issue: namely that being a woman also provides many *advantages* when it comes to health and the heart.

In most modern societies, women live an average of ten years longer than men. In the United States premenopausal women also have a ten-year lead over men in natural heart disease protection. A woman's natural protection is the built-in physiological advantage of estrogen, but there's more to a woman's edge than just her hormonal makeup. When it comes to longevity, what gives women such a stunning statistical advantage over her male peers?

There are many intriguing theories, including DNA repair afforded by women's additional "X" chromosome, her slower metabolism, and menstruation. But I believe there to be a mosaic of attributes that comprises what I call the "female advantage." We need to look beyond estrogen to consider the totality of what makes a woman who she is. For openers, women more often live "closer to their hearts" than do men. When it comes to making decisions—be they large or small—a woman is usually more mindful of weighing the risks and benefits to her emotional life or that of her loved ones.

Women also tend to be more flexible in their overall outlook on life and are more willing to risk "vulnerability" than men. I use this term in a very positive sense, to indicate an openness, flexibility, and capacity to bend and flow with the realities of different situations and personal relationships. True vulnerability is a calm, mature willingness to express your openness to life and others in a way that's balanced with a sense of knowing the appropriate time to reveal your "softer" human emotions, like love, sadness, and empathy.

To be "soft" is to be authentic, connected to oneself and to others—not wishy-washy, weak, or indecisive as some might interpret this trait. In contrast, "rigidity" signals a lack of capacity to feel and flow with one's own emotions and the emotions of others. Rigid people—men and women alike—store stress in different parts of their bodies, which results in blocked energy, constricted circulation, postural and musculoskeletal problems, and chronic illnesses. For example, someone whose held-in anger is carried in their back and shoulders often has hunched up shoulders—like a "monkey on your back."

Embracing the Joys and Hazards of Being a Woman

My massage therapist, Susan, says that women possess "Mother Earth" energy; because their bodies cycle with the moon and the passage of time, they remain connected to the natural rhythm of things in nature. My mentor, psychotherapist Dr. Alexander Lowen, often spoke of the ultimate joy that a woman experiences in the birth of her child. My wife Jan shared with me that the birth of her first child, Kristin, was the most profound experience of her life. Just looking into the face of her newborn daughter, she felt that she would literally explode. She felt an intense love and sense of wonder that made her feel as if her heart would burst with a joy she had never before experienced. She actually felt herself physically melt and fall in love with her little baby. And that feeling was no less intense when she later gave birth to her son, Greg.

Women are a bridge between nature and culture, and I believe that their femininity and their special life experiences make them more grounded in their biology.

Men are programmed to be harder from the time they are young boys, frequently molded by society and the energies of domineering men. Males in our society all too often have been programmed with messages like:

"Big boys don't cry"
"Don't cry or I'll give you something to cry about…"
"Real men never.…"

Men less often have the intuitive ability to take in support and wisdom from others. Few men my age that I know have developed their feminine sides at all; some just can't do it and others are afraid to even investigate it. And I will share with you two of the biggest fears men have about women: their intelligence and their sexuality. I learned this from running a men's psychotherapy workshop for many years. That's a secret that most of us men hope that we're keeping, but I'd bet that on an intuitive level, most women have already figured us out.

Now, if you know this secret and have learned how to work with it, then you're probably in touch with your intuitive side, your "gut" feeling. This is a great strength in women. In fact, I encourage you to embrace and appreciate this female attribute, and learn how to let it work for you.

The High Cost of Relinquishing "Softness"

Each culture has its own special rites of initiation and passage—personal processes and experiences that strengthen a member's identification with their "clan." It's striking how many cultures socialize a young man to be aggressive, with age-related rites of passage that involve forsaking the comfort of the "mother" figure to move out into the world, "toughen up," and conquer something, be it a team effort or a personal conquest.

In contrast, a young woman's initiations are more often signaled by changes in her interior physical world. Her rites of passage with her "clan" are often a quieter, more individual experience. Throughout her life, her most intimate life experiences—the onset of menstrual cycles, marriage and sexuality, childbirth, nursing—are often private moments about surrendering to the wisdom of her own body, and less about achieving specific standards in her external world. It is her very woman-ness that has the potential to render each woman her own female advantage—as long as she stays connected to it. I can't prove this theory with hard science but rather base it on observations from my twenty-five years of clinical experience. I have heard some very powerful stories while collaborating with women as their physician. I'd like to share the story of one woman who traded her softness and femininity for the illusion of success.

The Story of Barbara

I met Barbara many years ago at one of our psychotherapy workshops. She was a young woman who had thrown herself so completely into her corporate career that she had unwittingly sacrificed the essence of her female self. At the young age of twenty-eight she was working in the banking sector, then a business made up primarily of men. She was the only woman in a group of vice presidents. Her work atmosphere was crushingly stressful and bristling with competitiveness, unreasonable demands, a pervasive lack of trust and compassion, and an overriding pressure to dominate and win. (If it sounds to you like an old-line patriarchal business model, you're right.)

In this environment, and even at home, she felt it unsafe to expose any of her feminine attributes. To become successful, she became harder and tougher, stifling her own emotions and refusing to acknowledge them in others. By the time I met her, she even dressed and acted like a man. The *last* thing she would consider was allowing herself to cry. Adamantly denying herself the luxury of any emotional release that would feel "weak" or vulnerable to attack, she had unconsciously assumed the body stance of our culture's archetypal ideal-successful-corporate-male role model.

Barbara was devastated to find out that she had developed uterine cancer. She followed the standard treatment for this disease, agreeing to a total hysterectomy. Her uterus and ovaries were removed in an operation sometimes referred to as "female castration." One might speculate on the mind–body connection for her particular case of cancer development. My interpretation? By acting like a man and subjecting herself to years of heightened states of chronic stress—compounded by her betrayal of her inner personal strengths—she had denied her feminine self. After years of symbolic rejection of her own nature to survive in the corporate world, she was forced to give the ultimate sacrifice on a physical level. And of course with the loss of her ovaries and uterus she also lost her estrogen, menstrual cycle, and ability to become pregnant—all critical female attributes that have the potential to protect her from heart disease and other illnesses.

Barbara did break down and cry at that workshop, once she realized that she had betrayed herself as a woman. She got in touch with some of the unconscious needs that were fueling her drive, and why she had unwittingly believed that her success would buy her the approval, love, and security that she so desperately needed.

Barbara then made the decision to turn her life around and committed herself to do individual therapy to find her way back.

This woman's dilemma may sound extreme to you, but this scenario is not as unusual as you may think. I've had many conversations with women who have worked their way up the corporate ladder. Many have confided to me their secret fear: they were consciously aware that they shut down a part of themselves to survive, and they were afraid of what it might cost them later. The price tag on success is often very high, so it pays for all of us to be mindful about the choices we make. Now, I realize that women cannot abandon their careers, but there is a way out.

Many women, like Barbara, who shared their concerns with me have told me that with insight and personal growth they were able to discover a strength in themselves to rebalance their lives again. They explored the roots of their own driven behavior pattern and reconnected with their emotional selves. They were able to reinterpret and redefine their professional lives, often continuing to work in the same environment but without losing their connection to themselves. A few who realized that they were employed in businesses too toxic to support their emotional needs and personal essence chose to look elsewhere.

So while we know that cholesterol, diet, estrogen, and exercise are all important aspects of a woman's heart health, perhaps the most important key to the health of a woman's heart is staying in touch with her feminine side.

What Is the Feminine Side?
Cycles of Life: The Protective Benefits of Menstruation
The menstrual cycle holds many different meanings for women, and I'm acutely aware that, as a man, I can't even begin to know them as a woman can. But I do know that menstruation is fundamentally

about life, and a woman's deep connection to the energy of life. This monthly reminder that a woman's body is designed to nurture and give life also helps to reduce her risk of heart disease and may even contribute to her longevity. Some researchers speculate that the monthly shedding of the uterine lining reduces the amount of blood by about 10 percent, thus lowering the level of iron in the bloodstream. This may not only help prevent iron overload (discussed in Chapter 3), but may also reduce the formation of free radicals. From a bioenergetic standpoint, a woman's monthly menses provides a powerful, natural, and healthy release of blocked energy.

There is ultimately no difference between physical and emotional energy—the two freely translate into one another. As a result, the entire event of menses, including the emotionally charged time which frequently precedes it, releases a large amount of psychic as well as physical energy.

What Is the Significance of this Complex Hormonal Orchestration?

The release of blocked energy through menstruation discharges tension which, if held or blocked anywhere in the body, can cause physical changes or damage that contributes to a number of physical problems, including heart disease. In fact, stagnant energy anywhere in the body can set the stage for disease. Menstruation's release of energy extends well beyond the blood energy that is built up during the monthly cycle: it also encompasses other areas of stagnation that may have accumulated.

For instance, pelvic energy blocks may result from withheld anger, hurt, or other emotional trauma. These often reflect earlier sexual traumas like rape and incest, which are still all too common in our society. Other issues around sexuality may be stored as painful body-memories in the pelvic area, be it a psychically disturbing experience from childhood or later adult life, such as an abortion. Remember, any experience that causes the body to contract or shrink away from an outside stressor can be held in the body indefinitely as an energy block.

Tears Can Heal

During the premenstrual (postovulatory) part of the cycle, each woman's body changes to varying degrees. Some women report no changes at all while others report fluid retention, headache, or enlarged and tender breasts. The upside of the premenstrual period is often an incredible burst of physical energy which, though uncomfortable at times, can be channeled into creative outlets. My wife Jan has learned to reframe this experience, and so sets aside projects for herself that are better accomplished within the burst of energy she experiences during the premenstrual window. She also feels that planning ahead gives her a more positive outlook for the emotional surges she may feel.

But for many women, the premenstrual period can also be a time of mood swings alternating feelings of anxiety, euphoria, and depression. The good news is that the tearful episodes that may accompany tension, frustration, and enhanced sensitivity are actually healing to a woman's body—especially to the heart. I've watched Jan surrender and give herself permission to take time out and just cry for a few minutes when the anxiety is peaking and she is on the downslide into unexplainable sadness. She reports that, as a nurse-psychotherapist, she often does her most insightful work when menstruating.

Crying, which I consider a gift, is the most healing of all emotional outlets. The softening that occurs in the chest after deep sobbing is very protective to the heart and circulation. I have been surprised to learn that many women have as much trouble surrendering into crying as I once did. (I used to think that men had the corner on the market when it comes to rules like "big boys don't cry.")

You are blessed each month that your hormonal cycle brings you back into your body, whether you're ready or not, and takes you into healing spaces that men have yet to understand completely. I believe this monthly ritual has the power to keep women in touch with their bodies in a way that men may never know.

In fact, some cultures, such as Native Americans, believe that a woman is in her power during menses or "moon time," and that energy is so strong that she is encouraged to use the space to go off by herself, be still, and await messages and visions for her family and the community. This may be an ideal time to honor your body, your spiritual self, and your intuitive process. The softening that can occur before and during menstruation is a time to go inward, quiet the mind, and create a sacred space for yourself. Light candles, surround yourself with nurturing music, good books, or a warm bath and indulge in nurturing and listening to your inner voice. Give yourself permission to call "time out."

Menopause: Gateway to the Wisdom Years

Menopause—biologically the endpoint of a progressive failure of the ovaries to respond to the stimulation of "sex" hormones from the pituitary—typically occurs between forty-five and fifty-five years of age. As did her monthly cycle, menopause can offer a woman a time to pause, reflect, and take stock of where she is in her life as she transitions into her next physiological phase.

The onset of the perimenopausal period may be marked by hot flashes, copious sweating, muscular pains, and emotional swings. Christiane Northrup, MD, author of *Women's Bodies, Women's Wisdom* and editor of *Health Wisdom for Women* newsletter, notes that if a woman has unresolved psychological issues in her life, they may come forth to challenge her as she goes through this physiological "change." As a result, many women seek counseling during this time to come to terms with buried conflicts that may reemerge.

As we have discussed, after passing through menopause, a woman will lose the shield of menses as her estrogens dwindle. But remember, nature intended this to be a natural process, and a decline in hormones is normal. I believe that many aspects of a woman's aging involve a deeper softening—of her skin, her form, her psyche. If you are postmenopausal, this may be the time to explore new ways to honor your cyclical nature. Many women choose activities such as journaling, poetry writing, painting or sculpting, walking in nature, meditation, relaxation, and prayer to consciously enter into a healing space that encourages introspection and receptivity. The heightened awareness of the older woman, called the "crone" in many cultures, is a time of stronger, more deepened inner knowing: the result of time's teaching that is often referred to as the "wisdom years."

Women Are Emotionally Different From Men— And this Can Lower Your Heart Disease Risk

Since all emotional realities are underpinned by chemical and hormonal events, women have an innate ability to connect with others. This is a gift. Because women bear children, they've been equipped by nature to experience powerful emotional ties, to connect with and care for children. This is and always has been a matter of survival for the human species along with women's tendency to be more cooperative, team-oriented, and forgiving than men.

Now all of this doesn't mean that men can't develop strong emotional capacities, nor does it mean that women cannot excel in areas traditionally considered male domains, such as aggressiveness, strategic expertise, leadership, and physical strength. Obviously, women can do these things well. It also doesn't mean that women who are not connected with their feminine nature can't be rigid. But at a very primitive, basic, and biological level, women are designed to use their emotions very differently and much more forwardly than men, and this is a great strength.

Because men rarely express sadness, fear, or even rage outwardly, even when under extreme stress, their bodies produce and retain higher levels of stress hormones, such as adrenaline and cortisol. Since an overload of these dangerous chemicals plays a key role in heart disease; their inability to soften and to cry predisposes some men to cardiovascular disease.

I saw dramatic proof of this back in the 1980s in a workshop I facilitated on stress and its relationship to heart disease. In the workshop, which was attended by young cardiac men and their deeply concerned wives, both men and women went through the same stress-inducing experiences. At the end of the weekend program, we measured their levels of the stress hormone cortisol. The women in the workshop—most of whom didn't have heart disease—had much lower levels of cortisol than their cardiac spouses, suggesting that they were churning up and dumping out fewer stress hormones than the men.

Throughout the weekend, our team of therapists observed these women's ability to express their feelings outwardly—to cry or yell or release them rather than bottling them up. We speculated that their expressive nature might be a part of why none of these women had developed premature heart disease (under age forty-five) as had their spouses. The cardiac men had far higher cortisol levels and were described by their mates as especially inexpressive with their emotions.

Any woman who abandons her natural strength and becomes rigid and more like a man—psychologically and physiologically—also becomes more vulnerable to various diseases. One reason we are seeing a rise in heart disease among women over the past twenty years is that as our social structure changes and more women enter the work force, they are oftentimes encouraged to relinquish their "softness" and put up a tough facade, especially in professional arenas that are fiercely competitive. For both men *and* women, this can lead to toxic stress and heart disease.

For the woman blocked from experiencing her emotions, the healthiest thing she can do is to learn how to recapture her "softness" while being dynamic and assertive in her career, just as it would be healthier for a man to learn how to cultivate more compassion and team-building behaviors while pursuing his career. To learn to be able to move freely from being assertive to being open is a dynamic and important social skill, now widely called emotional intelligence. Like the expansion and contraction of the heart, this social skill ability is both constructive and healthy for oneself and those we love.

How a Daughter's Devotion Saved Her Mother's Life

Her mother had never been sick a day in her life. The only times that she ever received hospital care was to deliver her two children more than forty years before. Mary was a vibrant woman who had survived the death of her husband as a young wife and had gone on to raise her kids. And it was certainly no easy task back in the 1950s and 1960s when our family role model was based on the Nelsons, the Cleavers, and "Father Knows Best." There were few visible role models for women like Mary, but that was okay with her. She was no blushing rose....

Mary was a descendant of Thomas A. Edison. She holds a patent for a light switch and is a voracious reader. She raised her children with exuberance and instilled in them her beliefs, including her Native American heritage. Mary ran her own business as well as her home with a flair for the artistic and unusual. In fact, her daughter Ann is an artist herself, along with myriad other talents that keep her in touch with her true nature. But what was so impressive to me about this mother-daughter combination was the deep loyalty that had developed over the years.

When Ann looked at her vital mother, unconscious in a hospital intensive care unit, her gut feeling registered right off the Richter scale. This couldn't be right! Ann knew that intuitively. It had barely been days since Mary had moved herself into a trailer on their property while the fire damage in her house was being repaired. What the hospital staff was now evaluating as evidence of a decline in Mary's self-care and attributed to a downhill course in her health, Ann knew to be only the result of cramped and inadequate housing for the week before her admission.

When all medical treatments failed to bring her mother back to consciousness, Mary's doctors tried to convince Ann that it was time to let go and "pull the plug." But the daughter's response was a resounding "No!"—neither out of denial, nor any inappropriate overattachment to the outcome of her mother's illness. Ann was listening to her own inner voice, not that of the "experts," and she knew that this sudden turn of events in her mother's health just didn't ring true. She refused to give up... not yet!

Ann's intention was not to "save" her mother's life but rather to give her the opportunity to decide *whether or not to save her own*—to decide if she wanted to continue with her life or move on. Their Mohawk heritage is grounded in a belief about the tapestry of life and death, and the threads that weave in and out. Their basic axiom is this: If you save a life, you are responsible for that life for the rest of your own.

"My loving judgments were guided by that knowing and acknowledgment of the responsibility, as well as an understanding, that the situation was 'out of balance'... I felt that [Mary] was not given the opportunity because of the circumstances in that hospital. She was not able to exercise that choice-making, decision-making power. It is important that we all be allowed to make that decision, each in our own hearts, minds, spirits and use our death in a way befitting the nobility and dignity we have as human beings and as 'warriors.' Balance was what I was seeking...."

Ann turned for help to her brother, Bob, and they approached the doctors with an all-stops-out plan. Their efforts turned the tide and allowed Mary to return to consciousness... and eventually to making her *own* decisions about her life.

Trust Your Gut: The Choice Is Yours...

One woman's unshakable conviction regarding her mother's right to make her own choice gave her the motivation that made all the difference. It is my hope that this book will do the same for you. Every woman, if armed with the right information, has the right to make her own choices in her health care... and her heart care.

The women who allowed us to tell their stories in this book did so because they wanted to reach out and help other women. Many of them said that it was their personal hope that, by sharing what had happened to them, other women might not have to go through what they did to take care of their hearts. They hope that you will come away with the gift of more knowledge and insights than they had available at the time, and they feel strongly that this sharing will give more purpose and meaning to their experiences. All who shared positive outcomes did so to give you hope and faith that the "system" can work, and is more likely to do so when we ourselves become more engaged in ensuring the outcome.

It is our intention that this book arm you with the information that you need to be more engaged in your own health and your own heart. I have at times given you a lot of data—and a lot of cardiology. But I remind you that if you ever do feel confused about your best "choice," that you remember to surrender your head, go inside, listen contemplatively, and then trust your gut. When you follow the inner voice of your heart, behold the message... it will never lie to you.

APPENDIX A

A Guide to Diagnostic Testing for Women

Most diagnostic cardiac testing involves a thorough evaluation of the work capacity of the left ventricle (LV). An understanding of its attributes will enable you to better understand the diagnostic tests used to screen for heart disease. The life-sustaining blood pressure and energy requirements of the LV render it the primary chamber involved in most heart attacks; any shortage of oxygen supply (as occurs with a heart attack) will usually be felt first by the left ventricle, the veritable workhorse chamber of the heart.

Because it must generate enough strength to pump blood out of the heart against high pressure within the aorta, the left ventricle is the largest and thickest pumping chamber in the heart. As the most muscular and energetic part of the heart, the LV also demands the most oxygen and so has the richest blood supply. In fact, the heart's intricate circulatory system is organized so that— like all roads leading to Rome—all the blood vessels in the heart, no matter where they originate or what other part of the heart they serve, eventually end in the complex and overlapping tree of arteries of the left ventricle. It's the muscle most demanding of oxygen, but also usually the first chamber to sustain damage if there is a cutoff in blood flow to the heart.

Whether you are a man or a woman, *both angina and a myocardial infarction will signal a doctor to perform diagnostic tests* to evaluate how much heart muscle is in jeopardy and what steps can be taken to prevent further damage. But women who undergo standard diagnostic procedures must face the fact that most standard diagnostic tests for heart disease are at best inconsistent and at worst unreliable for many of them. Most of the diagnostic tests for men are more predictive and accurate.

The protocol for evaluating heart disease is a step-by-step process. Most of the information from diagnostic tests is indirect, with the exception of angiography. But from the results of preliminary screens, we can predict what's going on in the heart with varying degrees of reliability and specificity depending on the circumstances. But you will soon see for yourself why each one of these tools has its own limitations when it comes to evaluating women. *The truth is, even among cardiologists, there is still confusion about which is the best diagnostic tool for women.*

That's because women have more false/positive and false/negative tests when it comes to diagnosing heart disease. So choosing the right diagnostic test becomes critical. The major diagnostic tests include regular Exercise Stress Testing, Nuclear Stress Testing, Exercise Echo, PET Scanning, and the CT Scan for calcium deposits.

In my experience, the best noninvasive test to evaluate the possibility of heart disease in women is the Exercise Echo. But technology is changing daily, and when PET Scanning becomes available to more hospitals, it will provide an excellent noninvasive test. It is looking better and better for women as research findings come forth.

Another evaluation tool that's increasing in popularity is high frequency CT scanning as a way of detecting coronary calcification. The more calcium present, the greater the chance of arterial blockage.

We will take a look at each one of these tests—what they tell us, their strengths, and limitations—so that you can better understand the protocol and make sure that you are getting the best diagnostic workup possible.

First, however, we will look at the most basic tools that are usually employed in evaluating a woman's heart: electrocardiogram, bloodwork, chest X ray, echocardiogram, and Holter monitor.

The Electrocardiogram

The electrocardiogram (ECG or more commonly called the EKG from the German root word *kardio*) was developed by the Germans, who first figured out that there was electrical activity going on in the heart. They had the first EKG "patient" sit on a chair, with both hands and the left foot in pails of water while the right foot was left dry as the point of grounding. Early sensors, like those of today, used a stylus or pen to trace the currents and potentials that were going on in the heart. Using the sensors, these pioneers could look at the heart from six vantage points, dividing the heart muscle into electrical planes for viewing, sort of like walking around the various sides and angles of a car to get a 3D picture.

Years later, six more points of reference were added, starting at the right side of the chest and moving to the left and around the side of the heart. This enhanced reading is what we call the 12-lead EKG or ECG. Interpreting the cardiogram takes special training and years of experience. There are no leads to directly view the back, or posterior surface of the heart, so changes there must be deduced, or inferred, by changes in the leads that measure the front of the heart. Most of the electrical activity within the heart can be appreciated with 12 leads, some mirror images of what is happening in the opposite plane. Each lead provides information about a specific area of the heart, and some are overlapping. In this way, the ECG is an electrical blueprint about what's going on in the heart muscle and in which area.

The electrical pattern on the ECG gives us a lot of information about the heart:

❖ **RHYTHM:** The ECG, or even a single lead ECG on a cardiac monitor, is the only diagnostic tool that shows the rhythm of the heart, how regular or irregular it is, and from where the approximate sources of the arrhythmia are coming. Only the ECG gives us vital information about life-threatening arrhythmias including cardiac arrest, so that they can be diagnosed and treated.

❖ **RATE:** The ECG gives us a 100-percent-accurate assessment of the heart rate.   **HEART SENSE FOR WOMEN   13**

❖ **CONDUCTION:** The ECG alone provides the timing, in one-one hundredths of a second, of each impulse as it traverses the heart. Only the ECG gives vital information about conduction blocks: first-, second- and third-degree heart blocks and bundle branch blocks are all conduction delays resulting from a slowing in the electrical impulses in the heart. Frequently these conduction delays are a result of aging.

❖ **ISCHEMIA:** Ischemic changes signal that the heart is not getting enough blood flow. Prolonged ischemia can damage the heart muscle. Ischemia can be inferred by changes in the ECG. These changes can be very subtle and nonspecific or they can be very obvious when large areas of the heart appear to be compromised. A resting ECG may not pick up ischemia that is intermittent or occurs only when the heart is distressed or being challenged, such as during a stress test.

❖ **DAMAGE:** An ECG is fairly sensitive to identifying damage to the heart that is more than a few hours old. In fact, it is generally the ECG that signals the general area of the heart where the ischemia or damage has occurred. This allows cardiologists to speculate which arteries are probably involved and helps to put many puzzle pieces together.

Despite the fact that the cardiogram may not always be able to give a precise picture when someone is having a heart attack, it is an incredibly reliable tool that paints a picture of someone's heart and leads the trail on where to look next.

Blood Tests

If someone is being worked up in a hospital for a possible heart attack, the physician will order *blood tests* to see what's going on in the body and to add to the data collected from the ECG. The primary focus in analyzing the blood are the enzymes CPK (creatine phosphokinase) and LDH (lactate dehydrogenase), compounds that are released from cells whose walls are breaking down as they die. I won't go into exact lab values because different labs may have variable ranges for normal values of these enzymes. But the proportional amount and pattern of elevation gives the health care provider an idea whether an acute process is going on. We know that the CPK will elevate when there is muscle damage going on in the body, usually within the first twelve to twenty-four hours of the event, peaking within 72 hours before it heads back down to baseline when the storm is over. LDH, on the other hand, can take two to three days to elevate and not taper off until the fifth day.

And then there are the *isoenzymes*, a slightly more expensive blood test, but one that is specific for heart muscle. If a woman comes to the emergency room complaining of an intermittent symptom for the last twelve hours, the physician ruling out a heart attack will want to check her enzymes. But one dilemma is that an elevated CPK, for a man or a woman, tells us only that some muscle somewhere in the body is being injured. If the patient had a recent fall, muscle inflammation anywhere in her body, or even a recent intramuscular injection, their elevated CPK may not reflect heart muscle damage, but muscle damage elsewhere.

The isoenzyme level involves placing a radioactive dye in the medium that tags cardiac muscle specifically. It used to be that we went back and got an isoenzyme CPK on a sample only if a person's CPK was elevated, but now that we have thrombolytic agents ("clotbusters"), like TPA (tissue plasminogen activator and strep-tokinase, or SK) that need to be given within two hours of a heart attack, it is important to know the isoenzymes, as soon as possible, if a heart attack is suspected.

So, by analyzing the blood with these tools, we can usually get an estimate on the timing of heart muscle damage. An office physician may even order an LDH if he or she is given a history of symptoms or an ECG finding that indicates there may have been a heart attack in the past week. Now probably all of you know of someone who went to an emergency room to be evaluated for a possible heart attack but was sent home because the ECG and the blood work failed to show any abnormalities. Obviously, as helpful as these screening tools are, physicians are not infallible, and no test is 100 percent accurate.

The electrocardiogram and the blood are good indicators, but can take several hours to shift to reveal values suggestive of a heart attack. So my best advice to you is to trust your intuition. If you or someone you love has been sent home, but symptoms return, or something just does *not* feel right, trust your gut and bring the patient back to the emergency room or call your doctor. But things can get tricky here, because several disorders can mimic a heart attack, such as mitral valve prolapse and panic disorder (see Chapter 8).

Routine blood work such as a *chemical profile (CP)*, *complete blood cell count (CBC)*, *and electrolytes (LYTES)* are also usually done when evaluating anyone for a possible heart attack. Low potassium, for example, can make the heart more prone to irregularities of heart rhythm. Hypokalemia (low potassium) needs to be corrected to prevent possible life-threatening arrhythmias such as ventricular tachycardia (VTACH) and ventricular fibrillation (VFIB) which are more probable in the presence of ischemia, when the heart's electrical conduction system is unstable.

The Chest X-ray

A chest X-ray (CXR or chest roenterogram) may be done to evaluate the heart and lungs for a routine cardiology or a pre-operative assessment. Essentially, we evaluate a few key features including the size of the heart's silhouette on X-ray and its position. The heart should be fairly central and slightly to the left of the sternum. A large silhouette indicates an enlarged heart (cardiomegaly), most frequently seen with long-standing high blood pressure that has strained the heart muscle. We may also determine whether the left ventricle appears large or "dilated." In addition, the lung fields can be inspected for fluid, indicating the presence and extent of congestive heart failure. Findings from the chest X-ray are then compared with the clinical picture and the results of other tests, such as the Holter monitor and the echocardiogram.

Holter/24-hour Monitors

The Holter monitor is an ECG-recording device attached with electrodes and lead wires to an individual for about twenty-four hours. The recording device can be worn on a belt or strap. There are usually five adhesive chest leads that provide a continuous ECG recording from two sites. The patient wearing a Holter carries a diary and is asked to record medications and the times they are taken as well as symptoms with exertion and emotional stressors for the time of day they occurred.

At the end of the recording period, the tape is removed and analyzed. Some older equipment may print out twenty-four hours' worth of data to be hand-analyzed by a nurse and doctor. Newer computer programs do much of the processing by scanning the tape and are then reviewed and "over-read" and interpreted by trained professionals.

Holter monitors provide lots of information, and can be worn at home as well as at the hospital to give a "snapshot" of what is going on with daily activity. Computerized Holters give the best data on parameters also measured on ECG such as rate, rhythm, and conduction, so they are most frequently used to detect arrhythmias that are often missed on a routine ECG. Holters also record data about a person's highest and lowest heart rates for the twenty-four-hour period scanned, as well as count duration and frequencies of arrhythmias, and tell us the longest and shortest pause between heartbeats for the day. This information is then correlated with a person's activity, stress, medication, and other details so that we can look for events, precipitating factors, drug effects, and more.

Holter monitoring is a great tool for evaluating the effect of anti-arrhythmia medication. While not a first-line diagnostic tool for assessing ischemia, Holter monitors occasionally pick up ischemia not previously detected and can direct further testing. In unusual cases, where we miss an arrhythmia or a symptom that just failed to occur during the twenty-four-hour Holter test, we can order an event monitor. This device is usually given out for thirty days and can be hooked up when the individual is experiencing a symptom. Once attached to the Holter unit, the patient can relay via telephone lines into a receiving unit at a doctor's office where the heart's activity can be recorded during the symptom.

The Echocardiogram

Another noninvasive test is called echocardiography, in which a 3-D image of the heart is created using ultrasound waves in the same way that a sonogram is used to examine a pregnant woman's fetus. An echo takes about thirty minutes to perform. The patient lies on her left side to bring the heart closer to the chest wall. Jelly is applied to an echo transducer to make a good, sound seal with the skin.

Then the technician, who is trained and certified in ultrasonography, will slide the transducer sensor around, recording on tape the images being picked up by the bouncing of a sound wave against the heart. I have always found the echocardiogram to be a helpful tool to view the heart because it is *dynamic*—that is, we can see the structures of the heart as they move through space during each phase of the cardiac cycle. We watch as the heart stretches and surrenders to fill, and as it recoils and contracts energetically to pump blood forward; the heart's walls can be observed for how synchronously they work.

The healthy heartbeat looks like a wave moving from the top of the atria down to the bottom of the ventricles, as the chambers stretch, fill, and eject the blood through the tricuspid (right heart) and mitral (left heart) valves, down into the ventricles, which then contract with an even larger wave to propel the blood out into the lungs on the right, and the aorta on the left. We can visualize the four heart valves as they open and close. On some occasions the transducer may even be able to light up the base of the left main coronary artery. The echo does not give us direct information about the circulation, but abnormalities in movement of the heart walls may be noted. For example, a portion of the wall of the left ventricle may lag slightly behind the rest of the wall, instead of the 360-degree wall moving in harmony. The diagnostician, usually a board certified cardiologist, must analyze the abnormal pattern of wall motion to determine conditions such as an old heart attack, ischemia, or an aneurysm.

An echo is often done in the setting of an acute heart attack to assess what is called "myocardium at risk," or an area of tissue, usually around the vulnerable zone, which may be "stunned" by the ischemia and dragging behind. Fortunately, the damaged tissue may be salvaged with interventions such as clot-busters or emergency angioplasty or bypass surgery to restore blood flow.

In addition to the scarring or damage of an old heart attack, the echocardiogram can show whether or not the heart muscle itself has become enlarged, a critical risk factor for establishing a prognosis, or prediction, of someone's risk for future cardiac problems. Echos allow us to measure things like wall thickness, chamber size, valvular dimensions, and the estimated ejection fraction (the percentage of blood expelled from the left ventricle with each heartbeat) with high reliability. Like Doppler radar has increased the reliability of our weather forecasting, Doppler Echo allows us to hear heart sounds, just like a stethoscope, and record them so that they can be saved and interpreted for pitch, duration, location, and intensity. We can even turn up the volume to try to distinguish the different sounds better!

This is important information in assessing valvular disorders and making treatment decisions or planning surgical interventions. And a newer technique called Color Flow Doppler allows us to assign colors to different velocities of blood flow so that we can follow patterns of "jets" or turbulent areas in the heart. Color flow even helps clarify the direction of blood flow to further assess a "leaky valve" and how blood flow is being impeded.

All in all, echocardiography gives us a lot of data without actually going into the heart. In fact, many centers combine the echocardiogram with the stress test to get more anatomical information about what is happening to the heart during exercise. Again, this dynamic data adds another dimension to the clues we are evaluating.

While a routine echo is unable to show directly whether or not the coronary arteries are blocked, when combined with stress testing, the "exercise echo" just may be the best test to screen women for coronary artery disease, particularly those woman who can tolerate exercise, because the ultrasonic, real-time images allow us an appropriate visual window through which to view the heart as it pumps to meet an oxygen demand.

When employing the stress echo, the physician compares the echocardiogram taken pretest, at rest, with the echo ultrasound pictures taken during exercise. For those who cannot exercise, dobutamine may be injected intravenously to raise the heart rate. In fact, the television-like echo screen can be split on playback, allowing the viewer to watch pre- and post-test recordings simultaneously. If the left ventricular walls move energetically and synergistically at rest (a normal finding) but move sluggishly and/or out of harmony with the demands of exertion (a wall motion abnormality), then there is a good chance that the blood flow to the left ventricle is inadequate and that there is some ischemia. This finding on stress echo may warrant a more definitive test to further evaluate the competency of the heart, such as angiogram.

The Stress Test

The most common diagnostic test is the *exercise treadmill test* (ETT), in which the patient exercises on a treadmill while an electrocardiograph monitors the electrical activity of the heart at nearly its maximum capacity for energy. Stress testing may also be performed with an arm ergometer or stationary bike which is most commonly used for those who have trouble walking because of problems with gait, balance, knees, or arthritis.

The ETT is usually the first diagnostic test used to screen for heart disease, and while it has an accuracy rate of 70 percent in men, ETT yields false positive or false negative results in about 60 percent of women. A false positive is a test result that indicates heart disease when none is actually present, and a false negative is the opposite—a negative finding for heart disease when heart disease is actually present. To give you a frame of reference and understand false test results better, let me explain a healthy response to exercise.

First of all, when the body works physically, some shifting of blood flow occurs. Blood is shunted away from the gut and over to working skeletal muscle in order to deliver more nutrients, most notably oxygen. In order to accomplish this shift, the blood vessels in the working limbs widen or dilate to bring in more blood and remove the byproducts and toxins of increased metabolism, such as lactic acid. This means that the diastolic blood pressure (the lower number) may go down, or stay the same. To pick up the pace, a competent heart should be able to increase its rate of beating every minute in order to pick up the stroke volume and then the cardiac output to meet the demand. As the heart squeezes more forcefully, the systolic blood pressure (top number) should go up, incrementally and proportional to the workload, just like the heart rate.

Getting back to the stress test, the typical protocol is to start at a low level of work and increase the effort every three minutes. The average stress test lasts about six to twelve minutes, even less in those of advancing age or those who are just plain out of shape. We watch for an appropriate response to exercise; that is, the heart rate and systolic blood pressure go up while the diastolic blood pressure goes down. But we are looking at other parameters as well, such as changes in the ECG that indicate ischemia or arrhythmias with exertion that may or may not imply ischemia. A healthy response to exercise in the absence of ECG changes, arrhythmias, and symptoms implies what we like to see in stress testing: a "competent" left ventricle, able to meet the demands of exercise. The stress test may be ended for a variety of reasons, including but not limited to the following:

❖ The person has reached 85 to 90 percent of what would be considered a submaximal heart rate for someone their age, at which point the test has the best ability to detect coronary artery disease. (That's what is called the prognostic ability of the test.)
❖ The person is too fatigued or short of breath to go on.
❖ The person has requested to terminate the test.
❖ The supervising physician has determined that he has the results that he or she needs, be it a symptom or an end point that has been predetermined due to recent heart attack or another reason.
❖ The blood pressure response is too high or any arrhythmia has presented which make it unsafe to proceed.
❖ The ECG has shifted to a point that is either diagnostically positive or has justified stopping and proceeding with another diagnostic test, most commonly a nuclear test or an angiogram.

Getting back to the false test results, there are several factors that may cause the ECG to shift besides blockage of one or more coronary arteries, including a hypertensive blood pressure response, hyperventilation (most test centers do an ECG after hyperventilation before the stress test to screen for this), repolarization shifts with high heart rates, electrolyte abnormalities, MVP (mitral valve prolapse), IHSS (a condition called idiopathic hypertrophic subaortic stenosis—a mouthful just to say that there is too much heart muscle), sympathetic nervous system overdrive, and just being a woman. Let me explain.

When it comes to stress testing, we know that a woman's electrocardiogram (ECG) response to exercise stress may vary significantly from a man's—something not understood very well until recently. And because women are older than men when they develop heart disease, many female heart patients cannot perform the exercise for the test because of arthritis or other conditions. For women who cannot exercise because of limitations, we can fall back on the bicycle ergometer test if she can cycle, or another tool called the Persantine stress test, and nuclear testing which is performed at rest.

During a Persantine stress test, the drug Persantine is administered via an intravenous line while the woman (or man if he needs one) lies down on the table attached to the twelve lead ECG. Persantine acts similar to exercise in that it dilates the coronary blood vessels, shunting the blood around in the heart through a different mechanism of action. The woman is then given an additional injection of thallium or cardiolite isotope tracers, which can be picked up with a special SPECT camera. The isotope scan after any stress test takes about thirty minutes, and all the patient has to do is lie on his or her back while the camera above takes pictures of the heart from various angles and at various intervals.

Using a visualizing agent, such as thallium or cardiolite, raises what we call the predictive value of the stress test, so that the results have more reliability and specificity (ability to predict heart disease). For instance, a 90 to 100 percent maximal stress test (one where the heart rate reaches the maximal point for age) has about 85 to 90 percent validity to predict heart disease if it's truly present. But when we add imaging, the predictive value rises to 94 to 95 percent. Some of these imaging tests may be used with Persantine, to add the second dimension of an X-ray image of the heart to the reading of the ECG.

In these tests the tracer is picked up in the heart and "counted" as it is able to get through to the various regions of the heart muscle. A "cold spot," a region not perfused by the isotope, implies that there is obstruction to blood flow in that area.

And for a woman who can perform the exercise, a Thallium or Cardiolite stress test may be employed to assess the heart. For her the Thallium is injected at the peak of exercise or right afterward, a tiny amount of the radioactive thallium is injected into a vein, and the heart is monitored with an X-ray camera. If the amount of radiation given off by the thallium is too low, it indicates that not enough blood is reaching the heart muscle and that the coronary arteries are blocked. But, even though the thallium test is more accurate than the stress test alone, it is frequently less reliable for women. Why? Because their breast tissue may block the Thallium signals and distort the readings. This leads to more false positive and false negative results, and may give results that are uncertain. When the imaging is performed with Thallium-201, larger women have a higher reported rate of non-diagnostic results than do smaller women.

And there are a few other pitfalls when using the exercise ECG in women. The accuracy of the test is also problematic due to the lower prevalence of severe triple vessel disease for women, as well as reduced exercise capacity.

Another problem with exercise evaluation is that research has demonstrated that their statistical predictive values have been based on men. But, as you might expect, there are inherent problems with this. Men achieve higher ejection fractions than women when they are compared at maximum workloads even when the numbers are adjusted for aerobic capacities. And even at rest, women have a smaller end-diastolic volume—that is, there is less blood left in the left ventricle in reserve after systole, or contraction of the heart.

It involves a complicated computation in exercise physiology, but the bottom line is that *women use a different mechanism to move blood out into the aorta when there is an excess load placed on their hearts with exertion.* More than men, women increase their cardiac output by relying on something called the Frank–Starling effect. The basic premise of this mechanism is that each time a muscle contracts to meet a work demand, the heart adjusts its muscle fiber lengths so that the following contraction is even stronger. Essentially, these research findings suggest a fundamental physiological difference between the sexes and infer that there are inherent limitations when using the exercise evaluation to diagnose women.

But this is where the perfusion scan improves the predictive value of the exercise evaluation for females. Imaging should be an excellent tool for the cardiac assessment of women with known or suspected coronary artery disease, and this has actually been shown to be the case in several studies. And a real plus for women in terms of exercise testing with imaging is that the test's prognostic ability to show *stress-induced myocardial perfusion defects*, which have been well studied in men, appears to have equal if not better validity for women. The same predictive value holds true for women who have *normal* imaging studies, particularly those for whom abundant breast tissue does not create a diagnostic dilemma.

But the ultimate dilemma remains: Because of the reduced reliability of some of these preliminary noninvasive tests for women, they are less likely to be referred for an angiogram, the most accurate test for coronary artery disease. To sort through this quagmire of information, we now have PET and Ultrafast CT scanning, both of which offer great promise in the non-invasive assessment of coronary artery disease in women.

Positive Emission Tomography (PET)

Now, while most diagnostic tools for diagnosing heart disease have a built-in problem with nondiagnostic and false positive results, the high resolution, 3D images of the cardiovascular system that can be appreciated with positive emission tomography (PET) scanning offers new hope for diagnosing women. Unlike the gender-related differences in the left ventricle's response to physical exertion, there have been no demonstrable differences shown for the parameters being evaluated with PET: myocardial perfusion (the amount of blood being taken up by the heart muscle) and blood flow reserve (the amount of blood that can be made available to the heart from the vascular bed—capillaries—if needed).

The PET scan makes images of metabolic substances (usually glucose, ammonia, and nitrogen) in the heart that have been made radioactive and then injected into the circulation. Once in the bloodstream, a portion of this material will find its way to the heart, where it is naturally incorporated into the cells of the muscle. If the cells are reasonably functional and can pick up this tracer metabolite, it will accumulate enough for the PET scanner to detect. Failure of any area of the muscle to pick up this radioactive tracer material indicates that the cells are essentially no longer alive and active.

PET studies have been nicknamed "viability studies" because the manufacture of these substances is dependent upon the cells being alive. Ordinary studies also require an adequate flow of blood to the muscle to bring in the substance, such as Thallium, to "light up the heart." A defect in the ability of the heart muscle to show up on imaging may also indicate a blockage to blood flow, such as we see in heart disease. The trick in interpreting the PET scan is to differentiate dead heart muscle from that which is what we called "hibernating"; that is, alive and well, but in need of restoration of its blood supply. The physician reading the test must also be able to interpret "stunned myocardium," an area of the heart so injured that it cannot move much, such as after a heart attack or bypass surgery.

The bottom line of the PET interpretation, whether the cells are hibernating or stunned, is to assess the amount of myocardium that is capable of functioning and any areas in jeopardy, which might show a lack of blood flow that might be improved by medical intervention, whether it be drugs, angioplasty, or bypass surgery. The ultimate goal in deciding treatment is to preserve as much of the heart muscle as possible in order to prevent heart failure and enhance a woman's quality of life and survival. In theory, anyone about to undergo any cardiac surgical intervention should have this test to help to predict the success of the procedure. The problem is that a high percentage of cardiologists performing angioplasty and surgeons who perform CABS pay little or no attention to the benefits of having their patients go through this test.

PET scans have many advantages over other noninvasive tests, primarily because the images that are produced are corrected for breast attenuation. So far, PET is much better validated than MRI (myocardial perfusion imaging with SPECT) and the ultra-fast electron beam computed cinetomography (UFCT) as a clinical tool, but all three tests have offered enormous promise because of their outstanding spatial resolution and for combined images of left ventricular function, and perfusion at rest and with exercise.

The greater accuracy of PET offsets the greater initial cost of the test because it enables us to better diagnose and target treatment interventions, eventually reducing the overall cost of treatment. And, on a more ethical note, the PET scan offers a more accurate diagnosis, thereby reducing anxiety and suffering. Being able to swiftly and appropriately diagnose, or rule out, any medical disorder, has tremendous ramifications for patients and their loved ones in terms of reducing the stress of uncertainty and offer the benefit of early treatment, when needed. At the 1997 conference called "Heart Disease and Women," sponsored by the American College of

Cardiology, Dr. R. E. Patterson reported that the well-validated safety, convenience, and exceptionally high sensitivity and specificity of PET myocardial perfusion imaging justify terming it the "woman's test for coronary artery disease."

UFCT

The *ultra-fast electron beam computed cinetomography* (UFCT) offers another new development for imaging women who are at high risk for heart disease because of the presence of risk factors. This simple, ten-minute test may well be quite a useful assessment tool to diagnose early changes of CAD in women, even though their plaques have not reached the point of obstructing arterial flow. This means that the UFCT has the ability to detect calcified lesions before they have gotten far enough along to provoke some symptoms, a tremendous tool that allows us to evaluate high-risk women—such as those with strong family histories—and help them plan early interventions to protect themselves.

Not only is the UFCT scan a brief, cost-effective, noninvasive test, it doesn't require a large MRI-type of machine to perform the scan. The tubular, enclosed devices used for MRI create problems of claustrophobia for many people, but the CT scan involves merely lying on a table as the scanning table traverses the heart to take pictures, similar to the Thallium and SPECT imaging cameras. Also called electron beam computerized tomography (EBCT), the ultra-fast scanner can take pictures of the body in a fraction of a second.

A standard CAT scan is too slow, making pictures of the moving heart blurry and difficult to read. This new scanner takes pictures so fast that it actually freezes the heart in motion and produces images in three dimensions. By viewing these images, doctors can actually see evidence of early disease before a heart attack strikes.

What they see are calcium deposits in the coronary arteries, a common precursor to the plaque that can cause a heart attack.

The great thing about the test is that it gives incredible information about the heart without actual entry into the body, takes only a total of fifteen minutes and is relatively inexpensive ($400) compared to other noninvasive tests for the heart. Best of all, the UFCT can detect early heart disease about 85 to 95 percent of the time. In fact, the UFCT is one medical test where you do get a "grade"—we call it the Calcium Score, and it reflects the amount of calcium deposition picked up by the imaging equipment. A perfect score for this test is zero. The more your scores rise above zero, the greater the probability that there is calcium deposited in your arteries.

Further, studies have indicated even higher score accuracy in patients with advanced heart disease, so it offers a great way to track known heart disease without going inside with an angiographic catheter every time. The calcium scan is very beneficial in cases of positive stress test results: it can be used with some confidence to rule out a suspected false positive, or to confirm a true positive, before going on to the angiogram.

I find that the UFCT scan is also an appropriate and inexpensive screening tool if a woman is juggling her options for hormone replacement therapy. If she is at all unclear after weighing her risk of heart disease against her risk of breast cancer, then the calcium scan may give her the information she needs to make the HRT decision. If she has any calcification of the coronary arteries on this scan, then she should consider some form of HRT as an intervention to protect her high risk, as she already has an indication of the advanced changes of probable CAD. Ultra-fast CT images of the heart demonstrating calcification in women may be one of the best noninvasive tests to help a woman decide about hormonal replacement therapy.

The test does have its limitations: it will not detect any non-calcified plaque or any soft plaque—such as those made up of cholesterol streaks, dead red and white blood cells; and macrophages, fibrin, and blood clots, and other materials, which are also harbingers of coronary artery disease. Further, patients may have coronary heart disease even though there is no evidence of calcified arteries. So, a negative score on a Calcium Scan is not as predictive as a positive one.

The other downside to the UFCT Scan is its somewhat limited availability at this time. Accessing a hospital that has a UFCT scanner may mean traveling a distance, which is an obstacle for some. Despite its limitations, I am fully convinced that it is a very valuable tool for early detection of heart disease. And, since coronary calcium scores are indicative of potential heart disease, finding out that you have "scored highly" should be a red flag. It makes good sense to do some aggressive reduction of your other risk factors.

If coronary calcification is detected by high frequency CT scanning, it may suggest the greater need for hormonal replacement therapy in post-menopausal women in addition to increasing your motivation for a healthy lifestyle, including exercise, cessation of smoking, reduction in weight, and using targeted nutritional supplements.

For any woman who has symptoms of heart disease (chest discomfort, shortness of breath, etc.) and a high calcium score, the angiogram will disclose the location and severity of atherosclerotic lesions that may be obstructing blood flow. Hopefully, we will see this equipment more commonly in cardiac screening centers in the future.

The Angiogram: Window into the Heart
Now let's return to the angiogram or cardiac catheterization, the venerable "gold standard" for evaluating heart disease. Why don't physicians

just routinely order a cardiac catheterization for anyone suspected of heart disease? Well, for starters, the average angiogram costs about $10,000, so you can be sure that no insurance company is going to pay for one unless there has been some prior testing indicating that the probability for heart disease is high. But the major reason that physicians wait for preliminary test results before they consider angiography is that the angiogram is an invasive test—that is, we have to *enter* the body to perform it—and like any invasive procedure, it carries more risk than a noninvasive tool, such as a stress test, exercise echocardiogram, or PET Scan. Physicians, then, usually don't recommend an angiogram when these more preliminary tests fail to support a tentative diagnosis of coronary artery disease in a woman. The benefit of the angiogram is its high reliability in detecting blockages in the heart.

Angiography provides us with a real window into the heart and gives us such direct and accurate information that, in most cases, a negative result amounts to a dismissal of heart disease. An angiogram can also be used to evaluate the physical structure of the heart, such as chamber size and valvular composition. We can directly measure the pressure gradients across the four heart valves and how the valvular flaps are closing in order to assess valvular disorders or plan valve replacement surgery. Angiography also allows us to determine a precise assessment of the heart's *stroke volume* (SV) (the amount of blood ejected with each heartbeat) and its *cardiac output* (the volume amount of blood ejected per minute) as well as approximate the heart's *ejection fraction* with more reliability than the echocardiogram. The accuracy of the catheterization lies in the fact that it is not indirectly inferring this information from a point outside of the heart. The sensor tip of the angiography catheter is actually moving through the heart chambers and *in* the left ventricle at the time these measurement are taken.

Catheterization of the heart involves threading a thin tube (catheter) into an artery in the bend of the arm or in the crease of the groin (where the arteries are close to the surface and easy to access), and threading it carefully through the arterial system, guiding it into the heart. Once the catheter is placed at the source of the coronary arteries, a radio-opaque dye is injected, which lights up the heart like a Christmas tree, and makes it possible to see any blockages in the coronary arteries.

Unfortunately, angiography is sometimes a less accurate test for women. A woman's arteries may be so small that they are difficult to visualize and often appear normal on an angiogram, even though she may have some heart disease. Of the people who have angina serious enough to indicate an angiogram, but whose arteries appear normal, most are women. The Coronary Artery Surgery Study (CASS) found that *almost 50 percent of the women who underwent angiography showed normal arteries,* compared with only 17 percent of the men.

So for a woman, a "normal" angiogram is mostly but not always a clean bill of cardiac health as it is for a man. Some women may have other sources of chest pain, such as mitral valve prolapse, coronary artery spasm, or even panic disorder. Whenever a man or woman has symptoms suggestive of cardiac disease versus another medical problem, the protocol is always to rule out a problem with the heart first, as it has the most potential to be life-threatening.

Despite the statistics, in most cases, after a woman has normal findings on an angiogram, her doctor concludes that her symptoms are *not* the result of heart disease. *A negative angiogram usually forces the physician to conclude that there is no major heart disease,* reassure his patient, and re-examine other causes for her symptoms, such as esophageal spasm, gall bladder disease, and other noncardiac disorders.

I still use them to make a diagnosis. It is the gold standard, 95 to 97 percent effective with women. It is good, but carries some risk.

APPENDIX B

Testing Your Hormone Levels

For many women, salivary hormone testing helps take the guess-work out of hormone replacement therapy (HRT). Many women today are being overdosed with estrogen. This may not only make symptoms, like breast tenderness and weight gain, worse but also increases cancer risk. Keeping hormones at optimal levels balances a woman's body and reduces the risks and side effects of HRT.

Saliva Testing

There is a large population of women in their late 30s and 40s suffering from symptoms of estrogen dominance (levels of estrogen are high compared to progesterone levels), not deficiency, and many health professionals are not adequately checking both the estrogens (estradiol and estriol) and progesterone of their patients. Observations made by a few astute clinical labs over the years show that many women, both pre- and postmenopausal, are actually estrogen dominant. This is assessed by measuring their salivary estrogens (E2 and E3) and progesterone (P).

The goal is to rebalance estrogen (estradiol) and progesterone to levels that more closely match those that existed in the prime of life. This doesn't mean returning to having periods, but simply achieving a balance between the body's own natural hormones. This is not the case right now with thousands of women across the country. They are told that "estrogens" are needed to save their heart and bone. And now they are told they need "designer estrogens" for a more "selective" effect.

In addition to estrogen overdoses, women quite often have been using progesterone creams overzealously. A report in *The Journal of Alternative and Complementary Medicine* describes two women using very high strength (5 percent) progesterone creams. They developed symptoms such as water retention, increased body weight, breast engorgement, and mild to moderate depression. These symptoms were very gradual in onset (over six to nine months) such that the women (and their doctors) didn't associate the symptoms with the accumulation of progesterone. Salivary testing readily detects high progesterone levels. Dr. Bennett has had several cases in which the women using progesterone creams had salivary levels greater that 1,000 pg/ml in the first few days of use. After stopping, these women took many days to rebalance.

For the truly postmenopausal woman, one or two saliva tests can detect the ratio of estrogens to progesterone with great accuracy. For the cycling premenopausal woman or the woman with irregular or missed periods, it may take several salivary samples collected over a period of twenty-eight days to construct a more accurate picture of the estrogen/progesterone imbalance.

Catherine is a forty-seven-year-old cycling woman who was experiencing symptoms she assumed were related to the perimenopausal period. She had slight weight gain, bloating, some hot flashes, irregular periods, and some breast tenderness. In addition, she had an ongoing problem with insomnia that had gotten worse and was not relieved by melatonin. She also had headaches that were related to her periods.

It was recommended that she collect eleven salivary samples needed for the test and also record signs and symptoms each day to try and correlate the data to highs and lows of estradiol and progesterone. The test showed that Catherine is estrogen dominant and her symptoms correlate with fluctuating estradiol and progesterone levels. She experienced headaches on days one to ten of the cycle with hot flashes on days two, three, seven, and eight, and insomnia on days seven and eight.

Catherine is estrogen dominant and would not benefit from more estrogen. Instead, progesterone supplementation was recommended to balance out her hormones.

Blood Testing

Many conventional physicians have routinely used blood tests to assay sex hormone levels. This has been the "acceptable" standard of practice for years. Blood levels, however, can be misleading. Hormones are transported in the blood by carrier proteins, lipoproteins, and fatty acids. Therefore, the amount that is "free" and biologically active is very small compared to "bound" and biologically inactive. It is more difficult and costly to measure this "free" hormone in blood. Saliva, however, is used to measure this more directly.

The typical lab report gives "total" hormone unless the doctor directs the lab to do "free" levels. In the case of progesterone, very few labs are set up to do "free" progesterone levels in blood. Testosterone levels can also be reported as "free" or "total," with the latter being most common. Unless your report states "free" or "free fraction," it likely means "total."

Urine Testing

Some physicians use urine to assess hormone levels. There are several potential problems with using this biological fluid. The first is that urine reflects the end-products of metabolism. When the lab analyzes urine for specific sex hormones, interfering substances may confuse the picture.

Another reason urine is not suitable for clinical use is the lack of time specificity. The twenty-four–hour urine sample typically collected cannot determine circadian rhythms which most hormones exhibit. Testosterone, for example, is highest in the morning and lower in the evening. Urine values here are not as helpful as saliva. Also, urine does not reflect the biologically active "free fraction" discussed above. Urine data cannot duplicate saliva in plotting a women's cyclical highs and lows of estradiol and progesterone.

It is therefore more cost-effective and clinically relevant to use saliva for assessing sex hormone levels for women (and men).

Saliva testing gives women a scientific base to work from when it comes to knowing levels of estrogen, progesterone, and testosterone. If any woman becomes more symptomatic on HRT, with an unsatisfactory quality of life, saliva testing is one option that women can consider to get an accurate metabolic assessment of the situation. I am sure in the future more and more physicians will be considering saliva testing as a scientific basis to help balance a women's hormonal status which may give vital information regarding the type of therapy she wishes to regulate.

APPENDIX C

The Sinatra Modified Mediterranean Diet Seven-Day Meal Plan

Day One
BREAKFAST

½ whole wheat English muffin or 1 slice whole wheat bread

Phytoestrogen Shake (see page 365)

⅓ melon

LUNCH

1 4-ounce veggie burger with romaine lettuce, sliced tomato, and onion

2 slices whole wheat bread

1 cup coleslaw mixed with 1 tablespoon plain nonfat yogurt and 6 chopped walnuts

1 apple

DINNER*

1 6-ounce salmon steak

1 cup couscous

1 cup broccoli steamed with 2 tablespoons sesame seeds and a dash of fresh squeezed lemon

Sliced tomato salad with chopped onion, garlic, and 1 teaspoon olive or flax oil and a dash of balsamic vinegar

*Sprinkle salmon steak with ½ lemon and broil for 5 minutes. Use the other lemon half on the broccoli. Chop 1 small onion and 1 clove garlic for the sliced tomato salad and dress with oil and vinegar to taste.

Day Two

BREAKFAST

1 cup oatmeal

½ cup berries of choice

1 cup soy milk (½ cup in oatmeal, the other ½ cup as a beverage)

LUNCH

6 ounces sardines (or mackerel) in a sandwich topped with onion slices and 1 tablespoon low-fat mayonnaise (or substitute veggie burger)

2 slices of whole grain toast

2 cups tossed green salad with 1 tablespoon flax or olive oil mixed with fresh lemon juice or balsamic vineger to taste

2 plums

DINNER*

Stir-fried vegetables with 8 ounces chopped tofu

3 cloves garlic, chopped

1 tablespoon olive oil

2 tablespoons fresh Parmesan cheese

1½ cups cooked brown rice with chopped onion

★In a wok or large frying pan, steam 3 cloves chopped fresh garlic with chopped vegetables (1 small bunch broccoli, 12 mushrooms, 2 medium zucchini, 2 medium summer squash, peppers, etc.) in 3 to 4 ounces water. Toss in tofu. Drizzle oil and sprinkle cheese over veggies when tender. Serve over brown rice.

Day Three
BREAKFAST
Buckwheat Pancakes (see page 366)
½ cup chopped walnuts or almonds for topping
2 tablespoons real maple syrup

LUNCH
¾ chickpea hummus spread with sliced tomato, leafy green lettuce, and ½ sliced avocado on whole wheat pita
1 cup White Bean Salad (see page 368)
6 walnuts, chopped
1 peach

DINNER★
½ baked boned/skinless chicken breast
2 tablespoons mango chutney
1 cup new potatoes with 2 cloves chopped garlic, 1 small chopped onion, and 1 teaspooon olive oil
6 to 8 asparagus spears steamed and sprinkled with fresh lemon juice and a pinch of garlic salt

★Spread chicken with chutney and bake for 20 minutes in a 400 degree oven. Remove chicken from oven and keep warm. Combine chopped potatoes with garlic, onions, and oil, and bake for 25 minutes at the same temperature.

Day Four

BREAKFAST

Blueberry Bran Muffin (see page 365)

Phytoestrogen Shake (see page 365)

1 to 2 kiwis, peeled and sliced

LUNCH

1 cup low-fat cottage cheese served with ½ sliced cucumber and ½ sliced avocado mixed with 1 tablespoon flax or olive oil and 1 teaspoon lemon juice

½ baked acorn or butternut squash

1 peach

DINNER

8 ounces shrimp sautéed with 2 chopped garlic cloves, 1 chopped small onion, and 1 tablespoon olive oil served over 1 cup cooked brown rice

1 ½ cups spinach salad with one chopped garlic clove, 4 raw cauliflower florets, and 4 sliced strawberries served with Lemon-Honey Dressing (see page 365)

Day Five

BREAKFAST

2-egg omelet (use organic eggs or those from hens fed with flaxseed)

1 Bran Muffin (see page 365) with fruit spread (try a purée of your favorite fruit)

½ grapefruit

LUNCH

½ can white tuna (packed in water) drained and mixed with 1 cup

red kidney beans and 1 teaspoon balsamic vinegar
1 cup cooked tabouli with chopped tomato, mint, and 1 teaspoon
olive oil
3 to 4 fresh whole apricots

DINNER
Pasta Primavera (see page 367)
1 ½ cups Jerusalem artichoke or whole wheat linguine pasta
Small Caesar salad with two ground anchovies and mixed with 1
tablespoon olive oil, 2 tablespoons Parmesan cheese, and a dash of
fresh-squeezed lemon juice

Day Six
BREAKFAST
Wheat, bran, spelt, or kamut dry cereal (Arrowhead Mills/Nature's
Path brands can be found in your health food store)
1 ½ cups soy milk (½ on cereal, and ½ as a beverage)
½ cup berries or 1 banana, sliced

LUNCH
Antiguan Black Bean Soup (see page 366)
2 sliced multi-grain bread
1 shredded carrot salad with walnuts and 1 tablespoon low-fat
yogurt
Cherries

DINNER
Grilled Mediterranean Halibut (see page 368)
1 ½ cups Waldorf salad with romaine lettuce, pear slices, walnuts,
and Lemon–Honey Dressing (see page 365)
6 to 8 cauliflower florets, steamed

Day Seven

BREAKFAST

1 cup oatmeal mixed with 3 tablespoons low-fat or fat-free cottage cheese

½ cup berries of your choice

1 cup soy milk (½ on oatmeal, and ½ as beverage)

LUNCH

1 large portabello mushroom cap, sliced and sautéed in lite teriyaki sauce with 2 ounces chevre (goat or bleu cheese)

Sliced tomato and onion

2 slices whole grain bread or bun

Green salad with 1 chopped clove garlic

1 tablespoon olive or flax oil and fresh lemon juice

1 pear

DINNER

Lentil Stew (see page 369) served over 1 cup cooked brown rice

6 to 8 asparagus spears, steamed (when cooked add 1 teaspoon olive oil and a pinch of garlic salt)

2 to 3 cups raw, baby spinach salad topped with ¼ cup sliced strawberries, ¼ cup blueberries, 2 tablespoons chopped pecans and walnuts with a raspberry vinaigrette dressing

Mediterranean Recipes

PHYTOESTROGEN SHAKE

Flaxseed is considered one of the world's richest sources of omega-3s.

2 tablespoons organic flaxseed

8 to 10 ounces chilled soy milk

½ banana

4 strawberries or 2 tablespoons blueberries

Grind flaxseed in a clean coffee mill. Place in blender and add soy milk, banana, and berries and blend together.

LEMON-HONEY DRESSING

Juice of 1 large lemon

2 tablespoons honey

2 tablespoons olive oil

½ teaspoon dried basil

Freshly ground pepper to taste

Whisk all ingredients together in a small bowl.

BLUEBERRY BRAN MUFFINS

2 cups bran cereal

1 cup skim milk

1 tablespoon grapeseed oil

2 egg whites

1 tablespoon honey

⅓ cup molasses

1½ cups whole wheat flour or Soy Quik flour

½ teaspoon sea salt

1 cup blueberries

Preheat oven to 400 degrees.

In a medium bowl, mix bran cereal and milk and let stand 5 minutes. Stir in oil, egg whites, honey, and molasses. Stir in flour, sea salt, and blueberries. Pour in a muffin tin and bake for 15 minutes.

ANTIGUAN BLACK BEAN SOUP

2 tablespoons olive oil

½ green pepper, chopped

1 onion, chopped

½ clove garlic, minced

½ pound dried black beans cooked according to package directions, or two 16-ounce cans drained black beans

Freshly ground pepper

1 tablespoon red wine vinegar

1 bay leaf

2 quarts water

1 cup short-grain brown rice, cooked

Fresh parsley, chopped

In a large saucepan, combine olive oil, green pepper, 1½ tablespoons onion, and garlic. Sauté until tender. Stir in precooked or canned black beans, pepper, vinegar, and bay leaf. Add water and then simmer for 30 to 40 minutes. Remove bay leaf before serving. Top with remaining onion and brown rice. Garnish with parsley.

BUCKWHEAT PANCAKES WITH BLUEBERRIES

1 cup buckwheat flour

1 cup other whole grain flour

2 cups soy milk or water

2 eggs

1 tablespoon grapeseed oil

1 tablespoon honey
⅓ cup fresh unsweetened blueberries

Preheat a lightly oiled griddle.

Stir buckwheat and whole grain flour together in large bowl. Add soy milk, eggs, oil, and honey and mix briefly. Add blueberries and stir gently. Cook on griddle, turning once, until golden on both sides.

PASTA PRIMAVERA

2 cups fresh broccoli florets
1 cup fresh asparagus spears, chopped
1 tablespoon olive oil
2 to 3 cloves garlic, chopped
1 small onion, chopped
1 cup sun-dried tomatoes (not oil-packed)
2 small zucchini, chopped
1 cup grated carrot
2 cups Jerusalem artichoke or whole wheat linguine or angel hair pasta
1 cup chopped fresh parsley
2 tablespoons fresh Parmesan cheese

Steam broccoli and asparagus for 2 to 3 minutes in a vegetable steamer. In a large skillet, gently sauté the chopped onion and garlic in olive oil. Add sun-dried tomatoes, zucchini, and carrot and sauté for 5 minutes. (You may add 3 to 4 tablespoons water while sautéing, if necessary.) Add partially cooked broccoli and asparagus, and sauté for 1 minute.

Cook the pasta according to package directions. Mix with sautéed vegetables and gently toss with Parmesan cheese and chopped parsley.

WHITE BEAN SALAD

½ pound dry white beans (washed and soaked overnight) or 2 cans
cooked white beans, drained

3½ cups water

1 medium yellow onion

1 medium red or Vidalia onion, chopped fine

2 garlic cloves, chopped

1 yellow or red pepper, chopped

1 clove garlic, minced

1 tablespoon flax or olive oil

½ teaspoon dried mustard

1 bunch fresh parsley, chopped

Lemon juice and balsamic vinegar to taste

In a large pot, place the beans, water, yellow and red onions, and
2 chopped garlic cloves, bring to a boil, and simmer for 1½ hours or
until tender. Drain and reserve ¼ cup cooking liquid.

In a large bowl, mix pepper, minced garlic, oil, mustard, lemon
juice, vinegar, and the reserved cooking liquid. Add to warm beans
and toss with fresh parsley.

GRILLED HALIBUT MEDITERRANEAN STYLE
WITH LEMON-BASIL VINAIGRETTE

Juice of 1 lemon

2 tablespoons olive oil

3 garlic cloves, crushed

½ teaspoon grated lemon peel

3 tablespoons fresh basil or 3 teaspoons dried

2 teaspoons drained capers

One 4- to 6-ounce halibut steak, ¾-inch thick

Sea salt and pepper to taste

Vinaigrette: Whisk lemon juice, olive oil, garlic, and lemon peel in a small bowl. Stir in 2 tablespoons basil and capers. Season to taste with salt and pepper.

Preheat broiler or grill to medium-high heat. Season halibut steaks with salt and pepper. Brush fish with 1 tablespoon vinaigrette. Grill or broil halibut steaks until just cooked through, about 4 minues per side. Garnish fish with remaining basil and serve.

LENTIL STEW

1 cup uncooked red or green lentils

1 medium onion, chopped

2 garlic cloves, chopped

1 sweet potato or yam, chopped

¼ cup water

1 low-sodium vegetable boullion cube

1 stalk celery, chopped

2 leeks (white part only), sliced

1 medium zucchini, chopped

1 cup fresh parsley, chopped

1 tablespoon balsamic vinegar

Bring lentils to a boil and simmer until tender. (Green lentils take about twice the cooking time as red. Allow 45 minutes for green and about 20 minutes for red lentils.)

In a skillet or wok, sauté the onion and garlic for 1 minute. Add sweet potato (or yam) and sauté for 5 minutes. Add ¼ cup water, vegetable boullion, celery, leeks, and zucchini. Cover and steam for 5 minutes.

When vegetables are tender, mix in lentils, toss with chopped parsley and vinegar and serve.

Heart Healthy Extras

This seven-day meal plan has 1,700 calories per day. Snacks, beverages, and desserts are at your discretion. Try not to let more than four hours go by without at least a small, healthy snack.

SNACKS: Fresh fruits such as apples, peaches, plums, cherries, strawberries, kiwi, and rhubarb. Raw vegetables such as broccoli, cauliflower, celery. Also a handful of walnuts, pumpkin seeds, or almonds. All of the above will help to stop carbohydrate cravings.

BEVERAGES: Try to drink eight glasses of water or herbal tea per day. If you must drink fruit juice, have 4 ounces of juice diluted with 2 ounces of water per day. You may also drink 4 ounces of red wine each day.

DESSERTS: You may eat the fruits listed as snacks for a nutrious, sweet dessert. (For instance, strawberries are only 50 calories per cup and are high in phytonutrients, antioxidants, and fiber.) For a special treat, try dipping a banana in orange juice and 1 tablespoon finely chopped walnuts.

APPENDIX D

African American Women:
Increased Heart Disease Risk?

Incidence of Hypertension*

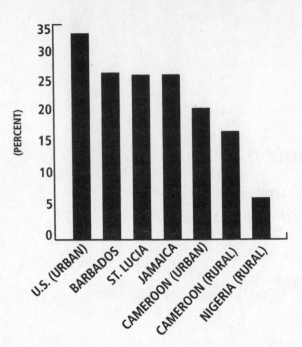

INCIDENCE OF HYPERTENSION, OR CHRONIC HIGH BLOOD PRESSURE, WAS ASSESSED IN AFRICANS AS WELL AS PEOPLE OF AFRICAN DESCENT IN THE U.S. AND CARIBBEAN. THE RATE DROPPED DRAMATICALLY FROM THE U.S. ACROSS THE ATLANTIC TO AFRICA, AND THE DIFFERENCE WAS MOST PRONOUNCED BETWEEN URBAN AFRICAN AMERICANS AND RURAL NIGERIANS. THE FINDINGS SUGGEST THAT HYPERTENSION MAY LARGELY BE A DISEASE OF MODERN LIFE AND THAT GENES ALONE DO NOT ACCOUNT FOR THE HIGH RATES OF HYPERTENSION IN AFRICAN AMERICANS.

*FROM COOPER, ET AL, THE PUZZLE OF HYPERTENSION IN AFRICAN-AMERICANS. ©1999 BY SCIENTIFIC AMERICAN, INC.

Body Mass Index*

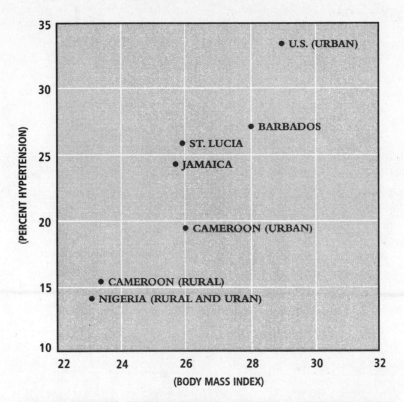

BODY MASS INDEX, OR BMI, MEASURES A PERSON'S WEIGHT-TO-HEIGHT RATIO. A BMI OVER 25 IS GENERALLY A SIGN OF BEING OVERWEIGHT. IN A STUDY OF PEOPLE OF AFRICAN DESCENT, A LOW AVERAGE BMI IN A POPULATION CORRESPONDED TO A LOW RATE OF HYPERTENSION IN THAT COMMUNITY. AS AVERAGE BMI INCREASED, SO DID THE PREVALENCE OF HYPERTENSION. THE FINDINGS SUPPORT THE VIEW THAT HIGH BMI CONTRIBUTES TO HIGH BLOOD PRESSURE.

*FROM COOPER, ET AL, THE PUZZLE OF HYPERTENSION IN AFRICAN-AMERICANS. ©1999 BY SCIENTIFIC AMERICAN, INC.

GLOSSARY

angina ("heart cramp")—chest pain, pressure, or discomfort; may also be accompanied by tingling of the legs, arm, jaw pain, shortness of breath, sense of indigestion, dizziness, sweating, and fatigue.

arrhythmia—irregular heartbeat.

bundle branch block—type of heart conduction delay resulting from a slowing of the electrical impulses of the heart as they pass through the ventricles.

cardiac insufficiency—also called ischemia, describing any of a number of situations in which reduced blood flow to the heart is causing symptoms such as angina. If blood flow to the coronary arteries is not restored within about four minutes, a heart attack can result.

cardiomegaly—enlarged heart.

cardiomyopathy—state in which the muscle tissue of the heart has become damaged, diseased, enlarged, or stretched and thinned, leaving the muscle fibers weakened; most often as a result of scarring from heart attacks, long standing high blood pressure, or valvular heart disease.

coronary angiogram (cardiac catheterization)—the "gold standard" for evaluating heart disease in men and women. Expensive (about $5000 to $10,000); usually not recommended unless preliminary tests strongly suggest presence of coronary artery disease. Involves threading a catheter into an artery in the bend of the arm or crease of the groin and threading it through the arterial system all the way to the heart. A radio-opaque dye is injected, lighting up the heart like a Christmas tree and illuminating any blockages around the heart.

coronary revascularization—a procedure performed by cardiac surgeons where leg or arm veins or the internal mammary arteries are used to "bypass" obstructions of coronary arteries. Blood flow is increased to the area in need.

CABG—coronary artery bypass graft surgery.

CVA—cerebral vascular accident or stroke from an obstruction in the carotid artery or in an artery in the brain.

diastolic dysfunction—progressive stiffening of the heart muscle that prevents it from stretching and filling properly.

ectopic beats—a heartbeat that originates from outside the normal conduction system.

ejection fraction—percentage of blood ejected from the left ventricle with each heart beat; normal range is 50 to 70 percent.

endothelium—innermost lining of the arteries; the smooth surface against which the blood flows. The endothelium is only one cell layer thick, a veneer so thin that it can be seen only under a microscope, but its cells exert a powerful influence on the functioning of the arteries. In response to stresses and chemicals produced by the body, the endothelium releases several substances called factors which cause the smooth muscle walls of the artery, just beneath the endothelial surface, to relax so the vessel can dilate and blood flow increases. The most important of these factors is **endothelial cell releasing factor (EDRF)**.

Estrogen Replacement Therapy (ERT)—when estrogen alone is given to a women.

exercise echo—perhaps the best noninvasive test to evaluate the possibility of coronary heart disease in women. An exercise stress test in which an echocardiogram is taken before (baseline), during, and after exertion.

fibrinogen—inflammatory product of blood coagulation, it can make the blood clot fast enough to trigger a myocardial infarction (heart attack). A high level is a serious risk factor in women.

free radical oxidative stress—a condition in the body when antioxidant defenses are overwhelmed by excessive free radical action.

homocysteine—"bad guy" amino acid, promotes oxidative stress and premature vascular disease. Forms in the blood as a result of eating too many foods high in methionine, such as red meat, avocados, sunflower seeds, wild game, poultry, and ricotta cheese, without enough B vitamins (especially folate, vitamin B6, or vitamin B12) to break down the methionine effectively. If you do not take in enough of these B vitamins, and you frequently enjoy red meat in your diet, you may be at risk of developing excess quantities of homocysteine. Congenital enzyme deficiency occurring in about 5 percent of the population also results in higher homocysteine levels.

Hormone Replacement Therapy (HRT)—When estrogen and progesterone are taken in combination.

hypokalemia—low potassium in the blood.

IHSS (idiopathic hypertrophic subaortic stenosis)—when excessive muscle in the heart causes obstruction of blood flow from the ventricles of the heart.

ischemia—reduced blood flow to the heart (see cardiac insufficiency).

lipid peroxidation—when oxidation of fats occurs such as oxidized LDL.

Lipoprotein(a)—although Lp(a) is technically considered a lipid, it is also considered a marker for thrombosis (clot formation) because it is structurally similar to plasminogen. Lp(a) is a unique lipid that appears to play a regulatory role in atherothrombosis. It is hypothesized to have blood-clotting properties because of its potential to directly inhibit endogenous fibrinolysis (thinning of the blood). Lp(a) is essentially an LDL particle whose proteins are linked by a disulfide bridge. Many factors influence the blood levels of Lp(a) with genetic factors perhaps playing the major role. The liver is also a source of Lp(a) production. A serious risk factor in women when Lp(a) is high.

microangina—pain from diffuse and widespread blockages in the smallest blood vessels in the heart.

MVP—mitral valve prolapse; a condition where the mitral valve "flops back" into the left atrium on occasion.

myocardial perfusion—the amount of blood being taken up by the heart muscle.

Positive Emission Tomography (PET)—high resolution, 3D imaging of the heart using metabolic substances that have been made radioactive and then injected into the circulation to evaluate blood flow in the heart muscle.

PTCA—percutaneous transluminal coronary angioplasty.

restenosis—when the dilation of the artery from a PTCA closes.

silent ischemia—reduced blood flow to the heart not perceived as painful or significant by the patient (see also cardiac insufficiency).

stents—hollow titanium wires that prevent mechanical recoil following balloon angioplasty, thereby eliminating geometric remodeling.

stroke volume (SV)—the amount of blood ejected with each heartbeat.

TIA—transient ischemic attacks, also called mini-strokes when blood flow is compromised in the brain.

Ultra-fast electron beam computed cinetomography (UFCT)—relatively new method of imaging hearts for evaluating heart disease risk in women and men; can detect calcified plaque lesions. Excellent for providing additional info to women with strong family history of heart disease who refuse to consider HRT or ERT

vascular remodeling—reshaping and potential loss of lumen diameter after a PTCA procedure.

ventricular fibrillation—effective rapid quivering of the heart; usually fatal event.

ventricular tachycardia—a serious accelerated heartbeat.

REFERENCES

Introduction: Unlocking the Mysteries of a Woman's Heart

Beery, TA. Gender bias in the diagnosis and treatment of coronary artery disease. *Heart and Lung.* 1995; 24(6):427–35.

Bonn, D. Gender differences abound in management after heart attack. *Lancet.* 1997; 350:343.

Coronary heart disease and stroke remain the leading causes of death of women in America. In Physicians Information. American Heart Association Website (www.americanheart.org); May 12, 1999.

Pert, CB. "Molecules of Emotion: Why You Feel the Way You Feel". New York; Scribner: 1997.

SECTION I: WOMEN AND HEART DISEASE: GETTING TO THE HEART OF THE MATTER

Chapter 1: Why Women are at Risk: Learn the Language of Your Heart

A Woman's Heart. *JAMA* (Patient Page). 1998; 280(16):1462.

Fruzzetti, F.; Ricci, C.; Fioretti, P. Haemostasis profile in smoking and nonsmoking women taking low-dose oral contraceptives. *Contraception.* 1994; 49:579–92.

Lidegaard, O. Oral contraception and risk of a cerebral thromboembolic attack: Results of a case-control study. *BMJ.* 1993; 306:956–963.

Marrugat, J.; Sala J.; Masia R.; et al. Mortality differences between men and women following first myocardial infarction. *JAMA*. 1998; 280(16):1405–10.

Schnatz, JD. Coronary heart disease and postmenopausal women. Lipid Education Service, Hoffman Heart Institute of Connecticut Website (www.stfranciscare.org) February 1, 1998.

Schwartz, LM.; Fisher, ES.; Tosteson, AN.; et al. Treatment and health outcomes of women and men in a cohort with coronary artery disease. *Arch Intern Med*. 1997; 157(14):1545–51.

Soucier, R.; Kosack, C.; Therrien, M.; Missri, J. Acute myocardial infarction in women: An observational study in a large academic hospital. *Journal of the Hoffman Heart Institute of Connecticut*. 1997; 3(1):2–5.

Wenger, N. Coronary heart disease in women: A "new" problem. *Hosp Pract*. 1992;27(11): 59–62.

Wenger, NK.; Speroff, L.; Packard, B. Cardiovascular health and disease in women. *N Engl J Med*. 1993; 329(4):247–256.

Chapter 2: Are You at Risk for Heart Disease? Take the Test

Allemann, YF.; Horber, F.; Colombo, M.; et al. Insulin sensitivity and body fat distribution in normotensive offspring of hypertensive parents. *Lancet*. 1993; 341:327–331.

Anderson, KM.; et al. An updated coronary risk profile: a statement for health professionals. *Circulation*. 1991; 83:356–352.

Barrett-Connor, EL; Cohn, BA.; Wingard, DL. Why is diabetes mellitus a stronger risk factor for fatal ischemic heart disease in women than in men? The Rancho Bernardo Study. *JAMA* 1991; 265(5):627–631.

Bittner, V. and Oparil, S. Hypertension. In Julian DG & Wenger NK (Eds). *Women and Heart Disease*. St. Louis: Mosby; 1997:299–327.

Bjornon, WM.; Fiore, MC.; and Logan-Morrison, BA. The growing problem of smoking in women. *Patient Care*. 1996; 30(13):142–165.

Castelli, WP.; Garrison, RJ.; Wilson, PW.; Abbott, RD.; Kalousdian, S.; Kannel, WB. Incidence of coronary heart disease and lipoprotein-cholesterol levels: the Framingham Study. *JAMA*. 1986; 256:2835–2838.

Castelli, WP. The triglyceride issue: A view from Framingham. *Am Heart J*. 1986; 112:432–437.

Castelli, WP. Cholesterol and lipids in the risk of coronary artery disease—the Framingham Heart Study. *Can J Cardiol*. 1988; 4(suppl):5A–10A.

Castelli, WP. Cardiovascular disease in women. *Am J Obstet Gynecol*. 1988; 158:1153–1160.

Castelli, W.P.; Anderson, K.; Wilson, P.W.; Levy, D. Lipids and risk of coronary artery disease: The Framingham Study. *Ann Epidemiol.* 1992; 2:23–28.

Castelli, W.P. Epidemiology of triglycerides: A view from Framingham. *Am J Cardiol.* 1992;70(19):3H–9H.

Charney, P.; Walsh, JM.; and Nattinger, AB. Update in women's health. *Annal Intern Med.* 1998; 129(7):551–8.

Dunlap, SH.; Sueta, CA.; Tomasko, L.; Adams, KF. Association of body mass, gender and race with heart failure primarily due to hypertension. *JACC.* 1999; 34(5):1602–1608.

Eckel, R.H. Insulin resistance: an adaptation for weight maintenance. *Lancet.* 1992; 340:1452–1453.

Ernst, E.; Matrai, A.; Scholzl, C.; Magyarosy, I. Dose-effect relationship between smoking and blood rheology. *Br J Haematol.* 1987; 65:485 467.

Glantz, AS.; Parmley, W.W. Passive smoking and heart disease. *JAMA.* 1995; 273:1047–1053.

Gordon, T.; Castelli, W.P.; Hjortland, MC.; et al. High-density lipoprotein as a protective factor against coronary artery disease: The Framingham Study. *Amer J Med.* 1977; 62:707–714.

Gueyffier, F.; Boutitie, F.; Boissel, JP.; et al. Effect of antihypertensive drug treatment on cardiovascular outcomes in women and men : A meta-analysis of individual patient data from the randomized, controlled trials. The INDANA Investigators. *Ann Intern Med.* 1997; 126:761–7.

Hennekens, C. Coronary Risk Intervention. In Julian DG & Wenger NK (Eds). *Women and Heart Disease.* St. Louis: Mosby; 1997:39–48.

Huang, Z.; Willet, W.C.; and Colditz, GA. Effect of weight on women's risk of hypertension. *Cardiol Review.* 1998; 15(10):1720.

Hully, SB. Epidemiology as a guide to clinical decisions. The associations between triglyceride and coronary heart disease. *N Engl J Med.* 1980; 302:1383–1389.

Hully, SB.; et al. Randomized trial of estrogen plus progestin for secondary prevention of coronary heart disease in postmenopausal women. Heart and Estrogen/progestin Replacement Study (HERS): Research Group. *JAMA.* 1998; 280(7):605 613.

Jacobs, DR.; Meban, IL.; Bangdiwala, SI.; et al. High density lipoprotein cholesterol as a predictor of cardiovascular disease mortality in men and women: The follow-up study of the Lipids Research Clinics Prevalence Study. *Am J Epidemiol.* 1990; 131:32–47.

Kannel, W.B.; D'Agostino, R.B.; Belanger, AJ. Fibrinogen, cigarette smoking, and risk of cardiovascular disease: insights from The Framingham Study. *Am Heart J.*

1987; 113:1006–1010.

Kannel, WB.; Wilson, P. Risk factors that attenuate the female coronary disease advantage. *Arch Intern Med.* 1995; 155:57–61.

Kawachi, I.; Colditz, G.; Stampfer; et al. Smoking cessation and decreased risk of stroke in women. *JAMA* 1993; 269(2):232–236.

LaRosa, JC. Triglycerides and coronary risk in women and the elderly. *Arch Int Med.* 1997; 157:961–8.

Lewis, SJ.; Moye, LA.; Sacks, FM.; et al. Effect of provastatin on cardiovascular events in older patients with myocardial infarction and cholesterol levels in the average range. *Ann Intern Med.* 1998; 129(9):681–9.

Lipids Research Clinics Program. The Lipid Research Clinics Coronary Primary Prevention Trial results: I: Reduction in incidence of coronary heart disease. *JAMA* 1984; 251:351–364.

Manson, JE.; Stampfer, MJ.; Hennekens, CH.; Willet, WC. Body weight and longevity: a reassessment. *JAMA.* 1987; 257(3):353–358.

Manson, JE.; Colditz, GA.; Stampfer, MJ.; et al. A prospective study of obesity and risk of coronary heart disease in women. *N Engl J Med.* 1990; 332:882–889.

Olivetti, G.; Giordano, G.; Corradi, D.; et al. Gender differences and aging: Effects on the human heart. *JACC.*

1995; 26(4):1068–79.

Ostlund, RE.; Staten, M.; Kohrt, WM.; et al. The ratio of waist-to-hip circumference, Plasma Insulin Level, and Glucose Intolerance as independent predictors of the HDL Cholesterol Level in older adults. *N Engl J Med.* 1990; 322:229–234.

Parrish, DM. Treatment of hypercholesterolemia in women: Equality, effectiveness, and extrapolation of evidence. *JAMA.* 1997; 277(16):1320–1.

Pearson, TA. and Myerson, M. Treatment of hypercholesterolemia in women: Equality, effectiveness, and extrapolation of evidence (Editorial). *JAMA.* 1997; 277:1320–1.

Pyorala, K.; Pederson, TR.; Kjekshus, J.; et al. Cholesterol lowering with simvastatin improves prognosis of diabetes with coronary artery disease: A subgroup analysis of the Scandinavian Simvastatin Survival Study (4S). *Diabetes Care.* 1997; 20:614–20.

Rexrode, KM.; Hennekens, CH.; Willett, WC.; et al. A prospective study of body mass index, weight change, and risk of stroke in women. *JAMA.* 1997; 277(19):1539–45.

Rich-Edwards, JW.; Manson, JE.; Hennekens, CH.; and Buring, JE. Risk factors in women: Which are unique? Which are shaped? In *Heart*

Disease and Women. American College of Cardiology and University of California, San Francisco School of Medicine. March 15, 1997: 1–9.

Rosenberg, L.; Palmer, JR.; Rao, RS.; Adams-Campbell, LL. Risk factors for coronary heart disease in African American women. *Am J Epidemiol.* 1999; 150(9):904–909.

Scandinavian Simvastatin Survival Study Group. Randomized trial of cholesterol lowering in 4444 patients with coronary heart disease: The Scandinavian Simvastatin Survival Study (4S). *Lancet.* 1994; 344:1383–1389.

Stamler, J.; Stamler, R.; and Neaton, JD. Blood pressure, systolic and diastolic, and cardiovascular risks. *Arch Int Med.* 1993; 153:598–615.

U.K. Prospective Diabetes Study 27. Plasma lipids and lipoproteins at diagnosis of NIDDM by age and sex. *Diabetes Care.* 1997; 20:168–7

Wenger, NK. CHD in women: A "new" problem. *Hosp Pract.* 1992; 27(11):59–67.

Wenger, NK. Coronary heart disease in women: Evolving knowledge is dramatically changing clinical care. In Julian DG & Wenger NK (Eds). *Women and Heart Disease.* St. Louis: Mosby; 1997:21–38.

Willett, WC.; Manson, JE.; Stampfer, MJ.; et al. Weight, weight change, and coronary heart disease in women: Risk within "normal" weight range. *JAMA.* 1995; 273(6):461–465.

Chapter 3: Beyond Cholesterol: New Millennium Risk Factors

Anzai, T.; Yoshikawa, T.; Shiraki, H.; et al. C-reactive protein as a predictor of infarct expansion and cardiac rupture after a first Q-wave acute myocardial infarction. *Circulation*; 96(3):778–84.

Anderson, RA. Nutritional factors influencing the glucose/insulin system: chromium. *J Am Coll Nutr.* 1997; 16:404–410.

Berk, BC.; Weintraub, WS.; Alexander, RW. Elevation of C-reactive protein in "active" coronary disease. *Am J Cardiol.* 1990; 65:168–172.

Boushy, CJ.; Beresford, SA.; Omenn, GS.; et al. A quantitative assessment of plasma homocysteine as a risk factor for vascular disease: Probable benefits of increasing folic acid intakes. *JAMA.* 1995; 274(13):1049–57.

Cantin, B. Lipoprotein(a) and ischemic heart disease. *Cardiol Rev.* 1999; 16(3):23–25.

Creamer, P.; Nagel, D.; Seidel, D.; et al. Consideration about plasma fibrinogen concentration and the cardiovascular risk: combined evidence from the GRIPS and ECAT Studies, Goettingen Risk Incidence and Prevalence Study. European Concerted Action on Thrombosis and Disabilities (letter). *Am J*

Cardiol. 1996; 78(3):380–381.

Ernst, E.; Resch, KL. Fibrinogen as a cardiovascular risk factor: a meta-analysis and review of the literature. *Ann Intern Med.* 1993; 118:956–963.

Graham, IM.; Daly, LE.; Refsum, HM.; et al. Plasma homocysteine as a risk factor for vascular disease. The European Concerted Action Project. *JAMA.* 1997; 277(22):1775–1781.

Grossman, E.; Messerli, FH. Diabetic and hypertensive heart disease. Review. *Ann of Intern Med.* 1996; 125:304–310.

Haider, AW.; et al. Serum lipoprotein(a) level is related to thrombin generation and spontaneous intermittent coronary occlusion in patients with acute myocardial infarction. *Circulation.* 1996; 94(9):2072–2076.

Haverkate, F.; Thompson, SG.; Pyke, SD.; et al. Production of C-reactive protein and risk of coronary events in stable and unstable angina. European Concerted Action on Thrombosis and Disabilities Angina Pectoris Study Group. *Lancet.* 1997; 349(9050):462–466.

Hayek, T.; Oiknine, J.; Dankner, G.; Brook, JG.; Aviram, M. HDL apolipoprotein A-1 attenuates oxidative modification of low-density lipoprotein: studies in transgenic mice. *Eur J Clin Chem Clin Biochem.* 1995; 33:721–725.

Hopkins, PN.; Wu, LL.; Wu, J.; et al. Higher plasma homocyst(e)ine and increased susceptibility to adverse effects of low folate in early familial coronary artery disease. *Arterio Thromb Vasc Biol.* 1995; 15(9):1314–20.

Hopkins, PN.; et al. Lipoprotein(a) interactions with lipid and nonlipid risk factors in early familial coronary artery disease. *Arterioscl Thromb Vasc Biol.* 1997; 17(11):2783–2792.

Juhan-Vague, I.; Pyke, SD.; Alessi, MC.; et al. Fibrinolytic factors and the risk of myocardial infarction or sudden death in patients with angina pectoris. ECAT Study Group. European Concerted Action on Thrombosis and Disabilities. *Circulation.* 1996; 94(9):2057–2063.

Kannel, WB.; Wolf, PA.; Castelli, WP.; D'Agostino, RB. Fibrinogen and risk of cardiovascular disease. The Framingham Study. *JAMA.* 1987; 258:1183–1186.

Kinlay, S.; Dobson, AJ.; Heller, RF.; et al. Risk of primary and recurrent acute myocardial infarction from lipoprotein(a) in men and women. *J Am Coll Cardiol.* 1996; 28(4):870–5.

Kostner, GM.; Gavish, D.; Leopold, B.; et al; HMG CoA-reductase inhibitors lowers LDL cholesterol without reducing Lp(a) levels. *Circulation.* 1989; 80(5):1313–19.

Kuller, LH.; Tracy, RP.; Shaten, J.; Meilahn, EN. for the MRFIT Research Group. Relationship of C-reactive protein and coronary heart disease in the MRFIT nested case-control study. *Am J Epidem.* 1996; 144:537–547.

Lawn, RM. Lipoprotein(a) in heart disease. *Scient Amer.* 1992:54–60.

Liuzzo, G.; Biasucci, LM.; Gallimore, JR.; et al. The prognostic value of C-reactive protein and serum amyloid: A protein in severe unstable angina. *N Engl J Med.* 1994; 331:417–424.

Malinow, MR. Hyperhomocysteinemia. A common and easily reversible risk factor for occlusive atherosclerosis. *Circulation.* 1990; 81:2004–2006.

Malinow, MR.; Nieto, J.; Szklo, M.; Chambless, LE.; Bond, G. Carotid artery intimal-medial wall thickening and plasma homocyst(e)ine in asymptomatic adults. The Atherosclerosis Risk in Communities Study. *Circ.* 1993; 87:1107–1114.

Marcovina, SM.; Koschinsky, ML. The effect of hormone replacement therapy on lipoprotein(a) levels in postmenopausal women. *CVR&R.* 1999; 387–394.

McCully, KS. Vascular pathology of homocysteinemia: implications for the pathogenesis of arteriosclerosis. *Am J Pathol.* 1969; 56:111–128.

Mosca, L.; et al. Antioxidant nutrient supplementation reduces susceptibility of low-density lipoprotein to oxidation in patients with coronary artery disease. *Am J Cardiology.*

1997; 30(2):392–399.

Mosca, L.; Rubenfire, M.; Tarshis, T.; et al. Clinical predictors of oxidized low-density lipoprotein in patients with coronary artery disease. *JACC.* 1997; 80:825–30.

Nguyen, TT.; Ellefson, RD.; Hodge, DO.; et al. Predictive value of electrophoretically detected lipoprotein(a) for coronary heart disease and cerebrovascular disease in a community-based cohort of 9936 men and women. 1997; *Circ.* 96(5); 1390–7.

Nygard, O.; Nordrehaug, JE.; Refsum, H.; et al. Plasma homocysteine levels and mortality in patients with coronary artery disease. *N Engl J Med.* 1997; 337:230–236.

Parthasarathy, S.; Barnett, J.; Fong, LG. High-density Lipoprotein inhibits the oxidative modification of low-density lipoprotein. *Biochem Biophys Acta.* 1990; 1044:275–283.

Pay, S.; Ozcan, N.; Tokgozoglu, SL. Elevated Lp(a) is the most frequent familial lipoprotein disorder leading to premature myocardial infarction in a country with low cholesterol levels. *Int J Cardiol.* 1997; 60(3):301–305.

Reaven, GM.; Chen, Y-DI.; Jeppesen, J.; Maheux, P.; Krauss, RM. Insulin resistance and hyperinsulinemia in individuals with small, dense low-density lipoprotein particles. *J Clin Invest.* 1993; 92:141–146.

Ridker, PM.; Manson, JE.; Buring, JE.; et al. Homocysteine and risk of cardiovascular disease among post-menopausal women. *JAMA*. 1999; 281(19):1817–1821.

Robinson, K.; Mayer, EL.; Miller, DP.; et al. Hyperhomocysteinemia and low pyridoxal phosphate: Common and independent reversible risk factors for coronary artery disease. *Circ*. 1995; 92(10):2825–30.

Salonen, JT.; Nyyssonen, K.; et al. High stored iron levels are associated with excess risk of myocardial infarction in Eastern Finnish men. 1992; *Circ*. 86(3):803–811.

Schwartz, SM.; Siscovick, DS.; Malinow, MR.; et al. Myocardial infarction in young women in relation to plasma total homocysteine, folate, and a common variant in the metylenetetrahydrofolate reductase gene. *Circ*. 1997; 96(2):412–7.

Selhub, J.; Jacques, PF.; Wilson, PWF.; et al. Vitamin status and intake as primary determinants of homocysteinemia in an elderly population. *JAMA*. 1993; 270:2693–2698.

Singh, RB.; Niaz, MA. Serum concentration of lipoprotein(a) decreases on treatment with hydrosoluble Q10 in patients with coronary artery disease. *Int J Cardiol*. 1999; 68(1):23–29.

Stacey, M. The fall and rise of Kilmer McCully. *The New York Times Magazine*. Aug 10, 1997:25–9.

Stein, JH.; McBride, P. Screening and managing patients with lipoprotein(a) excess. *Intern Med*. 1999; 20(6):9–21.

Sullivan, JL. The iron paradigm of ischemic heart disease. *Am Heart J*. 1989; 117(5):1177–88.

Superko, HR. Inherited disorders in the lipoprotein system. A common cause of premature heart disease. In Julian DG, Wenger NK, (eds). *Women and Heart Disease*. London: Martin Dunitz, 1997; 49–67.

Superko, HR. New aspects of cardiovascular risk factors including small, dense LDL, homocystinemia, and Lp(a). *Curr Opin Cardiol*. 1995; 10:347–354.

Wilhelmsen, L.; Svardsudd, K.; Korsan-Bengtsen, K.; et al. Fibrinogen as a risk factor for stroke and MI. *N Engl J Med*. 1984; 311:501–505.

SECTION II: HOW TO PREVENT AND HEAL HEART DISEASE: THE FOUR PILLARS OF HEALTH

Chapter 4: Nutritional Healing: Eat the Heart-Healthy Way

Albert, CM.; et al. Fish consumption and risk of sudden cardiac death. *JAMA*. 1998; 279:23–28.

Campbell, LV.; et al. The high monounsaturated-fat diet as a practical alternative to NIDDM. *Diabetes Care*. 1994; 17:177–182.

Christensen, J.; et al. Fish consumption, n-3 fatty acids in cell membranes and heart rate variability in survivors of myocardial infarction with left ventricular dysfunction. *Am J Cardiol*. 1997; 79:1670–1673.

deLorgeril, M.; et al. Effect of Mediterranean type of diet on the rate of cardiovascular complications in patients with coronary artery disease. *JACC*. 1996; 28(5):1103–8.

deLorgeril, M., et al. Mediterranean alpha-linolenic acid-rich diet in secondary prevention of coronary heart disease. *Lancet*. 1994; 343:1454–59.

deLorgeril, M., et al. What makes a Mediterranean diet cardio-protective? *Cardio Rev*. 1997; 14:15–21.

deLorgeril, M.; Salen, P.; Martin, JL.; et al. Mediterranean dietary pattern in a randomized trial: prolonged survival and possible reduced cancer rate. *Arch Intern Med*. 1998; 158:1181–1187.

Demrow, HS.; Slane, PR.; Folts, JD. Administration of wine and grape juice inhibits in vivo platelet activity and thrombosis in stenosed canine coronary arteries. *Circulation*. 1995; 91(4):1182–88.

Despres, JP.; Lamarche, B.; Mauriege, P.; et al. Hyperinsulinism as an independent risk factor for ischemic heart disease. *N Engl. J Med*. 1996; 334:952–957.

Foster-Powel, K.; Miller, JB. International tables of glycemic index. *Am J Clin Nutr*. 1995; 62:871S–893S.

Fraser, GE.; et al. A possible protective effect of nut consumption on risk of coronary heart disease. *Arch Intern Med*. 1992; 152:1416–1424.

Frost, G.; et al. Glycemic index as a determinant of serum HDL-cholesterol concentration. *Lancet*. 1999; 353(9158):1045–1048.

GISSI-Prevenzione Investigators. Dietary supplementation with n-3 polyunsaturated fatty acids and vitamin E after myocardial infarction: results of the GISSI-Prevenzione Trial. *Lancet*. 1999; 354:447–455.

Herman, W.; Biermann, J.; Kostner, GM. Comparison of effects of N-3 to N-6 fatty acids on serum levels of lipoprotein(a) in patients with coronary disease. *Am J Cardiol*. 1995; 76:459–462.

Hertzog, MC.; Feskens, EJ.; Hollman, PC.; et al. Dietary antioxidant flavonoids and risk of coronary heart disease: the Zutphen Elderly Study. *Lancet*. 1993; 342:1007–1011.

Hertzog, MC.; Feskens, EJ.; Kromhout, D. Antioxidant flavonols and coronary heart disease risk. *Lancet*. 1997; 349:699–700.

Howard, AN.; Williams, NR.; Palmer, CR.; et al. Do hydroxycarotenoids prevent coronary heart disease? A comparison between Belfast and Toulouse. *Inter J Vit Nutr Res*. 1996; 66:113–118.

Hu, FB.; Stampfer, MJ.; Manson, JE.; et al. Dietary fat intake and the risk of coronary heart disease in women. *N Eng J Med*. 1997; 337:1491–9.

Katan, MB. Fish and heart disease. (Editorial). *N Engl J Med*. 1995; 332:1024–1025.

Leaf, A.; Weber, PC. Cardiovascular effects of n-3 fatty acids. *N Engl J of Med*. 1988; 318:549–557.

Maxwell, S.; Cruickshank, A.; Thorpe, D. Red wine and antioxidants activity in serum. *Lancet*. 1994; 344:193–194.

Morris, MC.; Sacks, F.; Rosner, B. Does fish oil lower blood pressure? A meta-analysis of controlled trials. *Circulation*. 1993; 88:523–533.

Renaud, S.; de Lorgeril, M. Wine, alcohol platelets and the French paradox for coronary heart disease. *Lancet*. 1992; 339:1523–1526.

Sabate, J.; Fraser, GI. The probable role of nuts in preventing coronary heart disease. *Primary Cardiology*. 1993; 19(11):65–76.

Schacky, C.; Angerer, P.; et al. The effect of dietary w-3 fatty acids in coronary atherosclerosis: a randomized, double-blind, placebo-controlled trial. *Annals of Inter Med*. 1999; 130(7):554–562.

Simon, JA.; Fong, J.; Bernert, JT. Jr.; et al. Dietary alpha-linolenic acid lowers the risk of stroke. *Modern Medicine*. 1995; 63:45.

Siscovick, DS.; Raghunathan, TE.; et al. Dietary intake and cell membrane levels of long-chain n-3 polyunsaturated fatty acids and the risk of primary cardiac arrest. *JAMA*. 1995; 274:1363–67.

Visioli, F.; Bellomo, G.; Montedoro, GF.; Galli, C. Low density lipoprotein oxidation is inhibited in vitro by olive oil constituents. *Atherosclerosis*. 1995; 117:25–32.

Visioli, F.; Bellomo, G.; Galli, C. Free radical-scavenging properties of olive oil polyphenols. *Biochem and Biophys Res Com*. 1998; 247:60–64.

Willet, WC.; Stampfer, MJ.; Manson, JE.; et al. Intake of trans fatty acids and risk of coronary heart disease among women. *Lancet*. 1993; 341:581–585.

Wolk, A.; Manson, JE.; Stampfer, MJ.; et al. Long-term intake of dietary fiber and decreased risk of coronary heart disease among women. *JAMA*. 1999; 281(21):1998–2004.

Chapter 5: Vital Supplements: Unleash a World of Prevention

Ames, BN.; Shigenaga, MK.; Hagen, TM. Oxidants, antioxidants and the degenerative diseases of aging. *Proc. Natl. Acad. Sci*. 1993; 90:7915–7922.

Anderson, RA.; et al. Elevated intake of supplemental chromium improves glucose and insulin variables in individuals with Type II diabetes. *Diabetes*. 1997; 46:1786–91.

Baron, JA.; et al. Calcium supplements for the prevention of colorectal adenomas. Calcium Polyp Prevention Study Group. *N Engl J Med*. 1999; 349(2):101–107.

Binaghi, P.; et al. Evaluation of the cholesterol-lowering effectiveness of pantetheine in women of perimenopausal age. *Minerva Med*. 1990; 81(6):475–479.

Boushey, CJ.; Beresford, SA.; Omenn, GS.; Motulsky, AG. A quantitative assessment of plasma homocysteine as a risk factor for vascular disease: probable benefits of increasing folic acid intakes. *JAMA* 1995; 274:1049–1057.

Briggs, S. Magnesium: A forgotten mineral. *Health and Nutrition Breakthroughs.* 1977:18–19.

Demrow, HS.; Slane, PR.; Folts, JD. Administration of wine and grape juice inhibits in vivo platelet activity and thrombosis in stenosed canine coronary arteries.1995; *Circ.* 91(4):1182–1188.

Ewy, GA. Antioxidant therapy for coronary artery disease. *Arch Intern Med.* 1999; 159:1279–1280.

Folkers, K.; et al. Lovastatin decreases coenzyme Q10 levels in humans. *Proc Natl Acad Sci.* 1990; 87:8931–8934.

Gaddi, A.; Descovich, G.; Noseda; et al. Controlled evaluation of pantetheine, a natural hypolipidemic compound, in patients with different forms of hyperlipoproteinemia. *Atheroscl.* 1984; 50:73–83.

Gey, GF.; Puska, P.; Jordan, P.; et al. Inverse correlation between plasma, vitamin E, consumption and mortality from ischemic heart disease in cross cultural epidemiology. *Am J Clin Nutr.* 1991; 53:326S–334S.

Ghirlanda, G.; Oradei, A.; Manto, A.; et al. Evidence of plasma CoQ10 lowering effects by HMG-CoA-reduc-tase inhibitors. A double-blind, placebo-controlled study. *J Clin Pharm.* 1993; 33:226–229.

Giovannucci, E.; Stampfer, MJ.; Colditz, GA.; et al. Multivitamin use, folate, and colon cancer in women in the Nurses' Health Study. *Ann Intern Med.* 1998; 129(7):517–524.

Hankey, GJ.; Eikeboom, JW. Homocysteine and vascular disease. *Lancet* 1999; 354:407–413.

Hankinson, SE.; Stampfer, MJ. All that glitters is not beta-carotene. (Editorial). *JAMA* 1994; 272(18):1455–1456.

Hertzog, M.; Feskens, E.; Kromhout, D. Antioxidant flavols and coronary heart disease risk. *Lancet.* 1997; 349:699–700.

Hennekens, CH.; Buring, JE.; Manson, JE.; Stampfer, M.; et al. Lack of effect of long-term supplementation with beta carotene on the incidence of malignant neoplasms and cardiovascular disease. *N Engl J Med.* 1996; 334:1145–1149.

Homocysteine Lowering Trialists' Collaboration. Lowering blood homocysteine with folic acid based supplements: meta-analysis of randomized trials. *BMJ* 1998; 316:894–898.

Howard, AN.; Williams, NR.; Palmer, CR.; Cambou, JP.; Evans, AE.; Foote, JW.; et al. Do hydroxy-carotenoids prevent coronary heart disease? A comparison between Belfast and Toulouse. *Int J Vitamin*

Nutr Res. 1996; 66:113–118.

Itoh, K.; et al. The effects of high oral magnesium supplementation on blood pressure, serum lipids and related variables in apparently healthy Japanese subjects. *Br J Nutri.* 1997; 78(5):737–750.

Johnson, C.; Meyer, C.; Srilakshmi, J. Vitamin C elevates red blood cell glutathione in healthy adults. *Am J Clin Nutr.* 1993; 58:103–105.

Joosten, E. Metabolic evidence that deficiencies of vitamin B-12 occur commonly in elderly people. *Amer J Clin Nutr.* 1993; 58:468–476.

Kang, SS.; Wong, PW.; Cook, HY.; Norusis, M.; Messr, JV. Protein-bound homocyst(e)ine: a possible risk factor for coronary artery disease. *J Clin Invest.* 1986; 77:1482–1486.

Kushi, LH.; Folsom, AR.; Prineas, RJ.; et al. Dietary antioxidant vitamins and death from coronary heart disease in postmenopausal women. *N Engl J Med.* 1996; 334:1156–1162.

Lewis, SJ.; et al. Effects of Pravastatin on cardiovascular events in women after myocardial infarction: The Cholesterol and Recurrent Events (CARE) Trial. *JACC* 1998; 32:140–146.

Lichodziejewska, B.; Klos, J.; Rezler, J.; et al. Clinical symptoms of mitral valve prolapse are related to hypo-magnesemia and attenuated by magnesium supplementation. *Am J Cardiol.* 1997; 79:768–772.

Losonczy, KG.; et al. Vitamin E and vitamin C supplement use and risk of all-cause and coronary heart disease mortality in older persons: The established populations for epidemiologic studies of the elderly. *Am J Clin Nutr.* 1996; 64(2):190–196.

Malinow, RM.; Nieto, J.; Szklo, M.; Chambles, LE.; Bond, G. Carotid artery intimal-medical wall thickening and plasma homocyst(e)ine in asymptomatic adults: the Atherosclerosis Risk in Communities Study. *Circ.* 1993; 87:1107–1113.

McCarty, MF. Can correction of suboptimal coenzyme Q10 status improve cell function in type II diabetes? *Medical Hypothesis.* 1999; 52(5):397–400.

McCully, KS. Homocysteine and vascular disease. *Nature Med.* 1996; 2:386–389.

McLean, RM. Magnesium and its therapeutic uses: a review. *Am J Med.* 1994; 96:63–76.

Moore, AS.; Papas, AM. Biochemistry and health significance of Vitamin E. *J Adv Med.* 1996; 9:11–29.

Nesaretnam, K.; Guthrie, N.; Chambers, AF; Caroll, KK. Effect of tocotrienols on the growth of human breast cancer cell line in culture. *Lipids.* 1995; 30(12):1139–1143.

NIH Concensus Development Panel on Optimal Calcium Intake. *JAMA.* 1994; 272(24):1942–48.

Price, JF; Fowkes, FGR. Antioxidant

vitamins in the prevention of cardiovascular disease. *Eur Heart J.*
1997; 18:719–727.

Reaven, PD.; Khouw, A.; Belz, WF.;
Parthasarathy, S.; Witzum, JL. Effect
of dietary antioxidant combinations
in humans. *Arterioscler Thromb* 1993;
13:590–600.

Resnick, LM. Magnesium in the
pathophysiology and treatment of
hypertension and diabetes mellitus:
Where are we in 1997? *Am
Hyperten.* 1997; 10:368–370.

Rimm, EB.; et al. Folate and vitamin
B-6 from diet and supplements in
relation to risk of coronary heart
disease among women. *JAMA.*
1998; 279:359–364.

Serum carotenoids and coronary heart
disease. The Lipid Research Clinics
Coronary Prevention Trial and
Follow-up Study. 1994; 272:1439–41.

Shechter, M. Oral magnesium in coronary artery disease: fresh insight on
thrombus inhibition. *The Magnesium
Report.* 1999:1–4.

Shechter, M.; Merz, CN.; Paul-
Labrador, M.; Meisel, SR.; et al.
Oral magnesium supplementation
inhibits platelet-dependent thrombosis in patients with coronary
artery disease. *Am J Cardiol.* 1999;
84:152–156.

Simon, JA. Vitamin C and cardiovascular disease: a review. *J Am Coll Nutr.*
1992; 11:107–125.

Sinatra, ST. Alternative Medicine for
the Conventional Cardiologist.

Heart Disease. 2000; 2:16–30.

Sinatra, ST.; DeMarco, J. Free radicals,
oxidative stress, oxidized low density
lipoprotein (LDL) and the heart:
antioxidants and other strategies to
limit cardiovascular damage. *Conn
Medicine.* 1995; 59:579–588.

Sinatra, ST. "Optimum Health."
Bantam Books, New York, NY,
1997.

Sinatra, ST. Letters to the Editor:
"Care," Cancer and Coenzyme
Q10. *JACC.* 1999; 33(3):897–898.

Stamler, JS.; Osborne, JA.; Jaraki, O.;
Rabbani, LE.; Mullins, M.; Singel,
D.; et al. Adverse vascular effects of
homocysteine are modulated by
endothelium-derived relaxing factor
and related oxides of nitrogen. *J
Clin Invest.* 1993; 91:303–318.

Stampfer, MJ.; Hennekens, CH.;
Manson, JE.; et al. Vitamin E consumption and the risk of coronary
artery disease in women. *N Engl J
Med.* 1993; 328:1444–1449.

Stephens, NG.; Parsons, A.; Schofield,
PM.; et al. Randomized controlled
trial of vitamin E in patients with
coronary disease: Cambridge Heart
Antioxidant Study (CHAOS).
Lancet. 1996; 347:781–786.

The Alpha-tocopherol, Beta-carotene
Therapy Cancer Prevention Study
Group. The effect of vitamin E and
beta-carotene on the incidence of
lung cancer and other cancers in
male smokers. *N Engl J Med.* 1994;
330:1029–1035.

Thys-Jacobs, S.; et al. Calcium carbonate and the premenstrual syndrome: effects on premenstrual and menstrual symptoms. Premenstrual Study Group. *Am J Obstet Gynecol.* 1998; 179(2):44–52.

Ting, HH.; Creager, MA.; Ganz, P.; Roddy, MA.; Haley, EA.; Timimi, FK.; et al. Vitamin C improves endothelium-dependent vasodilation in forearm resistance vessels of humans with hyper-cholesterolemia. *Circ.* 1997; 95:2617–2622.

Verhoef, P.; Kok, FJ.; Kruyssen, DA.; et al. Plasma total homocystine, B vitamins, and risk of coronary atherosclerosis. *Atherioscler Thromb Vasc Biol.* 1997; 17:989–995.

Wald, NJ.; Watt, HC.; Law, MR.; Weir, DG.; McPartlin, J.; Scott, JM. Homocysteine and ischemic heart disease: results of a prospective study with implications regarding prevention. *Arch Intern Med.* 1998; 158:862–867.

Chapter 6: Get Moving! Exercise Can Save Your Life

Blumenthal, JA.; Matthews, K.; Fredrikson, M.; et al. Effects of exercise training on cardiovascular function and plasma lipid, lipoprotein, and apolipoprotein concentrations in premenopausal and post-menopausal women. *Arteriosclerosis & Thrombosis.* 1991; 11:912–917.

Featherstone, J.; Holly, R.; Amsterdam, E. Physiologic responses to weight lifting in coronary artery disease. *Am J Cardiology.* 1993; 71:287–292.

Horton, ES. Exercise and decreased risk of NIDDM. (Editorial). *N Engl J Med.* 1991; 325:196–197.

Kushi, LH.; Fee, RM.; Folsom, AR.; et al. Physical activity and mortality in postmenopausal women. *JAMA.* 1997; 277(16):1287–92.

Manson, JE.; Hu, FB.; Rich-Edwards, JW.; et al. A prospective study of walking as compared with vigorous exercise in the prevention of coronary heart disease in women. *N Engl J Med.* 1999; 341(9):650–658.

McCartney, N.; McKelvie, R.; Haslam, D.; Jones, N. Usefulness of weight lifting training in improving strength and maximal power output in coronary artery disease. *Am J Cardiology.* 1991; 67:939–945.

Mittleman, MA.; Maclure, M.; Tofler, GH.; et al. Triggering of acute myocardial infarction by heavy physical exertion. *NEJM* 1993; 329:1677–83.

Nelson, M.; Wernick, S. "Can Strong Women Stay Young." Bantam Books. New York, NY, 1997.

Pramik, MJ. Exercise may improve insulin sensitivity. *Med Tribune Diabetes.* 1996:7.

Reaven, PD.; McPhillips, JB.; Barrett-Connor, EL.; Criqui, MH. Leisure time exercise and lipid and lipoprotein levels in an older population. *J Amer Geriatric Society.* 1990;

38:847–854.

Sinatra, ST.; et al. Effects of continuous passive motion, walking, and a placebo intervention on physical and psychological well-being. *J Cardiopul Rehab.* 1990; 10(8):279–286.

Van Dam, SM.; Gillespy, M.; Notelovitz, Martin AD. Effect of exercise on glucose metabolism in postmenopausal women. *Amer J Obstet & Gyne.* 1988; 159:82–86.

Waller, BF.; Roberts, WC. Sudden death while running in conditioned runners aged 40 years or over. *Am J Cardiol.* 1980; 45(6):1292–1300.

Chapter 7: Emotional Healing, Stress Management, and Spiritual Healing

Benjamin, J.; Levine, J.; Fux, M.; et al. Double-blind, placebo–controlled, crossover trial of inositol treatment for panic disorder. *Am J Psychiatry.* 1995; 152(7):1084–86.

Byrd, RC. Positive therapeutic effects of intercessory prayer in a coronary care unit population. *Southern Med J.* 1988; 81(7):826–829.

Borysenko, J. "Minding the Body, Mending the Mind." Bantam Trade, 1988.

Boushey, CJ.; Beresford, SAA.; Omenn, GS.; Motulsky, AG. A quantitative assessment of plasma homocysteine as a risk factor for vascular disease: Probable benefits of increasing folic acid intakes. *JAMA.* 1995;

274:1049–1057.

Dossey, L. "Healing Words." New York: HarperCollins, 1995.

Eddy, MB. "Science and Health with Key to the Scriptures." Boston: The First Church of Christ Scientists, 1934.

Eliot, RS. "Stress and the major cardio-vascular disorders." Futura Publishing, Mount Kisco, NY. 1979.

Eliot, RS. "From Stress to Strength: How to Lighten Your Load and Save Your Life." Bantam Books, New York. 1994.

Friedman, M.; et al. Changes in the serum cholesterol and blood clotting time in men subjected to cyclic variation of occupational stress. *Circ.* 1958; 17:852–861.

Greene, WA.; Goldstein, S.; Moss, AJ. Psychosocial aspects of sudden death. *Arch Intern Med.* 1972; 129:725–731.

Guiley, RE. "The Miracle of Prayer." Simon & Schuster, New York, 1995.

Jacobs, SC.; Sherwood, JB. Heart & Mind: The practice of cardiac psychology: The cardiac psychology of women and coronary heart disease. *CVR&R.* 1997:32,37–44.

Joyce, CRB.; Welldon, RMC. The objective efficacy of prayer: a double-blind clinical trial. *J Chronic Disease.* 1965; 18:367–377.

Lynch, J. "The Broken Heart." Basic Books, New York, 1977.

Mittleman, MA.; Maclure, M.;

Sherwood, JB.; et al. Triggering of acute myocardial infarction onset by episode of anger. Determinants of Myocardial Infarction Onset Study Investigators. *Circ.* 1995; 92(7):1720–1725.

Nerem, RM.; Levesque, MJ.; Cornhill, JF.; et al. Social environment as a factor in diet-induced atherosclerosis. *Science* 1980; 208:1475.

Redford, W. Hostility and the heart. In: Goleman D, Gurin J. (Eds). *Mind/Body Medicine.* Consumer Report Books. Yonkers, New York, 1993:66–83.

Simon, SB.; Simon, S. "Forgiveness." New York; Warner Books, Philip Lief Group, 1990.

Sinatra, ST. Stress and the heart: behavioral interaction and plan for strategy. *Conn Medicine* 1984; 48(2):81–86.

Sinatra, ST. Stress: A cardiologist's point of view. *Postgrad Med.* 1984; 76(1):231–233.

Sinatra, ST.; Feitell, LA. The heart and mental stress, real and imagined. *Lancet.* 1985:223.

Sinatra, ST. Aortic dissection associated with anger, suppressed rage and acute emotional stress. *J Cardiopul Rehab.* 1986; 6:197–199.

Taggert, P.; Carruthers, M. Endogenous hyperlipidemia induced by emotional stress of race driving. *Lancet.* 1971; 1:16–22.

Thiel, HG.; Parker, D.; Bruce, TA. Stress factors and the risk of myocardial infarction. *J Psychosom Res.* 1973; 17:43–57.

Yawkes, ML. Emotions as a cause of rapid and sudden death. *Arch Neurol & Psychoanalysis.* 1936; 19:875–879.

SECTION III: COMMON CARDIAC CONDITIONS WOMEN ENCOUNTER

Chapter 8: The Great Pretenders: Conditions That Disguise Themselves as Heart Attacks

Benjamin, J.; Levine, J.; Fux, M.; et al. Double-blind, placebo-controlled, crossover trial of Inositol treatment for panic disorder. *Am J Psychiatry.* 1995;152(7)1084–86.

Cannon, RO. Chest pain with normal coronary angiograms. (Editorial). *N Engl J Med.* 1993; 328(23):1706–1708.

Giardina, EV. Syndrome X: Clinical characteristics and physiological considerations. *Clin Geriatrics.* 1997; 5(5):16–24.

Jeresaty, RM. "Mitral Valve Prolapse." Raven Press, New York. 1979.

Jeresaty, RM. *Journal of the Hoffman Heart Institute of Connecticut.* Vol. 1, No. 2, October 1995.

Kemp, HG.; Vokonas, PS.; Cohn, PF.; Gorlin, R. The anginal syndrome associated with normal coronary arteriograms: Report of a six year experience. *Am J Med.* 1973; 54:735–42.

Langsjoen, PH.; Langsjoen, A.; Willis, R.; and Folkers K. Treatment of cardiomyopathy with coenzyme Q10. *Mol Aspects Med.* 1997; 18(Suppl):s265–72.

Lanza, G. Unraveling the mystery of syndrome X. *The J of Myocard Ischemia.* 1994; 6:10–21.

Lichodziejewska, B.; Klos, J.; Rezler, J.; et al. Clinical symptoms of mitral valve prolapse are related to hypo-magnesemia and attenuated by magnesium supplementation. *Am J Cardiol.* 1997; 79:768–772.

Sarrel, PM.; Lindsay, D.; Rosano, GMC.; Poole-Wilson, PA. Angina and normal coronary arteries in women: Gynecological findings. *Am J Obstet & Gyne.* 1992; 167:467–472.

Wenger, NK.; et al. (eds.) "Coronary Heart Disease in Women." New York, Haymarket Doyma, 1987.

Chapter 9: Congestive Heart Failure and the Power of Coenzyme Q10: A Miracle in the Making

Baggio, E.; Gandini, R.; Placher, AC.; et al. Italian multicenter study on safety and efficacy of CoEnzyme Q10. *Mol Aspects Med.* 1994; 15:S287–294.

Barron, J.; Parrillo, J. Dilated cardiomy-opathy: management strategy. *Choices in Cardiology.* 1995; 6:205–208.

Chello, M.; Mastroroberto, P.; Romano, R.; et al. Protection by CoEnzyme Q10 from myocardial reperfusion injury during coronary artery bypass grafting. *Ann Thorac Surg.* 1994; 58:1427–32.

Chen, MR.; Chen, LT.; Gold, M.; Boyce, HW. Plasma and erythrocyte thiamin concentrations in geriatric outpatients. *J Amer Coll of Nutr.* 1996; 15(3):231–236.

Davini, P.; Bigalli, A.; Lamana, F.; Boem A. A controlled study on L-carni-tine therapeutic efficacy in post-infarction. *Drugs Exp Clin Res.* 1992; 18:355–365.

Folkers, K.; Langsjoen, PH.; Langsjoen, PH. Therapy with CoEnzyme Q10 of patients in heart failure who are eligible or ineligible for a transplant. *Biochem Biophys Res Commun.* 1992; 182:247–253.

Ghirlanda, G.; Oradei, A.; Manto, A.; et al. Evidence of plasma CoQ10 low-ering effect by HMG-CoA-reduc-tase inhibitors: A double-blind, placebo-controlled study. *J Clin Pharm.* 1993; 33:226–229.

Ioannis, K.; Rizos; Aristoteles, N.; et al. Hemodynamical effects of L-carni-tine on patients with congestive heart failure due to dilated car-diomyopathy. *JACC.* 1996; Abstract 339a.

Hoffman-Bang, C.; Rehnqvist, N.; Swedberg, K.; Astrom, H. Coenzyme Q10 as an adjunctive in treatment of congestive heart fail-ure. *Am J Cardiol.* 1992; Supp

19(3):216A.

Kelly, GS. L-Carnitine therapeutic applications of conditionally-essential amino acids. *Altern Med Rev.* 1998; 3(5):345–360.

Langsjoen, PH.; Folkers, K. Isolated diastolic dysfunction of the myocardium and its response to CoQ10 treatment. *Clin Invest.* 1993; 71:S140–4.

Langsjoen, PH.; Folkers, K.; et al. Long-term efficacy and safety of CoEnzyme Q10 therapy for idiopathic dilated cardiomyopathy. *Am J Cardiol.* 1990; 65:512–523.

Langsjoen, PH.; Langsjoen, AM. Overview of the use of CoQ10 in cardiovascular disease. *BioFactors* 1999; 9:273–284.

Leslie, D.; Gheorghiade, M. Is there a role for thiamine supplementation in the management of heart failure? *Am Heart J.* 1996; 131:1248–50.

Morisco, C.; Trimarco, B.; Condorelli, M. Effect of CoEnzyme Q10 therapy in patients with congestive heart failure: A long-term multicenter randomized study. In: Folkers K, Mortensen SA, Littarru GP, et al. (Eds): Seventh International Symposium on Biomedial and Clinical Aspects of CoEnzyme Q. *The Clinical Investigator.* 1993; 71:S134–S136.

Kobayashi, A.; Yoshinori, M.; Yamazaki, N. L-carnitine treatment for congestive heart failure: experimental and clinical study. *Jpn Circ J.* 1992;

56:86–94.

Singh, R.B.; Niaz, M.A.; Agarwal, P.; et al. A randomized, double-blind, placebo-controlled trial of L-carnitine in suspected acute myocardial infarction. *Postgrad Med J.* 1996; 72:45–50.

Singh, R.B.; Niaz, M.A.; Rastogi, SS.; Verma, SP. Coenzyme Q10 and Its Role in Heart Disease. *J Clin Biochem Nutr.* 1999; 26:109–118.

Sinatra, ST. Refractory congestive heart failure successfully managed with high dose CoEnzyme Q10 administration. *Mol Aspects Med.* 1997; 18(suppl):299–305.

Sinatra, ST. Coenzyme Q10: A vital therapeutic nutrient for the heart with special application in congestive heart failure. *Conn Medicine.* 1997; 61(11):707–711.

Sinatra, ST. "The CoEnzyme Q10 Phenomenon: The breakthrough nutrient that helps combat heart disease, cancer, aging and more." Keats Publishing, Inc., New Canaan, CT 1998.

Sinatra, ST. "L-Carnitine and the Heart." Keats Good Health Guides, Keats Publishing, Inc., New Canaan, CT 1999.

Sinatra, ST. CoEnzyme Q10—A Cardiologist's Commentary. *Natural Med J.* 1999; 2(2):9–15.

Chapter 10: High Blood Pressure: Overcome a Silent Killer

Burt, V.L.; Cutler, J.A.; Higgins, M.; et

al. Trends in the prevalence, awareness, treatment, and control of
hypertension in the adult US population; Data from the health examination surveys, 1960–1991.
Hypertension. 1995; 26:60–69.

Cooper, RS.; Rotimi, CN.; Ward, R.
The puzzle of hypertension in
African-Americans. *Scientific
American.*1999:56–60.

Duffy, SJ.; Gokce, N.; Holbrook, M.; et
al. Treatment of hypertension with
ascorbic acid. *Lancet,*1999;
354:2048–2050.

Ferrario, CM.; Yunis, C.; Mendys, P.; et
al. Control of hypertension and
blood pressure in the Southeast
region of the United States: a call
for action. *CVR&R.* 1999; 379–386.

Levinson, PD.; Iosiphidis, AH.; et al.
Effects of n-3 fatty acids in essential
hypertension. *Am J Hypertens.* 1990;
3:754–760.

Leviton, R. High blood pressue—lower
it naturally. *Alternative Medicine
Digest.* 1997:16.

Mori, TA.; Bao, DQ.; Burke, V.; et al.
Docosahexaenoic acid but not
eicosapentaenoic acid lowers ambu-
latory blood pressure and heart rate
in humans. *Hypertension.* 1999;
34(2):253–260.

Murray, M. "The Healing Power of
Herbs." Prima Publishing, 1995.

National Heart, Lung, and Blood
Institute. Morbidity and mortality:
1996 chartbook on cardiovascular,
lung, and blood diseases. *Mon Vital
Stat Rep.* 1996; 44:1.

Picot, SJ.; et al. Mood and blood pressure responses in black female care-
givers and noncaregivers. *Nurs Res.*
1999; 48(3):150–61.

Resnick, LM. Magnesium in the
pathophysiology and treatment of
hypertension and diabetes mellitus:
where are we in 1997? *Am J
Hyperten.* 1997; 10:368–370.

Rosenberg, L.; Palmer, JR.; Adams-
Campbell, LL.; Rao, RS. Obesity
and hypertension among college-
educated black women in the
United States. *J Hum Hypertens.*
1999; 13(4):237–241.

Seaton, K. Blood Pressure: understanding, preventing, and reversing hypertension. *JNMA.* 2000; in press.

Sinatra, ST. "CoEnzyme Q10 and the
Heart." *Keats Good Health Guide.*
Keats Publishing, Inc. New Canaan,
CT, 1998.

Singh, RB.; Niaz MA.; Rastogi, SS.; et al.
Effect of hydro-soluble CoEnzyme
Q10 on blood pressures and insulin
resistance in hypertensive patients
with coronary artery disease. *J Human
Hypertension.* 1999; 13(3):203–208.

Stamler, J.; Stamler, R.; Neaton, JD.
Blood pressure, systolic and diastolic, and cardiovascular risks. US
population data. *Arch Intern Med.*
1993; 153:598–615.

Tjoa, HI.; Kaplan, NM. Treatment of
hypertension in the elderly. *JAMA*
1990; 264:1015–1018.

Whelton, PK.; He, J.; Cutler, JA.; et al.

Effects of oral potassium on blood pressure. *JAMA* 1997; 277(20):1624–1632.

Yamagami, T.; Shibata, N.; Folkers, K. Study of coenzyme Q10 in essential hypertension. In: Folkers K, and Yamamura Y. (Eds). *Biomedical and Clinical Aspects of Coenzyme Q10.* Vol.1. Amsterdam: Elsevier, 1977:231–242.

SECTION IV: HORMONES, MENOPAUSE, AND YOUR HEART

Chapter 11: The HRT Dilemma: Should You Take Hormone Replacement Therapy?

Adlercreutz, H.; Hamalainen, E.; Gorbach, S.; Goldin, B. Dietary phyto-oestrogens and the menopause in Japan. *Lancet.* 1992; 339.

Baker, B. Natural hormones may offer effective alternative. *Internal Medicine News.* (Clinical Rounds) November 1, 1997.

Bennett, M. The replacements. *Nutr Sci News.* 1999; 4(8):373–378.

Bergkvist, L. Risk of breast cancer after estrogen and estrogen-progestin replacement. *N Engl J Med.* 1989; 321:293.

Bonn, D. Doses of tamoxifen used to prevent breast cancer may be too high. *Lancet.* 1999; 354:841.

Cauley, JA.; Seeley, DG.; Browner, WS.; et al. Estrogen replacement therapy and mortality among older women. The study of osteoporotic fractures. *Arch*

Intern Med. 1997; 157:2181–2187.

Chadhurz, N. Antioxidant and pro-oxidant actions of estrogens: potential physiological and clinical implications. *Seminars in Reproductive Endocrin.* 1998; 16(4):309–314.

Colditz, GA.; Hankison, SE.; Hunter, DJ.; et al. The use of estrogens and progestins and the risk of breast cancer in postmenopausal women. *N Engl J Med.* 1995; 332:1589–1593.

Colditz, GA.; Rosner, B.; for the Nurses' Health Study Research Group. Use of estrogen plus progestin is associated with greater increase in breast risk than estrogen alone. *Am J Epidemiol.* 1998; 147(suppl):64S.

Colditz, GA. Hormones and breast cancer: evidence and implications for consideration of risks and benefits of hormone replacement therapy. *J Women's Health.* 1999; 8(3):347–357.

Collaborative Group on Hormonal Factors in Breast Cancer. Breast cancer and hormone replacement therapy: collaborative re-analysis of data from 51 epidemiological studies of 52,705 women with breast cancer and 108,411 women without breast cancer. *Lancet.* 1997; 350:1047–59.

Corson, SL. A decade of experience with transdermal estrogen replacement therapy: overview of key pharmacologic findings. *Inter J*

Fertility. 1993.

Cummings, SR.; Eckert, S.; Krueger, KA.; et al. The effect of raloxifene on risk of breast cancer in post-menopausal women. *JAMA.* 1999; 281:2189–2197.

Delmas, PD.; Bjarnason, NH.; Mitlak, BH.; et al. Effects of raloxifene on bone mineral density, serum choles-terol concentrations, and uterus endometrium in postmenopausal women. *N Eng J Med.* 1997; 337:1641–7.

Douketis, JD.; Ginsberg, JS.; Holbrook, A.; et al. A reevaluation of the risk for venous thromboembolism with the use of oral contraceptives and hormone replacement therapy. *Arch Intern Med.* 1997; 157:1522–1530.

Ebeling, P.; Koivisto, VA. Physiological importance of dehydroepiandros-terone. *Lancet.* 1994; 343:1479–1482.

Espeland, M.; Morcovina, S.; et al: for the PEPI Trial. Effect of post-menopausal hormone therapy on lipoprotein(a) concentration. *Circ.* 1998; 97:979–986.

Evista, "PDR. 1999," Medical Economics, Co., Inc. Montvale, NJ:1576–1579.

Farish, E.; Spowart. K.; Barnes. JF.; et al. Effects of postmenopausal hormone replacement therapy on lipoproteins including lipoprotein(a) and LDL subfractions. *Atherosclerosis.* 1996; 126:77–84.

Gambrell, RD. Jr; Maier, RC.; Sanders, BI. Decreased incidence of breast cancer in postmenopausal estrogen-progestogen users. *Obstet Gynecol.* 1983; 62:435–443.

Genant, HK.; Lucas, J.; Weiss; et al. Low-dose esterified estrogen thera-py: effects on bone, plasma estradiol concentrations, endometrium, and lipid levels. Estratab/Osteoporosis Study Group. *Arch Intern Med.* 1997; 157:2609–15.

Grodstein, F.; Meir. S.; et al. Postmenopausal hormone therapy and mortality. *N Engl J Med.* 1997; 336:1769–1775.

Haines, C.; et al. Effect of oral estradiol on Lp(a) and other lipoprotein in postmenopausal women. *Arch Inter Med.* 1996; 156:866.

Herrington, D. Sex hormones and nor-mal cardiovascular physiology in women. "Women and Heart Disease," In: Julian, DG, Wenger NK, (eds). Martin Dunitz, Ltd, London. 1997:243–264.

Herrington, D.; Werbel. B.; et al. Individual and combined effects of estrogen/progestin therapy and lovastatin on lipids and flow medi-ated vasodilation in post-menopausal women with coronary artery disease. *JACC.* 1999; 33(7):2030–2037.

Hulley, S.; Grady, D.; et al. Randomized trial of estrogen plus progestin for secondary prevention of coronary heart disease in post-menopausal women. *JAMA.* 1998;

280:605–613.

Kabat, GC.; Chang, CJ,; et al. Urinary estrogen metabolites and breast cancer: a case controlled study. *Cancer Epidermiol Biomarkers Prev.* 1997; 6(7):505–509.

Kawano, H.; Motoyama, T.; Kugiyama, K.; et al. Gender difference in improvement of endothelium-dependent vasodilation after estrogen supplementation. *JACC.* 1997; 30(4):914–919.

Key, TJA.; Wang, DY.; et al. A prospective study of urinary estrogen excretion and breast cancer risk. *Brit J Cancer.* 1996; 73:1615–1619.

Knight, DC.; Eden, JA. A review of the clinical effects of phytoestrogens. *Obstet & Gynecol.* 1996; 87(#5, 2):897–904.

LaRosa, JC. Has HRT come of age?*Lancet.* 1995; 345:76–77.

Lee, JR.; Hopkins, V. "What Your Doctor May *Not* Tell You About Menopause." Warner Books, New York, NY. 1996.

Lerman, A.; Burnett, JC. Jr.; et al. Long-term L-Arginine supplementation improves small-vessel coronary endothelial function in humans. *Circulation.* 1998; 97:2123–2128.

Meade, TW.; Ruddock, V.; Stirling, Y.; et al. Fibrinolytic activity, clotting factors, and long-term incidence of ischemic heart disease in the Northwick Park Heart Study. *Lancet.* 1993; 342:1076–79.

Mikkolam, T. 17*B*-Estradiol stimulates prostacyclin but not endothelin-1 production in human vascular endothelial cells. *J Clin Endocrin & Metabol.* 1995; 80(6).

Morales, AJ.; Nolan, JJ.; Nelson, JC.; Yen, SSC. Effects of replacement dose of dehydro-epiandrosterone in men and women of advancing age. *J Clin Endocrinol & Metabolism.* 1994; 78(6):1360–1367.

Nachtigall, LE.; Nachtigall, RH.; Nachtigall, RD.; Beckman, EM. Estrogen replacement therapy, II: a prospective study in the relationship to carcinoma and cardiovascular and metabolic problems. *Obstet Gynecol.* 1979; 54:74–79.

Nachtigall, L.; Heilman, J. "Estrogen." Harper-Collins Publishers, New York, NY. 1991:16–38.

Norris, J.; Page, L. Peptide antagonists of the human estrogen receptor. *Science.* 1999; 285:744–46.

Persson, I.; Weiderpass, E.; Bergkvist, L.; et al. Risks of breast and endometrial cancer after estrogen and progestin replacement. *Cancer Causes Control.* 1999; 10:253–260.

Pike, MC.; Peters, RK.; Cozen, W.; et al. Estrogen-progestin replacement therapy and endometrial cancer. *J Natl Cancer Inst.* 1997; 89:1110–1116.

Pike, MC.; Spicer, DV.; Dahnoush, L.; Press, MF. Estrogens, progestogens, normal breast cell proliferation, and breast cancer risk. *Epidemiol Rev.* 1993; 15:48–65.

Rajkumar, C.; Kingwel, B.; et al.

Hormone therapy increases arterial compliance in postmenopausal women, *JAMA*. 1997; 30(2):305–356.

Rosano, GMC.; Patrizi, R.; Leonardo, F.; et al. Effect of estrogen replacement therapy on heart rate variability and heart rate in healthy postmenopausal women. *Am J Cardiol.* 1997; 80:815–818.

Sellers, TA.; Mink, PJ.; Cerhan, JR.; et al. The role of hormone replacement therapy in the risk for breast cancer and total mortality and women with a family history of breast cancer. *Ann Intern Med.* 1997; 127:973–80.

Schairer, C.; Lubin, J.; Troisi, R.; et al. Menopausal estrogen and estrogen-progestin replacement therapy and breast cancer risk. *JAMA*. 2000; 283:485–491.

Sourander, L.; Rajala, T.; Raiha, I.; et al. Cardiovascular and cancer morbidity and mortality and sudden cardiac death in postmenopausal women on oestrogen replacement therapy ERT). *Lancet.* 1998; 352:1965–1970.

Stampfer, MJ.; Willett, WC.; Colditz, GA.; et al. A prospective study of postmenopausal estrogen therapy and coronary heart disease. *N Engl J Med.* 1985; 313:1044–1049.

The Writing Group for the PEPI Trial. Effects of Estrogen or Estrogen/Progestin regimens on heart disease risk factors in postmenopausal women. The

Postmenopausal Estrogen/Progestin Interventional Trial. *JAMA* 1995; 273:199–208.

Wenger, NK. Coronary heart disease in women: Evolving knowledge is dramatically changing clinical care. In Julian DG & Wenger NK (Eds). *Women and Heart Disease.* St. Louis: Mosby; 1997:21–38.

Wenger, NK. The impact of estrogen and hormone replacement on cardiovascular disease. "Heart Disease in Women," from proceedings of the conference sponsored by the American College of Cardiology and the School of Medicine, UC, San Francisco, 1997:28–34.

Westerveld, HT.; Roeters van Lennep, JE.; et al. Apolipoprotein B and coronary artery disease in women: A cross sectional study in women undergoing their first coronary angiography. *Arteriocler Thromb Vasc Biol.* 1998; 18:1101–1107.

Whitcomb, H.; Bronson, P. Managing women's hormones naturally. *Altern Med. Digest.* 1999; 20:118–123.

Willett, WC.; Colditz, G.; Stampfer, M. Postmenopausal estrogens— opposed, unopposed, or none of the above. *JAMA*. 2000; 283(4):534–535.

Women's Health Initiative Group. Design of the Women's Health Initiative Clinical Trial and Observational Study. *Control Clin Trials.* 1998; 19:61–109.

Writing Group for the PEPI Trial.

Effects of estrogen or estrogen/progestin regimens on heart disease risk factors in women. *JAMA*. 1995; 273:199–208.

Chapter 12: Women's Choice: A Decision Tree

Anderson, LF.; Gram, J.; Skouby, SO.; Jespersen, J. Effects of hormone replacement therapy on hemostatic cardiovascular risk factors. *Am J Obstet Gynecol*. 1999; 180:283–289.

Grady; et al. Hormone therapy to prevent disease and prolong life in postmenopausal women. *Ann Intern Med*. 1992; 117(12):1016–1041.

Haines; C.; Chung, T.; Chang, A.; et al. Effect of oral estradiol on Lp(a) and other lipoprotein in postmenopausal women. *Arch Intern Med*. 1996; 156:866–872.

Hutchins, AM.; Lampe, J.; et al. Vegetables, fruits, and legumes: effect on urinary phytoestrogen and lignan excretion. *J Am Diet Assoc*. 1995; 95:769–774.

Muller, JL.; et al. Pharmaceutical considerations of common herbal medicine. *Am J Managed Care*. 1997; 3(11):1753–70.

Murray, MT. "The Healing Power of Herbs." Prima Publishing. Rocklin, CA. 1995.

Pepine, CJ.; Lewis, JF.; Limacher, MC.; et al. Interventions that may influence the course of CAD: Part II: Estrogens and antioxidant vitamins. *J Myocardial Ischemia*. 1995;

7(6):286–289.

Sinatra, ST. "CoEnzyme Q10 and the Heart." *Keats Good Health Guide*. Keats Publishing, Inc. New Canaan, CT. 1998.

Singh, RB.; Niaz, MA. Serum concentration of lipoprotein(a) decreases on treatment with hydrosoluble coenzyme Q10 in patients with coronary artery disease: discovery of a new role [In progress citation.] *Int J Cardiol*. 1999; 68(1):23–9.

Tham, D.; Gardner, CD.; Haskel WL. Potential health benefits of dietary phytoestrogens: A review of the Clinical, Epidemiological, and Mechanistic evidence. *J Clin Endocrinol Metab*. 1997; 83(7):2223–2235.

Willett, WC.; Colditz, G.; Stampfer, M. Postmenopausal estrogens— opposed, unopposed, or none of the above. *JAMA*. 2000; 283(4):534–535.

Xu, X.; Duncan, AM.; et al. Effects of soy isoflavones on estrogen and phytoestrogen metabolism in premenopausal women. *Cancer Epidemiol Biomarkers Prev*. 1998; 7(12):1101–1108.

SECTION V: HEART HEALTH FOR A LIFETIME

Chapter 13: Depression and Your Heart: How to Break Through

Bates, B. Depression in women predicts post-MI deaths. *Int Med News*.

1997:36.

Borysenko, J. "Minding the Body, Mending the Mind." Bantam Trade, 1988.

Denollet, J.; Sys, S.; Stroonbant; et al. Personality as independent predictor of long-term mortality in patients with coronary heart disease. *The Lancet*. 1996; 347:417–421.

Glass, R.M. Treating depression as a recurrent or chronic disease. *JAMA* 1999; 281(1):83–84.

Jiang, W.; Babyak, M.; Krantz, DS.; et al. Mental stress-induced myocardial ischemia and cardiac events. *JAMA*. 1996; 275(21):1651–56.

Kubetin, SK. Depression history may predict post-MI depression. *Internal Medicine News—Clinical Rounds*. Text. May 1, 1996.

LeBars, et al. A placebo-controlled, double-blind, randomized trial of an extract of Ginkgo Biloba for dementia. North American Study Group. *JAMA*. 1997; 278(16):1327–1332.

Levin, R.F. Heartmates: "A Survival Guide for the Cardiac Spouse." Prentice Hall Press. New York, NY, 1987.

Lieberman, J. "Light Medicine of the Future." Bear and Company Publishing, Santa Fe, New Mexico, 1991.

Linde, K.; Ramirez, G.; et al. St. John's Wort for depression: an overview and meta-analysis of randomized clinical trials. *Br Med J*. 1996;

313:253–258.

Mann, D. Chronic depression predictive of MI, mortality. *Medical Tribune-Cardiology Rounds*. Text. July 18, 1996.

Martinez, B.; Kasper, S.; et al. Hypericum in the treatment of seasonal affective disorders. *J Geriatr Psychiatry Neurol*. 1994; 7(suppl):S29–S33.

Mason, LJ. "Guide to stress reduction." Peace Press, Culver City, CA. 1980:116.

Murray, MT. "5-HTP—The Natural Way to Overcome Depression, Obesity and Insomnia." Bantam Books, 1998.

Ott, J. "Light Radiation and You." Devin-Adair Publishing, Greenwich, CT 1982.

Poldinger, W.; Calanchini, B.; Schwartz, W. A functional-dimensional approach to depression: Serotonin deficiency as a target syndrome in a comparison of 5-HTP and fluvoxamine. *Psychopathology*. 1991; 24:53–81.

Samson, KJ. Risk Factors for SAD Include Genetics. Geography. *Internal Medicine News—Clinical Rounds*. Nov. 15, 1996.

Study: Depressed women may face higher risk of osteoporosis. (Web posted: CNN) 1996.

Tubesing, DA. Kicking your stress habits. Whole Person Associates, Duluth, MN. 1981:15.

Walker, RJ.; Pomeroy, EC. Depression or grief? The experience of care givers of people with dementia. *Health Soc Work.* 1996; 21(4):247–254.

Whooley, MA.; Browner, WS. Association between depressive symptoms and mortality in older women. *Arch Intern Med.* 1998; 158:2129–2135.

Chapter 14: Cultivate the Mind-Body Connection

Allan, R.; and Scheidt, S. Group psychotherapy for patients with coronary heart disease. *Inter J Group Psychother.* 1998; 48(2):187–214.

Allan, R. and Scheidt, S. Psychosocial Factors. In "Clinical Trials in Cardiovascualr Disease: A Companion to Braunwald's Heart Disease." Hennekens CH (Ed.). Philadelphia; WB Saunders: 1999.

Lowen, A. "Bioenergetics." New York: Penguin Books, 1976.

Lowen, A. "Fear of Life." New York: Macmillan Publishing Company, 1980.

Lowen, A. "Love, Sex, and Your Heart." New York; MacMillan Publishing: 1986.

Northrup, C. "Women's Bodies, Women's Wisdom." New York: Bantam Books, 1994.

Reich, W. Character Analysis. New York; Farrar Straus and Giroux, 1969.

Sinatra, S. "Heartbreak and Heart Disease." New Canaan, CT; Keats Publishing: 1996.

Chapter 15: Secrets of Aging Gracefully: Staying Fit and Healthy for a Better Life

Barnes, S.; Peterson, TG.; Coward, L. Rationale for the use of genistein containing soy matrices in chemo-prevention trials for breast and prostate cancer. *J Cell Biochem.* 1995; 22:181–187.

Cauley, JA.; Seeley, DG.; Browner, WS.; et al. Estrogen replacement therapy and mortality among older women. The study of osteoporotic fractures. *Arch Intern Med.* 1997; 157:2181–7.

Folkers, K. Relevance of the biosynthesis of CoEnzyme Q10 and of the four bases of DNA as a rationale for the molecular causes of cancer and a therapy. *Biochem Biophys Res Commun.* 1996; 224(2):358–61.

Franklin, D. "The Healthiest Women in the World." Hippocrates, 1996:51–61.

Garnett, M. "First Pulse: A Personal Journey in Cancer Research." New York, 1998.

Ingram, D.; Sanders, K.; Kolybaba, M.; Lopez, D. Case-control study of phytoestrogens and breast cancer. *Lancet.* 1997; 350:990–994.

Kidd, P. Immunoceuticals—potentiating the body's offenses against cancer. *Total Health 21.* 1999:19–21.

Kilgore, C. Calcium enhances effect of anti-resorptive drugs. *Internal Med News.* 1997:16.

LeBoff, MS.; Kohlmeier, L.; Hurwitz,

S.; et al. Occult vitamin D deficiency in postmenopausal US women with acute hip fracture. *JAMA* 1999; 281(16):1505–1511.

Lemus-Wilson, A.; et al. Melatonin blocks the stimulatory effects of Prolactin on human breast cancer cell growth in culture. *Br J Cancer.* 1995; 72(6):1435–40.

Lissoni, P.; et al. Modulation of cancer endocrine therapy by melatonin: a Phase II study of Tamoxifen plus melatonin in metastatic breast cancer patients progressing under Tamoxifen alone. *Br J Cancer.* 1995; 71(4):854–856.

Lockwood, K.; Moesgaard, S.; Yamamoto, T.; Folkers, K. Progress on therapy of breast cancer with vitamin Q10 and the regression of metastases. *Biochem Biophys Res. Commun.* 1995; 212(1):172–7.

Longnecker, MP.; Newcomb, PA.; Mittendorf, R.; et al. Intake of carrots, spinach and supplements containing vitamin A in relation ro risk of breast cancer. *Cancer Epidemiol Biomarkers Prev.* 1997; 6:887–892.

Lu, LJW.; Anderson, KE.; Grady, JJ.; Nagamani, M. Effects of soya consumption for one month on steroid hormones in premenopausal women: implications for breast cancer risk reduction. *Cancer Epidemiology, Biomarkers & Prevention.* 1996; 5:63–70.

Marchand, LL.; Hankin, JH; Bach, F;

et al. An ecological study of diet and lung cancer in the South Pacific. *Int J Cancer.* 1995; 63:19–23.

Morris, DL.; et al. Serum carotenoids and coronary heart disease. *The Lipid Research Clinics Coronary Primary Prevention Trial and Follow up Study.* 1994; 272:1439–1441.

Nestel, PJ.; Pomeroy, S.; Kay, S.; et al. Isoflavones from red clover improve systemic arterial compliance but not plasma lipids in menopausal women. *J Clin Endocrinol Metab.* 1999; 84(3):895–898.

Packer, L.; et al. Alpha lipoic acid as a biological antioxidant. *Free Radic Biol Med.* 1995; 19:227–250.

Persky, V; Van Horn. L. Epidemiology of soy and cancer: perspectives and directions. *J Nutr.* 1995; 125:709S–712S.

Rock, CL.; Saxe, GA.; et al. Carotenoids, vitamin A and estrogen receptor status in breast cancer. *Nutrition and Cancer.* 1996; 25(3).282–296.

Seddon, JM.; et al. Dietary carotenoids, vitamins A, C and E and advanced age-related macular degeneration. *J Am Med Assn.* 1994; 272:1413–20.

Setchell, KDR.; Zimmer-Nechemias, L.; Cai, J.; Heubi, JE. Exposure of infants to phyto-oestrogens from soy-based infant formula. *Lancet.* 1997; 350:23–27.

Suzuki, YJ. et al. Alpha-lipoic acid is a potent inhibitor of NT-kappa B activation in human T cells. *Biochem Biophys Res Commun.* 1992; 189:1709–1715.

Tiwari, RK.; et al. Selective responsiveness of human breast cancer cells to Indole-3-Carbinol, a chemopreventive agent. *J Natl Cancer Inst.* 1994; 86(2):126–31.

Voelker, R. Study examines stress—immune system links in women with breast cancer. *JAMA.* 1997; 278(7):534.

Walters, R. "Options—The Alternative Cancer Therapy Book." Paragon Press, New York. 1993:105–119.

Chapter 16: The Female Advantage: Stories of Healing and Hope

Northrup, C. "Women's Bodies, Women's Wisdom." New York: Bantam, 1994.

Sinatra, ST. Stress and the heart—behavioral interaction and plan for strategy. *Conn Med.* 1984; 48:81–86.

Sinatra, ST.; Kurien, A.; Hatch, H.; Montano, G.; et al. A stress management program with biochemical assay. *Conn Med.* 1982; 46:370–372.

Sullivan, JL. The iron paradigm of ischemic heart disease. *Am Heart J.* 1989; 117(5):1177–88.

Appendix A: A Guide to Diagnostic Testing for Women

Julian, DG.; and Wenger, NK. (Eds.) Women and heart disease. Mosby. St Louis, MO. Pepine, Original review D (1997).

Heart disease in women. Pamphlet for preconference. American College of Cardiology. March 15, 1997. Anaheim, CA

Heart disease treatment. Aired February 28, 1998. Your Health: CNN Transcripts. Http://www.CNN.com.

Wayne, HH. Living longer with heart disease: The noninvasive approach that will save your life. Proof copy. Health information Press. Los Angeles, CA, (1998).

Appendix D: African American Women: Increased Heart Disease Risk?

Cooper, RS.; Rotimi, CN., Ward, R. The puzzle of hypertension in African-Americans. *Scientific American.* 1999; 56-62.

RESOURCES

Compounding Pharmacies

Apex Pharmacy
1223 Dixwell Avenue
Hamden, CT 06514
203-287-3132

Hopewell Pharmacy
1 West Broad Street
Hopewell, NJ 08525
609-466-1960
800-792-6670
Fax: 800-417-3864

Women's International Pharmacy
5708 Monoma Drive
Madison, WI 53704
800-279-5708
608-221-7800

Environmental Lighting Products

American Environmental Products
800-705-5559

Environmental Lighting Concepts
800-842-8848

Labs

Antibody Assay Laboratory
Reference Laboratories, Inc.
1715 E. Wilshire, Suite 715
Santa Ana, CA 92705
800-522-2611
Fax: 714-543-2034

Great Smokies Diagnostic Laboratory
63 Zillicoa Street
Asheville, NC 28801-1074

828-253-0621
800-522-4762
Fax: 828-252-9303

MetaMetrix
Medical Research Laboratory
5000 Peachtree Ind. Blvd.
Suite 110
Norcross, GA 30071
770-446-5483
800-221-4640
Fax: 770-441-2237

Newsletter Subscriptions
HeartSense
Stephen T. Sinatra, M.D., F.A.C.C.
7811 Montrose Road
P.O. Box 61350
Potomac, MD 20859-1350
800-861-5970

Heart Wisdom for Women
Christine Northrop
7811 Montrose Road
Potomac, MD 20859-1350
800-804-0935

Nutritional Supplements
Optimum Health International,
L.L.C.
483 West Middle Tpke.
Manchester, CT 06040
800-228-1507
860-647-9729
Fax: 860-533-9747

ACKNOWLEDGMENTS

This book has been a work in progress for more than five years. It's been a true team effort, and I wish to acknowledge those who contributed to its creation.

My deepest thanks, love, and gratitude must first go to my wife and coauthor, Jan DeMarco Sinatra, RN, MSN, for her ongoing and brilliant contributions to this book. Her feminine perspective and energy immeasurably enriched the text, as she continuously taught me how to really listen to a woman.

To my coauthor and chief editor, Bobbie Lieberman, my gratitude for taking on the challenge of transforming the technical subject of heart disease and hormone replacement therapy into the book you now hold in your hands.

My heartfelt thanks go out to all of the women who shared their stories with us, motivated solely by a sincere desire to reach out to other women and spare them some of the pitfalls on the road to diagnosis and recovery. Your stories have deeply touched our hearts as you have stretched out your arms to the many women who will benefit from your candor.

I owe a huge debt of gratitude to Susan Graham, LPN, master massage therapist and herbalist, for her research, writing, editing, and creativity throughout this project. I deeply appreciated her assistance in helping us sort through the riddle of hormone replacement therapy. Her own story is a testament to persistence and the blending of conventional and complementary methods to heal the whole person.

To Donna Chaput, for her countless hours typing and retyping the manuscript as well as helping me prepare the bibliography.

To Dr. Robert Lang, a Connecticut endocrinologist, who helped with the final editing of the HRT section, shedding light in those dark areas of complex endocrine physiology.

To Michael Bennett, PhD, a California pharmacologist and an incredible resource on natural estrogen and progesterone therapies found in plants, who helped shape the HRT section. His depth of experience and a profound understanding of drug therapy, phytoestrogens, and saliva testing have been an outstanding asset to this book.

To Tom Phillips, and my friends and colleagues at Phillips Publishing and Doctor's Preferred, including Karen Berney, Donna Engelgau, Robert Kroening, Erica Bullard, Glory Kneass, Bob Austen, Robert DiFato, David Sokoloff, Richard Stanton Jones, and Kevin Donoghue—my thanks for all you have done.

To Stan Jankowitz, Mel Rich, David North, Raj Chopra, and Ken Hassen for supporting me through my mission in anti-aging and preventive medicine.

To my "team" at Regnery Publishing: Marji Ross, publisher extraordinaire, and my editor, Erica Rogers, for their inspiration and professionalism.

To Anne Sellaro, my publicist, for your enduring faith and enthusiasm for my work.

To Jo-Anne Piazza, my executive assistant, for keeping me on track with humor and grace.

To all of my staff at the New England Heart Center, for your patience, forbearance, and unflagging support throughout this project.

To Greg and Maile Pouls for their warm nurturing.

To our animal friends, Chewie, Charlie, and Kuma, for teaching us the value of play, the meaning of unconditional love, and for keeping our spirits up when the going got rough.

To my ex-wife Susy Sinatra, who supported me in my earlier years.

To my children Marchann, Step, Drew, and Donna, Kristen, and Greg—I love you all unconditionally!

And finally, to all of my patients, past and present, for keeping me humble and putting me back in touch with the true nature of healing.

INDEX